ADVANCE PRAISE FOR *THE ALZHEIMER'S ACTION PLAN*

"Dr. Doraiswamy has done a masterful job of communicating what the layman should know on the treatment, the caregiving, and, most important, the prevention of Alzheimer's. It was gratifying to learn about the mountain of evidence that what is good for your heart is also good for your brain."
> —Arthur Agatston, M.D., cardiologist and #1 *New York Times* bestselling author of *The South Beach Diet*

"Memory does matter. Adults across the life cycle are asking questions, many questions! The authors answer these questions for the educated public, family members who encounter memory loss in a loved one, and even adults who believe they are experiencing early memory loss. The answers are comprehensive and understandable, no small accomplishment given the plethora of new information available—information that at times is not only confusing but also conflicting."
> —Dan G. Blazer, M.D., Ph.D., former Dean of Medical Education at the Duke University School of Medicine and past president of the American Geriatrics Society

"If you and your family face the specter of Alzheimer's disease, run—don't walk—to get Lisa Gwyther's help. She combines many years of experience with empathy and respect for the patient. That results in the most sensible, compassionate, and practical advice. . . . She is my hero."
> —Naomi S. Boak, executive producer of the Emmy Award–winning PBS special *The Forgetting: A Portrait of Alzheimer's*

"This book is the most comprehensive and up-to-date guide for the diagnosis and management of Alzheimer's disease. Whether you are a health-care professional or have Alzheimer's in your family or are simply interested in living to an old age, this book is a must-read."
> —Deepak Chopra, M.D., *New York Times* bestselling author of *Perfect Health: The Complete Mind/Body Guide*

"I love this book! A powerful and vital resource for people who need it the most. Dr. Doraiswamy is that unique blend of medical expertise mixed in with warmth and compassion and topped off with humility that makes him rare and wonderful."
> —Leeza Gibbons, Emmy Award–winning TV host and founder of Leeza's Place and the Leeza Gibbons Memory Foundation

"Lisa Gwyther is a national treasure. She has been a pioneer in providing innovative care and education for Alzheimer's patients and their families for many years. Lisa's long experience helping families cope with the challenges of memory loss and Alzheimer's disease makes her uniquely qualified to co-author this book. Families experiencing the new world of memory loss and Alzheimer's couldn't ask for a better companion for the journey. Her warmth, compassion, and wisdom shine through, and will help light the way."
> —Pat Lynch, Director of Communications for the Alzheimer's Center Program, National Institute on Aging

"*The Alzheimer's Action Plan* provides a clear and compelling message that there is something we can all do about Alzheimer's disease. The book presents accurate, up-to-date information and step-by-step recommendations that people with the disease, their families, and friends can use now to reduce the potentially devastating effects of Alzheimer's disease."
> —Katie Maslow, M.S.W., Associate Director of Quality Care Advocacy for the Alzheimer's Association and winner of the 2003 ASA Award from the American Society on Aging

"Most of us will either get Alzheimer's or care for a loved one who has it. This action plan can empower you to make a difference."
— **Mehmet C. Oz, M.D., co-author of the #1** *New York Times* **bestseller** *You: The Owner's Manual*

"A readable, informative, and thorough guide to the early stages of Alzheimer's disease. I highly recommend it."
— **Peter Rabins, M.D., co-author** *of The 36-Hour Day: A Family Guide to Caring for Persons with Alzheimer's Disease, Related Dementing Illnesses, and Memory's Loss in Later Life*

"Dr. Murali Doraiswamy, one of America's top memory and Alzheimer's specialists, has packed this book with expert advice and compassionate wisdom, creating an indispensable guide for anyone concerned about their own memory or that of a loved one. Both accessible and comprehensive, this is a must-read not just for families, but for their doctors as well."
— **Gary Small, M.D., director of the UCLA Center on Aging and author of** *The Memory Bible* **and** *The Longevity Bible*

"The authors speak authoritatively, providing sound evidence for the points they make that is based on the current understanding of Alzheimer's disease, but the language they use and the tone of the book will make their advice and guidelines for Alzheimer's care and treatment readily accessible to the public. . . . Bravo on a job so well done!"
— **John Q. Trojanowski, M.D., Ph.D., director of the Alzheimer's Disease Center, the University of Pennsylvania**

The Alzheimer's
ACTION PLAN

The Alzheimer's
ACTION PLAN

▶ **THE EXPERTS' GUIDE TO THE
BEST DIAGNOSIS AND TREATMENT
FOR MEMORY PROBLEMS**

P. Murali Doraiswamy, M.D.
and Lisa P. Gwyther, M.S.W.
with Tina Adler

ST. MARTIN'S PRESS   NEW YORK

www.stmartins.com

Book design by Maura Fadden Rosenthal /Mspace

ISBN-13: 978-0-312-35539-5
ISBN-10: 0-312-35539-4

First Edition: April 2008

10 9 8 7 6 5 4 3 2 1

To my grandparents, Dr. P. K. Kalyanaraman and Dr. K. A. Kalyanam, who inspired my medical career; my family, P. K. Doraiswamy, Uma Doraiswamy, Anu, Shivaraman, and Aditya, for their love and support; and to Saraswati, the goddess of learning.

—PMD

For Naomi, Selwyn, Miriam, Bob, Marni, and Ryan for their unwavering commitment to meaningful work, and for Emma, Avery, Elena, and Aidan with fervent hope that the prevention and treatment of Alzheimer's will enhance the quality of their lives.

—LPG

To Doug for his support and encouragement, to Mikaela and Ella for their patience and good humor, and to Mary Jo and Hans for everything.

—TA

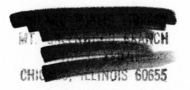

NOTE TO READERS

Medicine is an ever-changing science, and as new research or clinical experience increases our knowledge, it may change diagnosis and treatment. The authors have checked with sources believed to be reliable, at the time of writing, in their efforts to provide information. However, the authors are not engaged in rendering medical or any professional services in this book, and the information in this book is not intended as a substitute for advice from your doctor. It is impossible to list every risk or benefit associated with diagnostic tests, medications, lifestyle changes, and herbal and alternative medicines, and individual experiences may vary. Individual readers are solely responsible for their own health-care decisions; the authors and the publisher do not accept responsibility or liability for any adverse effects individuals may claim to experience, whether directly or indirectly, from the information contained in this book.

The fact that an organization or Web site is listed in the book as a potential source of information does not mean that the authors or publisher endorse any of the information they may provide or recommendations they may make.

The stories in this book are fictional accounts based on the experiences of many individuals. Similarities to any person or persons are coincidental and unintentional.

CONTENTS

INTRODUCTION

"What Would You Do If She Were Your Mother?" (Answer: Take Action!)

Imagine this scenario: You're a career woman with a family. You've noticed that your mother's memory has been going downhill for a couple of years. She mixes up the names of some of her friends, she's missed two bill payments, and she recently dropped out of her weekly bridge club, saying she prefers being at home. She denies any memory problems and takes pleasure in saying, "Even my family doctor said I was in great shape at my last physical three weeks ago."

You take a day off and bring her to the doctor, who sees her privately for about twenty minutes. The doctor then invites you to join them and says that your mother may have a mild memory problem (which you already knew!) but that it's not Alzheimer's. Your mother, relieved, smiles at the doctor and gives you an "I told you so" look. You are too uncomfortable to ask the doctor what tests she did, how accurate the tests are, and whether you should seek a second opinion. Back at home, you say to your mother, "Looks like you aced the tests the doctor gave you. Were they difficult?" Your mother answers, "All I had to do was draw a round clock. I passed, so don't bother me about my memory anymore."

Nearly two years after that visit, your mother's short-term memory has gotten much worse. She repeats herself often, as though she has forgotten what she said just minutes ago. She has also stopped reading her favorite magazines, and her hairdresser says she is show-ing up for "appointments" that she never made. A family friend calls to say that your mother got lost on her way to their house even though she had been there many times before. You take your mother back to the doctor, and this time the doctor orders a brain scan and blood work. When the doctor calls back a few days later, she says your mother has early Alzheimer's disease and should try a medica-tion. The doctor does not tell you the test results or refer you to a specialist but does transfer you to the clinic's social worker, who sug-gests you call the local Alzheimer's Association chapter.

When you hang up from the call, you're stunned and you don't know where to begin. You have no one to help you decide whether you should tell your mother the diagnosis, whether she can live on her own, what will happen to her next. Is it a definitive diagnosis? Should you take her for another evaluation? Should she take any medications?

Your questions are beginning to snowball. You vaguely remember hearing about promising treatments on the news, and you've seen newspaper ads seeking participants with Alzheimer's for a clinical trial—but how do you make sense of this information? Bewildered by the differing options for treatment and care, and worried about your own future, you wish you could ask a top doctor: "What would you do if she were your mother?"

That is just the question we want to answer in this book. As a doctor who specializes in treating and studying Alzheimer's disease, and a social worker with years of experience teaching people how to live with and care for those with the illness, we are grounded in the latest advances in the field as well as the inside information you need to take charge. We want to help you create a plan of action to get the best diagnosis and treatment for the person in your life who has or may have Alzheimer's. That action plan will also help you find the best support for the person with Alzheimer's and the person taking care of him or her.

In fact, the idea for our book arose when Dr. Doraiswamy realized that he was repeatedly asked the very question posed by the daughter in this scenario. In lectures delivered to medical and lay audiences alike, the most poignant and common query was, "What would you do if your mother was starting to have memory problems?"

Embedded in that question, he understood, was people's belief that expert physicians provide a higher level of medical care for their immediate family members or close friends than for routine patients. To test that perception, he conducted a survey of more than a hundred Alzheimer's experts and found his intuition was correct. In each of several questions posed—whether about treatment options for early memory problems or the types of diagnostic tests doctors said they'd prescribe—the physicians said they would indeed order better, more sophisticated tests and treatments for "their own" than for the average patient.

The idea that a doctor's family and friends might get better care than others is neither surprising nor fair. But it is a reality we'd like to change. Our intent is to open up that expert knowledge base to anyone diagnosed with Alzheimer's or its precursors and to those who care for them so that you can get the most from your doctors, from your local chapter of the Alzheimer's Association, the leading and the oldest Alzheimer's support and research organization, and from other community resources.

In a few pages, we'll return to the mother and daughter, and show how having extra knowledge would have improved her treatment. But let's start with a quiz to see how much you already know about Alzheimer's.

Which of these statements are true and which are false? (The answers follow the statements.)

1. Some people get Alzheimer's in their forties or fifties.
2. Dementia is the same as senility or aging.
3. If your mother developed Alzheimer's in her eighties, you have a 95 percent chance of getting it as well.
4. Alzheimer's brain changes may start years or decades before memory problems become fully apparent.
5. Specialists can tell with up to 90 percent accuracy whether or not someone has Alzheimer's.
6. A depressed mood or a vitamin deficiency can impair one's memory.
7. There is no approved medication for treating Alzheimer's symptoms. The only options are experimental drugs.
8. High blood pressure or obesity may increase one's risk for dementia.
9. Being socially involved and keeping one's mind active may postpone Alzheimer's.

10. All clinical research studies involve taking risky experimental drugs.

Answers: **1.** T **2.** F **3.** F **4.** T **5.** T **6.** T **7.** F **8.** T **9.** T **10.** F

If you're like most people, you could use some help separating the facts about Alzheimer's from the myths. The following chapters will provide a wealth of knowledge, as well as encouragement and support for handling the many complexities of early- and middle-stage Alzheimer's. You will find:

- Information on the diagnosis and treatment of early- and middle-stage Alzheimer's, including numerous new developments that your doctor may not know about

- Coverage of the earliest warning signals of Alzheimer's, such as mild cognitive impairment (MCI) and cognitive impairment no dementia (CIND), conditions that may be precursors to Alzheimer's disease or a related disorder

- Detailed descriptions of why and when a person needs a medical evaluation, how to find the best doctors, and when to get a second opinion—including eye-opening examples of missed opportunities to get help at early to moderate stages of the disease

- State-of-the-art advice on the medical treatment of early- to middle-stage Alzheimer's, including the latest studies of treatments approved by the Food and Drug Administration (FDA) and so called off-label prescription treatments, where a drug is used for a purpose not specified by the FDA

- Expert advice on psychotropic drugs for treating depression, anxiety, insomnia, and behavioral problems in people in the early and middle stages of Alzheimer's, including the latest information on both prescription and nonprescription treatments, as well as their adverse effects

- The newest information about the growing links among heart and vascular disease, stroke, diabetes, and Alzheimer's, and how to take advantage of this information to assess—and reduce—the risk of memory impairment

- Clear, compassionate, and practical answers to questions about living with Alzheimer's in its early and middle stages, as well as about nondrug approaches that promote quality of life

- Unique coverage and explanation of clinical trials, with information specific to Alzheimer's

- Sound advice on lifestyle factors and complementary treatments for Alzheimer's disease, including herbs, exercise, diets, vitamins, and mental activities

- A look at the future of Alzheimer's disease and other memory disorders, including new treatments and diagnostic techniques now being tested

THE STATE OF ALZHEIMER'S

Here are some facts and statistics about Alzheimer's in the United States:

- Alzheimer's is the most common cause of dementia in the elderly, and the number of people with Alzheimer's has doubled since 1980 as people live longer. There are now about 5 million people with Alzheimer's and 3 to 4 million people with MCI.

- Every seventy-two seconds someone develops Alzheimer's.*

- About half a million people have early-onset dementia.*

- Almost 10 million people are caring for someone with Alzheimer's.*

- For about 60 percent of people with early Alzheimer's, the condition is either not recognized by their family or not evaluated by a doctor.

- Medical risk factors for memory loss—including diabetes, heart disease, high blood pressure, and depression—are present in more than a third of all adults and seniors.

- Most people with Alzheimer's still come to the attention of the medical community only when damage to the brain has already advanced to the moderate stage.

*Source: Alzheimer's Association 2007 Report

Unfortunately, even having access to the latest scientific research on Alzheimer's and the finest, most caring medical team doesn't guarantee you'll receive the best treatment. Because of this, we also provide insider tips, good ideas that are available to people who already know a doctor, nurse, or social worker. The tips should get you around the typical roadblocks to timely, appropriate care. We firmly believe that everyone—not just the lucky few—deserves access to this kind of information so they can develop their own action plan for making the most of their lives when Alzheimer's enters the room.

By the way, while we are hopeful about the expanding state of knowledge in Alzheimer's prevention, delay, diagnosis, and treatment, we are also realists, familiar with the day-in, day-out difficulties of caring about and for a person with Alzheimer's. So besides giving you lots of cutting-edge information, we discuss what you are going through if you are living with or caring for someone who has Alzheimer's. We help you answer the question many of us have asked ourselves: "Am I getting Alzheimer's myself?" We do this through stories and examples of real people living with or caring for those with the disease, as well as some humor and perspective— ingredients that are vital to living with, instead of just coping with, Alzheimer's.

Now let us return to the mother and her daughter. The scenario probably has a familiar ring to it, and you don't want any version of it to happen to you.

Getting an early and accurate diagnosis is crucial, for a number of reasons. The sooner you get the right diagnosis, the better your chance of starting treatment early, when it is most effective, or gaining access to cutting-edge research studies. In addition, people with early-stage Alzheimer's retain all or most of their capacity to state reasoned preferences and values, which enables them to make crucial treatment decisions for themselves.

Unfortunately, as mentioned, this is also the stage where diagnosis is often missed. In this case, the doctor made several common mistakes:

- Failed to recognize MCI or Alzheimer's at the first visit
- Relied too much on one memory-screening test
- Should have spent more time getting the daughter's input, or gathering background information on the woman's condition

- Should have more fully discussed the findings and options with the family

Based on our long experience in the area, we know that learning about these problems and how to ask about them can truly make a difference in diagnosis and treatment.

► A WORD ON THE MEDICAL SYSTEM

One reason we are so passionate about sharing this information is that we know the medical system well. Like any system, it is flawed and imperfect. On the topic of Alzheimer's, the system, particularly until recently, had too few scientific facts and too many misunderstandings. The old medical model—which holds that patients have no rights—still pervades parts of the system. While that model has been successfully challenged over the past two decades, it lingers in places. Unfortunately, the debilitating nature of Alzheimer's tends to reinforce the model's notion of patients as helpless victims.

In addition, good, well-intentioned nonspecialists are unfamiliar with the latest advances in Alzheimer's treatment and care, as the story of the mother illustrates. It isn't their fault: They are required to stay abreast of an enormous number of diseases, and they face multiple societal and professional pressures and expectations. Moreover, some of today's physicians went to medical school in an era when standard medical textbooks covered Alzheimer's in a paragraph or two. Because of such factors, the Alzheimer's Association describes the primary-care environment as a place with "many recognized barriers" to the successful diagnosis and treatment of Alzheimer's.

Indeed, even having specialty training in areas related to Alzheimer's might not be enough. Being a psychiatrist, neurologist, geriatrician, pharmacist, psychologist, or social worker per se, for example, doesn't guarantee you'll have an in-depth knowledge of Alzheimer's. Until recently, many doctors received only a few lectures on Alzheimer's during a four-year residency; even now, the average psychiatrist or neurologist may have seen only a dozen Alzheimer's patients by the end of his or her training. Yet these doctors are expected to be the specialists in their communities the minute they start practicing.

As experts in the area, we can provide you with accurate information as well as a way to make sense of it all. We are advocates who believe that people with Alzheimer's have the right to access the best, most personalized care possible.

Because knowledge is power, we want you to become advocates, too. To this end, we will conclude by sharing a concept first proposed by the renowned bioethicist Nancy Dubler in 1987 called "The Rights of Alzheimer's Families." Dr. Doraiswamy has expanded these rights several times so that now they include not only the person with memory loss but also family members at risk for future disease or health problems that arise as a result of caring for someone with Alzheimer's.

These rights are similar to those used for years in other diseases, including cancer, heart disease, and AIDS. We hope they will soon be the norm in Alzheimer's care as well.

THE RIGHTS OF ALZHEIMER'S PATIENTS AND PEOPLE AT RISK

1. The right to get the latest, best, and most appropriate diagnostic tests at the earliest onset of memory loss

2. The right to know one's diagnosis as well as the results of all tests

3. The right to start treatment before additional brain functions are lost

4. The right to get the best and newest treatments

5. The right to access the best support services and complementary therapies

6. The right to plan for assets and your future

7. The right to participate in clinical trials and research studies

8. The right to receive care consistent with the values of you and your family

We also recognize that any set of rights needs to placed in the proper context. While our rights were framed primarily from the patient's point of view, if there are conflicts of interest between the individual and the family, then the rights of the family member also become important. Further, a right to good care assumes that everyone has equal access to care and that all care providers are obligated to provide treatment. This may not hold true if someone lacks adequate health insurance coverage. Further, critical aspects of caring such as family support and respite care can be hard to access since they are very underfunded. The right to access the latest treatments or clinical trials also presumes that these treatments are proven clinically effective and that one is being protected from harmful trials. Lastly, while everyone has a right to transfer their assets to prepare for public funding of long-term care, this raises larger societal justice issues. Within this context, it is our hope that these rights will form a template for future discussions about optimal care.

A final note: We and other Alzheimer's experts believe that Alzheimer's is now at the point where heart disease was two decades ago. There is still no cure, but a number of existing and promising treatments are helping to ease the burden of the disease compared to even ten years ago. Moreover, we believe an explosion of new knowledge about Alzheimer's and its risk factors holds great potential for more targeted treatments as well as future prevention.

That is promising news indeed, and we hope you can learn through this book what we have learned from the thousands of people with memory loss we've known throughout our careers. What we say here may upset some professionals who work in this field, from primary-care doctors to specialists, from pharmaceutical supporters to herbalists. It is our view that as long as all sides are equally mad at us, we are well positioned to serve the public: you.

Throughout the book, our goal is simple: to tell you what we would do if we, or someone close to us, were concerned about memory lapses or had recently been told he or she might have Alzheimer's.

PART ONE

► **EARLY AND ACCURATE DIAGNOSIS:
HOW TO GET IT AND WHY IT MATTERS**

CHAPTER ONE

COULD IT BE ALZHEIMER'S?

Inside every older person is a younger person
wondering what the hell happened.

—MARK RUSSELL

Jane, fifty-seven, managed a large sales force. She prided herself on being good at names, and introductions were easy for her—until last spring when she referred to Barbara as Betty at a meeting and had to correct herself. She started noticing that her memory wasn't as dependable as it once was—she had to really try to remember names and dates. Her mother had developed Alzheimer's in her late seventies, so Jane entertained a wide array of worries: Is this just aging? Is it because of menopause? Is it early Alzheimer's? Did her coworkers or family notice her slips? Should she ask them? Should she see a doctor, and if so, which doctor? Would she really want to know if she was getting Alzheimer's? Would she lose her job, health insurance, or friends if she did have Alzheimer's?

As it turns out, Jane did not have Alzheimer's. She consulted a doctor, who, in docspeak, told her that the passage of time (getting older) had taken a slight toll on her once-superquick memory. She was slowing down a little, and if she relaxed, the name or date or other bit of information she needed would come to her soon enough. She was still good at her job and home life. She had simply joined the ranks of the worried well.

Normal brain aging, beginning as early as the forties in some people, *may* include:

- Taking longer to learn or remember information
- Having difficulty paying attention or concentrating in the midst of distractions
- Forgetting such basics as an anniversary or the names of friends
- Needing more reminders or memory cues, such as prominent appointment calendars, reminder notes, a phone with a well-stocked speed dial

Although they may need some assistance, older people without a mental disorder retain their ability to do their errands, handle money, find their way to familiar areas, and behave appropriately.

How does this compare to a person with Alzheimer's? When Alzheimer's slows the brain's machinery, people begin to lose their ability to

- remember recent events or conversations, yet they retain old memories. They may remember where they were born or their first job, but they won't remember that they told you about both in some detail a few minutes earlier.
- plan, start, or organize tasks
- find the right words or name everyday things, such as a clock or a stove
- comprehend or follow even simple directions
- keep track of the time and where they are

The severity and the speed of the memory loss distinguishes aging from Alzheimer's, yet the line between where normal aging ends and Alzheimer's begins is as unclear as the memories of a person with Alzheimer's. Even the changes that occur in the brain during Alzheimer's are just a more severe version of the changes we see in the aging brain. Indeed, some scientists argue that Alzheimer's is a form of accelerated but otherwise normal aging.

But to the family members of someone with Alzheimer's, the differences between normal aging and Alzheimer's are real and in their face. In contrast to their healthy older friends, people in the early stage of Alzheimer's have more problems with shopping, handling money, or getting to familiar places. If someone has become a little uneasy driving and finds alternative routes to avoid major highways, that's not a sign of Alzheimer's. If a person avoids being alone in the car because he or she is getting lost, that could very well be Alzheimer's.

Alzheimer's is more than memory loss. People with the disease have trouble behaving appropriately. Even though they desperately want to appear like their normal selves, their brains aren't up to it. Healthy individuals without Alzheimer's or other forms of dementia still have that choice.

DEMENTIA VERSUS ALZHEIMER'S

Dementia is the broad general diagnosis given to a person whose thinking, particularly memory, is so impaired it affects day-to-day functioning. Not all dementia is due to Alzheimer's, but everyone with Alzheimer's has dementia. However, the term *Alzheimer's* is often used incorrectly to refer to different types of dementia that impair memory and occur in older individuals. More than a hundred different disorders cause dementia, and their different symptoms depend on what parts of the brain they attack.

► WHAT CHANGES IN ALZHEIMER'S?

Alzheimer's is about change. If you are wondering if a family member has Alzheimer's, think about how he has changed. It's the decline that is telling. For example, your father may remember all sorts of interesting facts or stories, but when you think about it, you realize he's actually become forgetful *for him*. Some people never knew the name of their senators, but a lobbyist forgetting a senator's name could be a sign of serious memory loss. If your mother loves to read, has always forgotten the name of the author, and now finds the name slipping more often, she's probably fine. If she is losing her interest in reading, she's not.

Alzheimer's is gradual, but not as gradual as normal aging. It comes on more slowly than some kinds of dementias. If you ask family members when they noticed the changes, they will have difficulty saying. If there is a sudden onset of memory loss or confusion, it is likely due to another cause, such as a stroke, medication side effects, or an infection that is disturbing the person's thinking or mood. When these conditions are treated, memory sometimes improves as well.

Personality and mood shift as well in people with Alzheimer's. We aren't talking about normal changes in response to events or big decisions, such as retiring, falling in love, or losing a loved one. We mean, "Have you noticed how Dad is so sullen all the time?" or "What has gotten into Dad?" or "Why is he so irritable and suspicious?" Not all Alzheimer's-induced mood and personality changes are for the worse. Some people become more accepting or spontaneous.

It's not unusual for a person with Alzheimer's to seem almost fine one day and do something quite out of character the next day. Symptoms seem to come and go. As the disease progresses, the variability continues, but the good days become less frequent and less good.

Eventually, Alzheimer's can become quite intrusive. If a person doesn't get proper help, Alzheimer's can seem to undermine all aspects of life at work and at home.

► WHAT DEFINES ALZHEIMER'S

To be diagnosed with the disease, there have to be signs that the person's memory has declined *along with* one other cognitive or "thinking" function, such as language, sense of time, judgment, reasoning, or executive function, which includes the ability to plan, organize, and start or stay on task. The defining characteristics of Alzheimer's are:

- A subtle onset followed by a slow decline in memory (not caused by reversible conditions such as thyroid imbalance)

- A slow decline in one other mental function, such as language
- Having problems in daily functioning as a result of the mental changes

These and other criteria are what doctors use to make a clinical diagnosis that someone has "probable Alzheimer's." If the person only partially meets these criteria, he or she has "possible Alzheimer's." A definitive diagnosis of Alzheimer's is usually made only during an autopsy, by examining the brain tissue.

DEMENTIA SCREENING INTERVIEW

If you are worried about whether your relative is developing Alzheimer's, answer the following questions. Put a yes by the ones that describe *a change* that you've seen in your relative in the last several years, if you think the change is caused by thinking and memory problems. So if he has always had trouble remembering appointments but hasn't gotten any worse, it's not a yes. Or if he now has trouble with his financial affairs because he is losing his eyesight and is too stubborn to get someone to read him his financial documents, it's not a yes, either (yes, it's annoying; no it's not necessarily dementia). Try to answer the questions quickly, without dwelling on the accuracy of your answers.

1. Problems with judgment (e.g., problems making decisions, bad financial decisions, problems with thinking)
2. Less interest in hobbies/activities
3. Repeats the same things over and over (questions, stories, or statements)
4. Trouble learning how to use a tool, appliance, or gadget (e.g., VCR, computer, microwave, remote control)
5. Forgets correct month or year
6. Trouble handling complicated financial affairs (e.g., balancing checkbook, income taxes, paying bills)
7. Trouble remembering appointments

(continued)

8. *Daily* problems with thinking and/or memory

Scoring: If you put a yes next to none or just one, your relative probably does not have any kind of dementia. The questionnaire can't rule out cases of very early dementia, nor is it perfect, so don't hesitate to get help for your relative if he or she continues to worry you. If you answer yes to two or more, you do need to get your relative assessed promptly by a specialist.

Source: Adapted with permission from J. E. Galvin et al., "The AD8, a Brief Informant Interview to Detect Dementia," *Neurology* 65 (2005): 559–64.

► BRAIN CHANGES

Although we don't know exactly how Alzheimer's arises in the brain, we believe it involves a buildup of so-called plaques and tangles. Plaques are clumps of a protein called beta-amyloid, which start accumulating in the front of the brain and gradually spread to other parts. Tangles are twisted knots of another protein called tau that arise from inside cells. Tangles start near the hippocampus, the brain's memory center, and spread through the brain.

There may be different types of beta-amyloid plaque, researchers are now discovering. Just like there is good and bad cholesterol, it appears that we have good and bad beta-amyloid. Scientists are trying to develop drugs that get rid of the bad plaque.

Other theories on how Alzheimer's damages the brain implicate inflammation, ministrokes, free radicals, a glucose deficit, and more. We also don't know when Alzheimer's starts in the brain: Some new studies suggest that it may have a long incubation period. Indeed, brain changes may start decades before diagnosis.

► ALZHEIMER'S MEMORY TARGETS

Brain cells communicate with one another through chemical and electrical signals. These signals form a sort of "wiring" (called synapses) that connect the different parts of the brain. One theory is that

Alzheimer's gradually clogs up that connective wiring over time. The good news is that different parts of the brain handle different functions, and Alzheimer's does not damage all of them at the same time or rate. So a person's sense of humor may be intact while the storage unit for remembering what just happened takes a big hit, or a person remembers some arcane facts of art history but not how many children he or she has.

The brain has multiple warehouses for storing memory. People with very early Alzheimer's can sometimes use the brain's temporary notepad that holds information that we are going to retain for only a short period, such as directions to the nearest gas station, fairly well. But then they stumble when it comes to transferring important information to longer-term storage, probably because Alzheimer's early on damages the memory center (the hippocampus) and nearby areas. Other areas of the brain damaged in the beginning stages of Alzheimer's handle learning, math, language, drawing skills, sense of place, and more.

Shortfalls in short-term memory occur early on in Alzheimer's. Remembering what you ate for lunch or where you are going, for example, requires a good short-term memory. A part of short-term memory called *episodic memory* holds daily events and encompasses verbal and visual memory. Loss of episodic memory causes people with Alzheimer's to repeat questions and stories frequently. *Verbal memory* stores words you just heard, such as the name of someone you just met or a news item on the radio. *Visual memory* enables you to recognize people or places—to remember what something looks like.

Semantic memories are the memory of meanings and concepts as opposed to specific experiences. Semantic memory stores the information you need in order to do your job, whether it's being a doctor or a store manager, or to pursue a hobby, whether it's gardening or golf, poker or Polish history. The strength of the semantic memory depends in part on a person's age and education. In people with Alzheimer's, semantic memory fails usually after episodic memory fails.

The memory function that is next affected by Alzheimer's is *procedural memory*, which stores information that is below awareness, tucked securely in the subconscious. It's the memory for how to do something that has become almost automatic. Procedural memory lets people with Alzheimer's play the piano when they can no longer learn or read new music. It (unfortunately) enables them to drive a car even if they can't remember how they got to their destination. As Alzheimer's spreads in the brain, procedural memories and skills are also lost.

Surprisingly, people with early Alzheimer's can sometimes re-learn how to do a procedure that once was automatic, such as making coffee. But the new skill is very limited. For example, they can use only the type of coffeepot that they practiced on and only if it's in the same location where they practiced.

Long-term memory, which stores information from more than two to five years ago, is also initially somewhat resistant to Alzheimer's. A first job, a mother's bedtime song, or something funny that happened at high-school graduation are all in long-term memory storage. Stories of traumatic or powerful events that people retell, such as experiences related to war, discrimination, and immigration, are also well preserved. Some people with Alzheimer's forget a recently deceased spouse yet remember well their parents who died many years earlier. (For more on how Alzheimer's travels through the brain, check out "Inside the Brain: An Interactive Tour" at www.alz.org/brain.)

► HOW THE BRAIN AGES

Autopsies reveal that the brain usually begins to show signs of age in our fifties and sixties. The brain continues to change over time, either gradually or more dramatically if Alzheimer's is at work. Genes and lifestyle contribute to wide variations in how our brain ages. Here is what you can expect a "normal" brain to undergo:

- The connections throughout the brain start slowly malfunctioning.
- Levels of chemicals that promote communication within the brain, called neurotransmitters, are dropping.
- Cholesterol plaque is clogging up small blood vessels that get oxygen to the brain.
- Amyloid plaque is accumulating outside brain cells.
- Growth factors that help strengthen the brain are decreasing.
- Inflammation is increasing and damaging useful cells.

- The brain can no longer successfully fight off cell-damaging molecules.

The Alzheimer's-afflicted brain changes more than the healthy brain. But what's interesting is that the brains of some people who appeared free of Alzheimer's while alive actually show significant signs of the disease. We clearly need to better understand what causes Alzheimer's and what protects people who have brain changes associated with the disease from becoming forgetful.

► WHAT ALZHEIMER'S FEELS LIKE: AN INSIDER'S VIEW

We talk a lot about what Alzheimer's looks like to doctors, family members, and friends. But what does the person with early symptoms of Alzheimer's experience? Most people with the disease do recognize changes in themselves, but they often attribute them to stress or other causes, or say they don't know what's wrong. For example, while the husband notices stains on his wife's clothes, she thinks of herself as the natty dresser she always was. A grandfather considers himself the safe driver he once was and doesn't understand why his children won't let him drive the grandkids. Sadly, this lack of self-awareness often goes hand in hand with Alzheimer's-related apathy and indifference.

On the other hand, about half of all people with Alzheimer's know something is wrong with their behavior or thinking. Those who are aware of their memory loss and can talk about it, report feeling

- perplexed, unsure, uneasy, or uncertain
- fearful of making mistakes
- intermittently aware of their own memory loss
- fuzzy or foggy

Self-awareness of memory impairment hits everyone at different times:

- One woman felt angry at her toaster and coffeepot for not working, yet on some level she knew she had just forgotten how to use the appliances.

- Another woman knew that the reports she wrote for her boss didn't make sense, but she didn't know how to fix the problems.
- A scholar was acutely aware that his concentration was failing him.
- Not surprisingly, the first symptom that a technology buff noticed was a decline in his computer skills.

► WHAT FAMILIES SEE VERSUS WHAT THE PERSON WITH ALZHEIMER'S EXPERIENCES

How people with Alzheimer's feel and how they view their own behavior can be quite at odds with their family members' impressions of them. In a small study of people with Alzheimer's and their families, people with the disease said:

- Daily tasks, such as getting dressed, are really frustrating and upsetting.
- Physical problems, such as arthritis, poor vision, or physical disabilities, are more serious than their memory shortfalls.

The family members reported that the person with Alzheimer's

- gets frustrated by daily tasks, yet also forgets the incidents quickly
- worries a lot, obsessively checks for missing things, or asks repeatedly for reassurance with such questions as "Do I have an appointment?" or "Is this where I should be?"
- avoids situations that would make him or her look foolish
- denies that something is difficult
- gets defensive about his or her disabilities

In another study, the chief complaints of the people with early Alzheimer's were:

- Difficulty in handling money
- Getting lost
- Forgetting what they just did

The family members said the person was forgetful and

- unusually quiet
- withdrawn
- apathetic

"When I finally confronted my husband about being so crabby, he finally admitted he felt like he was losing his mind. He was exhausted trying to hide his forgetfulness."

▶ PEEK IN THE PANTRY

Sometimes snooping around can tell you a lot about how your relative is doing. When one out-of-town daughter visited her mother after a six-month absence, she was very surprised to discover that her mom's kitchen was in disarray. Spoiled food was in the refrigerator and an opened carton of milk was in a cupboard. The mother didn't remember how long the milk had been there, and she was uncharacteristically unconcerned about these lapses in food safety—a complete about-face from her formerly fastidious ways. The mother had sounded okay on the phone with her daughter, and friends reported that Mom was fine. But the mother was operating on "social autopilot" during her brief encounters with neighbors and friends. Meanwhile, she was entering the early stage of Alzheimer's. (For excellent information on how to check in from afar, read "So Far Away: Twenty Questions for Long-Distance Caregivers" at the National Institute of Aging's Web site, at www.nia.nih.gov.)

What You Might Notice in Yourself if You Have Early Alzheimer's

- You are having trouble learning new information, concentrating, or remembering recent events. You may have always joked about being "an old dog" who can't learn how to use new gadgets, but now you can't even remember how to use the old gadgets.

- You feel sluggish. You are thinking in slow speed. Your brain feels as if you are driving with the parking brake on.
- You're making more than just "dumb mistakes." You left the stove on—again. You got lost in your own neighborhood—again.
- You avoid crowds and cocktail parties.
- You're worrying and checking yourself more.
- It's taking longer to do everything and you're uncertain of yourself, especially at work.
- Repairs that used to be easy for you are taking forever or are left unfinished.
- Planning meals for family or guests has become harder for you.
- People mention that you are repeating yourself.
- You answer questions by making jokes or changing the subject because you don't know the answer.

▶ WHEN ALZHEIMER'S STRIKES EARLY

Soon after Harriet turned fifty-two, she began accusing her husband, John, a prominent physician, of having an affair with their neighbor, a much older married woman. At the same time, the volunteers at the hospital gift store, which Harriet had founded and run successfully for many years, told John that she was making many accounting errors. John was worried, in part because Harriet's mother had died in her late fifties in a mental hospital of what was then called "organic brain syndrome." Harriet refused to go to a doctor and instead insisted on marriage counseling, but the counselor said Harriet needed a psychiatric evaluation. Soon after, Harriet had a car accident. When the police came, she seemed almost delusional and was hospitalized, which—finally—led to a full medical workup. The diagnosis: early-onset Alzheimer's disease.

She responded well to Alzheimer's medications, and her distrust of her husband gradually subsided. She refused to get any help or go to an adult day program, but the hospital volunteer director engaged some of her friends to work in teams with her at the gift store, so she continued "working" for a year after her diagnosis. Her husband noted that

her friends and volunteers at the hospital were far more accepting of her
once they learned that she had a "brain disorder."

As many as half a million Americans have early-onset Alzheimer's,
which means that their memory problems start before the age of
sixty-five.

Many are still working and some are still raising children. Their
colleagues and family members may be attributing the changes they
see to stress, a family conflict that has left the person disgruntled, or
just an ever-souring personality. A survey of people age fifty-five to
sixty-four with early-onset dementias found that it took an average
of one year from the time they sought medical attention to the time
they received a diagnosis. Along the way, many received multiple incorrect diagnoses.

Early-onset Alzheimer's looks and sounds much like the Alzheimer's
that strikes in the later years, but studies suggest it may progress
more quickly. Also, early onset appears to run in families that have an
inheritable abnormality in their genes (called mutations) that leads to
development of memory problems even in people as young as their
mid-thirties. We now have tests that can often detect these genetic
mutations. Early-onset memory loss can also result from a severe head
injury, Down syndrome, stroke, or vascular disease.

Moreover, other health conditions can masquerade as early-onset
Alzheimer's, including alcohol abuse, malnourishment, HIV, syphilis,
herpes, thyroid deficiencies, and more. Other less common dementias, such as frontotemporal dementia (which leaves the memory
somewhat intact but causes inappropriate social behaviors, changes
in mood and judgment, and an inability to find the right words when
speaking), can also start before age sixty-five.

Given how insidious memory loss is, how difficult it is to pinpoint
when memory loss started, and how long it can take to get a diagnosis, the designations early onset and late onset may soon be discarded.

Even if they are diagnosed correctly, people with early-onset
Alzheimer's face a host of emotional, social, and financial hurdles.
They may get fired and lose valuable work benefits, or lose their busi-
nesses before they are eligible for Medicare. Others take on less complex jobs, only to discover that the learning curve for any new job is
compromised by the progress of their disease. Moreover, these lower-
paying jobs with less responsibility typically offer poorer disability

benefits. Finally, even though they are routinely denied disability pay, it's critical that anyone diagnosed with early-onset Alzheimer's apply for it immediately and appeal any rejections.

In one study, people with early-onset Alzheimer's who were still in the early stage of the disease reported that some of their earliest symptoms were emotional changes, including irritability, anger, agitation, and fatigue. They also noticed that they were

- losing things
- forgetting how to do things that were previously automatic and easy
- forgetting coworkers' names
- having difficulty completing tasks
- getting lost driving
- forgetting words

Prior to being diagnosed, they blamed their problems on stress, overwork, menopause, depression, small strokes, getting older, or going crazy. Many said their doctors came up with the same explanations, until finally they were correctly diagnosed as having early-onset Alzheimer's.

► IN SUMMARY: WARNING SIGNS OF ALZHEIMER'S

None of these problems alone qualifies a person for an Alzheimer's diagnosis (or else we'd all be card-carrying Alzheimer's patients). However, each of the following problems is a red flag *if* it represents a change from how the person has been in the past and if the problem has steadily worsened over the last six to twelve months.

Memory Shortfalls

- Difficulty learning and holding on to new information
- Trouble with step-by-step reasoning, such as following directions or figuring out in a logical fashion why something won't work

- Repeating themselves
- Forgetting recent conversations or events
- Not knowing where to look for misplaced things, because they can't retrace their steps or remember where they might have had something last
- Inability to remember the normal words, so they substitute general words for specific names, such as "the girls" for a wife and daughter or "the cleaner" for the vacuum. They may also use words that don't quite sound right but make sense to them. For example, a math teacher began to say, "That doesn't correlate," whenever she was confused.
- Reading and rereading instructions without understanding

Poor Judgment Calls

- Bad financial decisions, such as falling for a get-rich-quick scam that previously they would have known to avoid
- Excessive generosity with money
- Going out alone at night in a dangerous area

Confusion

- Getting lost in familiar places
- Misinterpreting what they hear
- Repeatedly asking what they are supposed to be doing now
- Struggling to make simple decisions or choices
- Mistaking the past for the present, such as believing they still pay their bills on time as they once did, or trying to go to their former office
- Not knowing how to respond if something unexpected happens, such as being faced with a detour when driving
- Getting confused by tasks that require using numbers, such as making change or paying bills

Behavior Changes

- Dropping their normal routines and social activities
- Changing their preferences in both food and dress
- Losing interest in hobbies, family, friends, or work
- Repeating the same action, such as dusting the same spot, or never completing a task because they forget what they set out to do
- Difficulty starting, planning, or organizing meals, trips, or any event that was once routine, in part because they are easily distracted
- A shortened attention span; wanting to leave an event soon after arriving
- Trouble driving or doing routine activities
- Visuospatial problems, such as overreaching for objects or misjudging the distance between cars
- Disregarding polite rules of conduct
- Obsessively checking things, such as whether the doors are locked
- Hoarding things of little value, such as tissue boxes
- Refusing treatment for other conditions, especially depression

Hazel spent months planning a surprise weekend in Washington, D.C., for her husband, Bobby, who had never been to the nation's capital but had always wanted to go. She even mapped out a lovely walking tour for them of the city's historic monuments. When the big weekend came, Bobby was so worried about getting lost, he would hardly leave the hotel. Hazel was in tears by the end of the weekend.

Personality

These attributes are important only when they represent a clear change from a person's accustomed personality. For example, being passive isn't a sign of Alzheimer's, but becoming passive or more passive than normal may be.

- Becoming passive and less animated
- Resisting change or anything new
- Becoming silly, moody, generous, or trusting
- Being argumentative, especially at work and at home
- Becoming easily frustrated or angry
- Taking unusual risks
- Acting impulsively, without regard for the feelings of others
- Misunderstanding sarcasm, humor, or subtleties
- Becoming obstinate, stubborn, insensitive, tactless, suspicious, threatening, or accusatory
- Responding poorly to any kind of change, whether it's going on a trip, staying in the hospital, or switching bedrooms

Alzheimer's can sometimes change people's facial expressions and even the look in their eyes. Patti Davis, daughter of Ronald Reagan, wrote in 1995 that as her father developed Alzheimer's, his eyes seemed to "shimmer across some unfathomable distance, content to watch from wherever his mind alighted."

Ask Yourself

Here's a series of questions for anyone worried about Alzheimer's. If you answer yes to even one of these and you wouldn't have just a few months ago, then it's time to talk to your doctor. You can also apply these questions to a relative you are worried about.

- Do you repeat things that you say or do more now than in the past? Are you forgetting conversations or appointments or where you put things more now than you used to? (What's at risk: learning and remembering new information.)
- Do you have trouble performing tasks that require many steps, such as balancing a checkbook or cooking a meal? (What's at risk: ability to handle complex tasks.)

- Do you have trouble solving everyday problems at work or home, such as knowing what to do if the bathroom is flooded? (What's at risk: reasoning ability.)

- Do you have trouble driving or finding your way around familiar places? (What's at risk: spatial ability and orientation.)

- Do you have trouble finding the words to express what you want to say? (What's at risk: language skills.)

- Do you have trouble paying attention? Are you more irritable or less trusting than usual? (What's at risk: ability to control your behavior.)

CHAPTER TWO

WHAT LOOKS LIKE ALZHEIMER'S AND FEELS LIKE ALZHEIMER'S BUT ISN'T ALZHEIMER'S

The question is not what you look at but what you see.
—HENRY DAVID THOREAU

At one time, when an older person first became forgetful or confused, family members would say the person was becoming senile, which literally means "old" and was synonymous with confused and forgetful. If memory failures began before someone had actually reached old age, a woman might blame it on her "change of life," and a man might wonder if he should cut back on the booze or the overtime at work.

Nowadays, when we lose our keys or misplace our glasses, the first thought that jumps to mind is: Could it be Alzheimer's? But many conditions other than Alzheimer's—some of them treatable—can impair memory. Even people with Alzheimer's need to be checked out to see if something such as a thyroid imbalance or depression could be making their Alzheimer's symptoms worse. In fact, autopsies often show that people who were diagnosed with Alzheimer's also had other diseases that changed their brains, such as strokes, Parkinson's disease, or vascular dementia, the second most common cause of dementia. Vascular dementia is the result of not enough oxygen getting to the brain. For example, the brain gets shortchanged on oxygen during strokes and, more gradually, from chronic high blood pressure or clogged arteries.

Whether you are worried about your own memory or someone else's, you should know that in some cases confusion, memory loss, and impaired thinking can be treatable or even reversible. There is no guarantee, of course: The cause of most serious memory loss is indeed Alzheimer's or a combination of Alzheimer's and another disorder. Studies of older people with dementia show that at least 50 percent probably have Alzheimer's and 15 to 25 percent have vascular disease or a combination of vascular disease and Alzheimer's. But in about 10 to 25 percent of people the cause is neither of those conditions. We'll explore these other causes of memory loss in this chapter.

If It's Not Alzheimer's, It Might Be . . .

- *Depression* can interfere with the ability to remember information by upsetting concentration and attention. The information can't get laid down in memory if the brain never picked it up in the first place. Depression occurs in about 50 percent of people who have had a major stroke and is sometimes confused with Alzheimer's. (On the other hand, sometimes a first episode of depression can be an early sign of Alzheimer's.)

- *Thyroid deficiency* weakens concentration and slows thinking.

- *Diabetes* can cause problems with blood vessels that weaken blood flow to the brain and increase the risk of memory problems.

- *Heart, lung, or circulation problems*, such as having heart bypass surgery, increase a person's risk of having ministrokes and memory loss.

- *Vitamin deficiencies*, particularly B_1 (thiamine), B_{12}, or folate, interfere with brain function.

- *Liver failure* can cause hallucinations and delirium, which may be mistaken for Alzheimer's.

- *Heavy drinking* depletes thiamine levels, which is hard on nerve cells. Susceptibility to alcohol and its toxic effects varies considerably among individuals. For example, differences in the enzymes that metabolize alcohol can determine how quickly alcohol leaves the body. Having a poor diet also makes a person more susceptible to alcohol poisoning.

- *Hearing and vision loss* can make people appear to have early Alzheimer's or even believe they have it, because such losses are exhausting and distracting. In addition, people may miss out on valuable information and then think they just forgot it. So if you didn't hear your spouse ask you to pick up some tomatoes, and then you come home without them, she may think you just forgot them.

- *Delirium*, temporary but serious confusion, is caused by infections, poor nutrition, dehydration, hormone disorders, and other conditions. Hospital staff often misdiagnose delirium as Alzheimer's in older people.

- In addition, an array of conditions such as *infections* (e.g., herpes), *cancer*, and *inflammation* can cause memory loss.

▶ OTHER TYPES OF DEMENTIA

As we have discussed, Alzheimer's is just one kind of dementia. Others include:

- Vascular dementia
- Dementia with Lewy Bodies (DLB)
- Parkinson's dementia
- Frontotemporal lobar dementia, which includes Pick's disease, progressive supranuclear palsy (PSP), and primary progressive aphasia (PPA)
- Creutzfeldt-Jakob disease
- Alcoholic dementia, which includes Wernicke-Korsakoff syndrome

- Huntington's disease
- Down syndrome
- Toxic dementias
- Hashimoto's encephalopathy

Vascular Dementia

As we mentioned above, poor blood flow to the brain can cause vascular dementia. If the blood flow blockage is sudden, the dementia will occur suddenly. If the blood flow blockage is only partial, the dementia will become apparent more gradually. Having high blood pressure, high cholesterol, or diabetes—all of those conditions are bad for your heart—can increase your risk of developing vascular dementia. You don't have to have a stroke to develop vascular dementia.

The blood vessels in the brain are like a tree; big vessels feed blood to the brain, and smaller vessels coming off the larger ones supply the smaller corners of the brain. Any of these vessels can get blocked, and the effects on memory and behavior will vary depending on what area of the brain is deprived of the blood. What's clogging the vessels? The blood vessels that carry blood away from the heart develop plaque, and pieces of the plaque, called clots, break loose and travel to the brain. When seen on autopsy, the brains of most people with vascular dementia also have Alzheimer's-like changes in their brains. Indeed, the two conditions often overlap. Doctors often use the same medications to treat Alzheimer's and vascular dementia. Compared with Alzheimer's, vascular dementia can be prevented or at least kept from getting worse more successfully. You need to follow a heart-healthy lifestyle, including a low-fat diet, exercise, and medications, if necessary, to keep your blood pressure and cholesterol in check.

Tabitha, a sixty-four-year-old social worker with diabetes, was accustomed to a hectic schedule that took her into some very deprived households. But she managed to keep her emotions and, most of the time, her blood sugars in check. After having heart bypass surgery, however, she found herself forgetting appointments and crying about cases that would previously have left her just shaking her head. She underwent special testing, which showed that her memory and her ability to plan, such as thinking out projects, were slightly below normal for a woman her age and educational level. A brain scan found evidence of multiple tiny strokes in the parts of her brain that are key to memory and emotional processing.

The neurologist diagnosed her as having vascular cognitive impairment, which is a type of mild cognitive impairment (MCI) seen in people with vascular disease. She started on stronger hypertension medication, an antidepressant for her tearfulness (which often accompanies strokes), and a medication called donepezil to try to improve her memory. For the first time, her daughter took on the role of medication manager, making sure Tabitha didn't run low on any of her pills. Tabitha's cognitive abilities improved slightly and then stabilized.

The usual culprits increase the risk of developing vascular dementia: smoking, high blood pressure, high cholesterol, diabetes, or a stroke. But you can have none of these risks and still develop vascular dementia or Alzheimer's.

Unlike Alzheimer's, vascular dementia generally does not start gradually. Family members can usually tell doctors the month or time of year when they first noticed that something was wrong. Also unlike the steady decline seen with Alzheimer's, vascular dementia plateaus and then gets worse rather noticeably. The early stages of vascular dementia differ from Alzheimer's in the following ways. People with vascular dementia are generally more likely to

- have high blood pressure, high cholesterol, and other conditions that increase the risk of having a stroke
- have a history of heart attacks, strokes, or other coronary problems
- have more problems with planning and organizing than with memory
- respond well to reminder cues or hints (people with Alzheimer's don't store the new information in memory, so cues to retrieve it are not so useful)
- develop depression, sleep problems, and physical complaints, yet show fewer personality changes

- remember recent events or something they were told
- have slurred speech or trouble with language
- be more emotional and have poor social skills
- have poor balance

PREVENTING STROKES MAY HELP PREVENT DEMENTIA

About six hundred thousand strokes occur in the United States each year, plus an additional 10 million silent strokes (detected through brain scanning). Treating high blood pressure can reduce the risk for strokes by about 30 percent. Treating that high blood pressure also reduces the risk of vascular dementia by about 50 percent—or by 10 percent, or not at all, depending on which study you read. Likewise, treating high cholesterol levels can reduce the risk of strokes, but we don't yet have any clear evidence that it reduces the risk for vascular dementia. So at present our recommendations are based on what makes sense, given our knowledge of how the brain works and what studies are at least hinting at.

Dementia with Lewy Bodies (DLB)

Another major cause of dementia in the United States, DLB leads to a gradual decline in thinking and memory, much like other dementias. It is best thought of as a cross between Alzheimer's and Parkinson's and was formerly referred to as Alzheimer's plus Parkinson's. People with DLB develop the physical and memory problems at the same time, whereas in Parkinson's the memory problems come later. Compared to other dementias, with DLB people's mental abilities seem to fluctuate, causing them to "space out" or lose consciousness for periods of time and have trouble staying focused. Tasks that require visual and spatial skills, such as putting on a seat belt, can prove particularly difficult.

Clumps of proteins, called Lewy bodies, that form inside nerve cells and disrupt brain function cause the symptoms of DLB.

(Dr. Friederich H. Lewy discovered the clumps.) However, we don't know why these clumps form. Autopsy studies suggest that more people have DLB (or Alzheimer's along with DLB) than are being diagnosed. It is not easy to diagnose and usually takes a specialist.

Some experts think that people with DLB may respond better than people with Alzheimer's to drug treatment. However, doctors and families must focus on managing the symptoms, which can be difficult. DLB causes visual hallucinations, muscle stiffness, tremors, a slow shuffling walk, and a stiff "poker face." Delusions, such as believing that a dream is real or that bugs are crawling on them, are also common, but thankfully the delusions don't seem to be frightening. What can be scary for people with DLB and their companions is that they sometimes appear to lose consciousness and faint or fall. In fact, REM sleep disorder, in which people act out vivid nightmares, is one possible early sign of DLB.

It's very important to get an accurate diagnosis if a person has DLB and to distinguish it from Alzheimer's. For one thing, unlike people with Alzheimer's, people with DLB can sometimes have an extremely bad reaction to certain popular antipsychotics, such as Risperdal and Haldol. However, their thinking and behavior may improve or temporarily stabilize when they take Alzheimer's drugs called cholinesterase inhibitors—this has been best demonstrated with the drug Exelon. Therefore, drugs like Exelon, while not approved for treating DLB, are often the first choice of medication treatment for both the memory and behavior problems of DLB.

When Bertrand's daughter got a call from the police about her father, she laughed at first, assuming he had been speeding. Now that he was widowed, he was driving his sports car as fast as he wanted. But when Bertrand got on the phone, he was in tears. He had been walking at the mall and fainted. A security guard tried to help him back to his car, but he couldn't remember where he'd parked. Then the big surprise: The police told her that they knew him, because he had called a few times in recent months when he thought strangers had broken into his house. She had noticed he was shuffling when he walked and he did space out at times, so the fall didn't surprise her—but calling the police?

She brought him to his regular doctor, who thought he had Parkinson's, but a neurologist whom they consulted for a second opinion diagnosed Lewy Body Dementia. Bertrand's condition was stabilized on an Alzheimer's medication, and physical therapy improved his walking and balance.

Parkinson's dementia is similar to DLB, but the dementia starts as long as ten years after the muscle stiffness and tremors that characterize Parkinson's disease. About 20 percent of people with Parkinson's develop dementia, usually after the age of seventy. About 750,000 people in the United States have Parkinson's dementia. For the dementia, they often take the same medications that people with Alzheimer's use, such as Aricept and Exelon.

Frontotemporal Lobar Dementia (FTLD)

FTLD refers to a few different types of dementia. Like Alzheimer's, they are degenerative brain disorders that cause dementia, but they impair thinking and behavior before striking memory. Symptoms can start as early as the mid-forties but not after about age seventy-five, and people usually die from the disease in an average of eight years. About 40 percent of the approximately 250,000 people in the United States who have FTLD have a relative who had it. Unlike Alzheimer's, FTLD doesn't initially ruin a person's ability to keep track of where he is, how much time has elapsed, or what's going on in his daily life. But FTLD does usually cause noticeable social, behavioral, psychiatric, and language problems. As a result, people are sometimes misdiagnosed with schizophrenia or bipolar disorder. Eventually memory does falter, as the disease marches through the brain. The different forms of FTLD each harm distinct areas of the brain and, therefore, have their own unique effects on behavior. One type gradually destroys balance, eye movements, speech, and swallowing.

Pick's disease is one form of FTLD, named after the neurologist who identified the abnormal particles in the brain that characterize this disorder. Pick's usually starts as subtle behavior changes, including being unusually apathetic or indifferent at times, or being impulsive and having trouble with attention, planning, and judgment. As it progresses, it can cause more severe behavior changes, including excessive eating or drinking and loss of inhibition or impulse control.

These behavior problems usually precede memory loss, and that is one way doctors differentiate this disease from Alzheimer's. They also use brain scans to look for a particular pattern of shrinkage in the brain, and they can use neuropsychological tests to uncover significant problems with organization and planning. Although researchers have identified genetic links, Pick's is usually not inheritable. It can start at a much younger age than Alzheimer's does, and tends to progress steadily over five to fifteen years. No cure or proven treatment exists, but psychiatric drugs (and some non-drug interventions) help ease the out-of-control behavior and depression. Newer types of brain scans may be able to diagnose the disease at earlier stages and speed up the development of new therapies.

When Helen, a fifty-three-year-old economist, became uncharacteristically aggressive and deceptive, her doctor diagnosed her as having early-onset Alzheimer's and she had to resign from her job. Her speech and vocabulary steadily worsened, yet her memory remained surprisingly intact. After running some more tests, her doctor rediagnosed her with Pick's disease. By the time she was sixty-eight, she was still able to live at home but only with constant supervision. Thankfully, she had purchased long-term care insurance, which helped to cover the costs of hiring aides to come to her home. The insurance had some loopholes and didn't cover everything, but it made a difference.

People with FTLD may

- become very uninhibited—for example, swear or undress in public, be sexually inappropriate, shoplift
- become either very apathetic or grandiose and silly
- drink or smoke excessively
- become mute, talk compulsively, or repeat words or phrases
- develop a strong preference for sweets
- have unusually poor hygiene
- be unaware of their limitations or how their behavior affects others

Creutzfeldt-Jakob Disease (CJD)

Caused by an unusual and unstoppable protein called a prion, classic CJD is a very rare and rapidly progressing brain disease that proves fatal within a year. Usually striking people around the age of sixty, CJD can cause very rapid mental decline, aggressive physical behavior, tremors or jerky movements especially during sleep, loss of appetite, seizures, poor muscle coordination, and headaches. Sometimes insomnia, anxiety, depression, and symptoms of mental illness are the first signs of CJD.

People with CJD have gone to their office in the middle of the night thinking it was normal work hours, called their children strange names, banged on a neighbor's door insisting it was their house, and much more. Although prions cause both diseases, classic CJD is not associated with mad cow disease (also called bovine spongiform encephalopathy). However, a type of CJD, called variant CJD, has been linked to mad cow disease.

> After the death of her youngest son to AIDS, Ruthie, who was in her late fifties, became forgetful, quiet, and unusually clumsy. She couldn't figure out how to turn a doorknob in her own home, and she lost weight, insisting she was not hungry. The family at first attributed these changes to grief, but after further discussion realized that she hadn't been "normal" for some time and had probably been getting more help than they realized from her husband and the son's aides, who had been around constantly. Her husband took her to a local doctor, who initially attributed her changes to Alzheimer's disease.
>
> Yet her husband couldn't reconcile his wife's unusual physical changes and rapid mental decline with what he knew about Alzheimer's. He sought a second opinion at an Alzheimer's Disease Research Center, where she underwent special tests and was diagnosed—this time correctly—with CJD. He was told that she would require more nursing care soon, as her motor symptoms, language, and memory would decline rapidly. Indeed, she lived only nine months after her diagnosis.

Normal Pressure Hydrocephalus (NPH)

This is a buildup of spinal fluid on the brain, which causes unstable walking, bladder accidents, and dementia. It is a rare disorder, affecting primarily people over age sixty. A surgical procedure that involves putting a shunt in the brain to drain off excess spinal fluid can prove quite successful in some patients and let them go on to live normal lives, particularly if they are treated when they're in the early stages of the disease. Although the cause of NPH is not always known, risk factors include anything that may obstruct the flow of spinal fluid, including a head injury or infection.

Nutritional Dementia (Wernicke-Korsakoff)

This is a brain disorder caused by a thiamine (vitamin B$_1$) deficiency. Long-term heavy drinking interferes with the body's ability to absorb and use thiamine, and alcoholism is the most common cause in the United States of thiamine deficiency. Crash diets, malnourishment, dialysis, and absorption problems (such as those due to bowel surgery) can also sometimes lead to thiamine deficiency. If the disorder is detected early, the symptoms usually stop getting worse if the person is treated with thiamine injections and stops drinking. Otherwise, the damage may be irreversible. Alcohol damages the brain in other ways as well. The liver damage caused by heavy drinking can worsen mental confusion. Memory problems, unsteadiness, numbness, uncontrolled rapid eye movements, and delirium are all features of a person suffering from alcohol-induced dementia. Personality changes and hostility are common and may continue even if the person stops drinking.

Huntington's Disease

Huntington's is a fatal disease that affects people in their late thirties to forties, destroying their ability to control their movements. The disease causes dementia, depression, irritability, apathy, and anxiety. Inheriting a faulty gene causes this disease.

Down Syndrome

This disease is the most common cause of developmental disabilities, and it often leads to symptoms of Alzheimer's by age forty. Around this time, people with Down syndrome may become progressively more forgetful and unable to carry out their daily activities or to care for themselves.

Toxic Dementias

These occur rarely and are the result of direct exposure to a nerve poison, such as pesticides or lead, usually in the workplace. The poisoning causes a variety of neurological symptoms that rapidly disable the person. The symptoms stop getting worse, but don't usually improve, when the exposure stops.

Hashimoto's Encephalopathy

This is another very rare condition that causes memory problems, disorientation, headaches, and muscle jerks and weakness. It is often mistaken for Alzheimer's or a psychiatric disorder. It is treatable with steroids.

► WHAT'S THE DIFFERENCE BETWEEN ALZHEIMER'S AND MILD COGNITIVE IMPAIRMENT (MCI)?

A diagnosis still used primarily by specialists and researchers, MCI is worse than normal age-related memory loss yet not bad enough to qualify for the dementia or Alzheimer's label. Researchers disagree about whether it truly is a separate condition or just an early stage of Alzheimer's, so stay tuned for new definitions. MCI can take different routes in the brain, impairing memory and language skills *or* planning and organizational skills. When memory is the victim, the condition is called amnestic MCI, and that's the best-studied version. MCI is also sometimes called preclinical Alzheimer's or prodromal Alzheimer's.

Amnestic MCI and Alzheimer's share some features. Both are noticeable to family and friends and, to some extent, the person with the condition. They also cause poor performance on memory tests. Yet people with amnestic MCI retain their normal language, judgment, and reasoning skills, and can accomplish their daily activities without much extra help.

Like Alzheimer's, the cause of amnestic MCI is not yet known. Some pathologists consider MCI a very mild form of Alzheimer's, because they see Alzheimer's-like changes in the brains of people who died with amnestic MCI—but only about a third as many cells are damaged or dead.

The good news is that some people with MCI do get better. Among those who decline, approximately 60 percent have about three years before they progress to Alzheimer's. Hence, a diagnosis of MCI offers an earlier opportunity to pursue lifestyle interventions and clinical trials, which we describe later, to preserve the brain's nerve cells. This is also the stage at which patients can make crucial treatment decisions for themselves.

What's the bottom line? While patients with MCI are at higher than average risk of developing Alzheimer's, they are also ideal candidates for Alzheimer's prevention, delay, and treatment strategies through clinical trials or working with a specialist.

► SYMPTOMS THAT MAY SUGGEST IT'S NOT ALZHEIMER'S

Memory loss that begins and progresses very quickly or that starts before age thirty-five is probably not due to Alzheimer's. Here is a list of conditions that suggest memory loss may be due to a condition other than Alzheimer's:

- Tremors, tingling, or numbness of hands and feet
- Slurred speech
- Urinary leakage
- Lack of balance
- Muscle weakness or muscle twitches
- Having just had a stroke, uncontrolled high blood pressure, or diabetes
- Profound apathy, excessive worrying, thoughts of death
- Loud snoring or gasping for breath during sleep
- Extreme sensitivity to cold

- Bizarre or disinhibited behavior, excess drinking
- Very fast deterioration, sudden onset of memory problems
- Hallucinations in a high-functioning person
- Recent heart or lung surgery
- Recent infections
- Irregular heart rate

The cause of early memory loss doesn't always become clear at your first doctor's visit—or second or third! You will need to be monitored over time by a specialist. It's like following a developing news story: The first day's headline might be the most dramatic but not the most accurate. Or a story might be small and on page seven, but within a few weeks it's all over page one.

▶ MEDICATIONS TO WATCH FOR

Certain medications can cause people to be somewhat fuzzy-headed, particularly if they are over age sixty-five. In fact, there is an entire class of drugs that should be avoided when possible by seniors. The drugs, called anticholinergics, block acetylcholine, the very brain chemical that Alzheimer's medications increase and that helps with learning and memory. Anticholinergics include Elavil, which treats depression, and Benadryl, which is an allergy medicine. Dozens of commonly used compounds to treat dizziness, depression, allergies, incontinence, diarrhea, and Parkinson's are anticholinergics or have some anticholinergic effect. (See the partial list below or go to www.dcri.duke.edu/ccge/curtis/beers.html for a complete list.)

Researchers testing new memory medications sometimes induce transient Alzheimer's symptoms in healthy volunteers by giving them large amounts of anticholinergic drugs. The researchers then measure the effect of the new Alzheimer's drugs on the volunteers' temporarily impaired memory. Anticholinergic drugs are so common (and useful for certain conditions) that nearly one in five older people is taking them, despite doctors' efforts to find substitutes.

What to do? If you or family members have problems with thinking or memory, see whether you are taking any of the drugs known to have anticholinergic effects. The drug may be essential, so don't stop any treatments without consulting your doctor. You can also ask your pharmacist to review the medications to see how many of them have an anticholinergic effect. Then take this information to your doctor to find out which are optional and which have alternatives.

Potentially Inappropriate Drugs for Older People, Including Those with Memory Disorders

The drugs listed below are not equally problematic—some are worse than others, some cause problems for some people and not for others. Plus, their negative side effects vary. For example, Indocin may cause an ulcer or bleeding. Elavil may raise the risk for heart or memory problems. (This is a partial listing of the drugs. For the complete list, see Donna M. Fick et al., "Updating the Beers Criteria for Potentially Inappropriate Medication Use in Older Adults," *Archives of Internal Medicine* 163, no. 22 (2003). 2716–24.)

Painkillers

propoxyphene (Darvon) and combination products (Darvon with aspirin, Darvon-N, Darvocet-N), indomethacin (Indocin and Indocin-SR), pentazocine (Talwin), naproxen (Naprosyn, Avaprox, Aleve), oxaprozin (Daypro), and piroxicam (Feldene), ketorolac (Toradol), meperidine (Demerol)

Anti–Nausea Drugs

trimethobenzamide (Tigan) (in high dosages)

Muscle Relaxants and Antispasmodics

methocarbamol (Robaxin), carisoprodol (Soma), chlorzoxazone (Paraflex), metaxalone (Skelaxin), cyclobenzaprine (Flexeril), oxybutynin (Ditropan), cyclandelate (Cyclospasmol)

Older Psychiatric Drugs (sleeping pills, antidepressants, and antianxiety medications)

- *Antidepressants*: amitriptyline (Elavil), chlordiazepoxide-amitriptyline (Limbitrol), perphenazine-amitriptyline (Triavil), doxepin (Sinequan), meprobamate (Miltown, Equanil)
- *Anxiety medications*: alprazolam (Xanax), triazolam (Halcion), flurazepam (Dalmane), chlordiazepoxide (Librium), chlordiazepoxide-amitriptyline (Limbitrol), clidinium-chlordiazepoxide (Librax), diazepam (Valium), quazepam (Doral), halazepam (Paxipam), chlorazepate (Tranxene); all barbiturates (except phenobarbital) except when used to control seizures
- *Tranquilizers*: thioridazine (Mellaril), mesoridazine (Serentil), chlorpromazine (Thorazine)

Heart Medicines

disopyramide (Norpace, Norpace CR), digoxin (Lanoxin), short-acting dipyridamole (Persantine), methyldopa (Aldomet), methyldopa-hydrochlorothiazide (Aldoril), amiodarone (Cordarone), orphenadrine (Norflex), guanethidine (Ismelin), guanadrel (Hylorel), cyclandelate (Cyclospasmol), isoxsuprine (Vasodilan), nitrofurantoin (Macrodantin), doxazosin (Cardura)

Diabetes Medicine

chlorpropamide (Diabinese)

Stomach Drugs

dicyclomine (Bentyl), hyoscyamine (Levsin, Levsinex), propantheline (Pro-Banthine), belladonna alkaloids (Donnatal and others), clidinium-chlordiazepoxide (Librax)

Anticholinergics and Antihistamines

chlorpheniramine (Chlor-Trimeton), diphenhydramine (Benadryl), hydroxyzine (Vistaril, Atarax), cyproheptadine (Periactin), promethazine (Phenergan), tripelennamine, dexchlorpheniramine (Polaramine)

CHAPTER THREE

WHY TO SEEK A DIAGNOSIS *NOW*

You may delay, but time will not.

—BENJAMIN FRANKLIN

If you or someone you care about is having memory problems, you may be wondering when is the right time to get them checked out. The answer is clear and simple: ***Go now!*** If you were feeling short of breath, you probably wouldn't hesitate to call the doctor. Your brain deserves the same type of attention.

Despite the public's awareness and fear of Alzheimer's, most people wait years before consulting with a doctor about memory lapses. Sadly, more than 90 percent of people with mild cognitive impairment or the earliest symptoms of Alzheimer's don't get diagnosed until their disease worsens. But those who go early have an advantage.

> *"Before diagnosis, I was worried and agitated a lot. After, we came to treat the Alzheimer's as a manageable disability and I stopped thinking about it."*
>
> *—A person with early Alzheimer's*

▶ WHY YOU NEED AN EARLY DIAGNOSIS

There are many benefits to an early assessment and diagnosis. One of the first and most clear-cut is that you may find treatable conditions that could be causing the memory loss or confusion. Treating ailments such as depression, stress, thyroid imbalance, or vitamin deficiencies could return your memory to normal. Even if you do end up with a diagnosis of Alzheimer's or another serious dementia, it's still important to find out if you have any conditions that could be making the dementia symptoms worse. (However, we will warn you against spending too much time finding a "better news" diagnosis just to make your relatives happy.)

Of course, if you do have Alzheimer's, the real benefit of early diagnosis is early treatment. Various medications offer the hope of slowing the disease, reducing symptoms, and reducing the effects of the disease on day-to-day functioning. Treating the disease early may buy several months of extra time and may postpone the emergence of disturbing behavioral changes (such as hallucinations). Alzheimer's begins damaging the brain decades before symptoms appear, especially in people who are genetically vulnerable to the disease. By the time you notice problems, Alzheimer's has already affected your brain. But you can do a lot to ease the stress and take control of your life if you get diagnosed early. You can:

- Take medications and make dietary and lifestyle changes that may help slow some of the cognitive losses expected from the disease and maintain you at a higher level of daily functioning than would have been otherwise possible.
- Find out which medications work best for the most difficult symptoms of Alzheimer's, such as depression, anxiety, and agitation.
- With help from family, find a new sense of "normal" (lots more on this later).
- Participate in studies that will keep you up-to-date on the latest Alzheimer's treatments, plus provide you with thorough and usually excellent medical care.

Another reason for getting an early diagnosis—and maybe the only one you need—is that even if the disease is unavoidable, some of its practical consequences—including financial woes and endangering yourself or others—can be prevented.

Having unrecognized and untreated Alzheimer's increases your risk of having an accident, losing valuables, and embarrassing yourself and others. Because early Alzheimer's impairs reasoning skills, you are at risk for safety hazards, such as injuring yourself with equipment or tools, being exploited, and getting lost. Knowing you have Alzheimer's allows you and your family members to put in safeguards.

For example, family members can call you to remind you to take your medications. Such reminders reduce the likelihood of adverse reactions from taking the wrong dose or the wrong drug. You and a neighbor can agree to check in on each other once a day. You may want to hire a nephew to do the riskier chores that you once handled, such as a plumbing project.

An early diagnosis helps you retain control over your future. You can make sure your family knows your preferences, values, and priorities. You can plan for where you want to live and find the right level of supportive housing or network of family and friends to see you through the upcoming years. To make the best use of the time you have bought with an early diagnosis, you may enlist the help of social workers, counselors, support groups, and groups like the Alzheimer's Association. You may also want to join one of the increasing numbers of groups that are springing up to help others newly diagnosed with Alzheimer's.

NO JOKING

When a middle-aged person jokes with his longtime family doctor that he feels as if he has "a Teflon brain," the doctor may do little more than laugh. But if the same man joked about having a pea-sized bladder, the doctor would insist on checking his prostate and probably refer him to a specialist. Prostates are important, but we like to think our brains are, too. Don't joke your way out of a memory checkup.

Keep in mind that if you wait until the disease has progressed, you will have trouble understanding and participating in a range of decisions that will affect your future. With an early diagnosis, you have time to select a substitute decision maker for financial and health-care decisions, to put all of your wishes in writing, and to make sure the document is in the hands of people you trust to abide by it. Make sure everyone close to you knows your wishes. Early detection prevents your having to make a hasty decision about where you should live, what to do with your finances, and other important matters. Alzheimer's disease usually progresses gradually, so getting diagnosed early gives you and family members time to fully investigate options.

Another benefit of early diagnosis is that it frees you from trying to cover up your memory and behavior lapses—a common *and* exhausting effort. You and your family need time to learn to blame the disease for your mistakes, to increase your tolerance for unimportant mistakes or repetition, and gradually to replace any perfectionist standards with greater flexibility.

► THE ONLY GOOD DIAGNOSIS IS A THOROUGH DIAGNOSIS

Getting a quick McDiagnosis is like buying a house after doing a casual walk-through or buying a car after just kicking the tires. Early-stage diagnoses are tricky because symptoms of early-stage Alzheimer's are similar to normal aging. Someday there may be foolproof diagnostic procedures that detect Alzheimer's-like changes in the brain years before memory loss sets in, but those tests are still in development. So get an accurate diagnosis; go to an experienced doctor and get a thorough assessment. (Later we discuss exactly what is involved in a thorough assessment.)

That said, not everyone needs the same degree of testing to get an accurate diagnosis, nor is knowing everything about the person's memory and mental functioning equally important to all families. Early-stage Alzheimer's is harder to diagnose than later stages and requires more sensitive and potentially longer testing. Doctors can diagnose later stages with fewer tests. Knowing one's precise mental capacities is not equally important for all people. A nursing home resident who has many people looking out for him or her and a very regular daily schedule may be less concerned about getting a thorough assessment than someone who is still working or raising children.

> Ted, a sixty-year-old divorced salesman, was often running late, not showing up at all, or showing up at the wrong time for appointments, including family occasions at his brother's and children's homes. One evening, he called his oldest and closest friend in tears to say he was lost on the way to the friend's home for their weekly poker game. Finally, his friend, brother, and children talked with one another and compared notes, then met with him. Ted acknowledged that his sales commissions were way off, and he was losing valuable time obsessively checking his work. He was only too aware of the specter of Alzheimer's, having lost both parents to Alzheimer's and vascular dementia. He agreed to get a thorough memory evaluation at a university Alzheimer's research clinic, where the doctors would meet with him and his family members to explain the results.
>
> To no one's surprise, Ted was found to have early Alzheimer's. Despite his grief at having his fears confirmed, he was incredibly relieved as well. He didn't have to blame himself; he could stop "just trying harder." Moreover, he applied successfully for disability, so he could ease out of his difficult and frustrating job. He had time to decide "what next?" and eventually move to an affordable smaller condo near his children. He had time to learn his way around his new place and the children's homes before his disease progressed.
>
> Most important to Ted and his family, he could take time while he was still healthy to travel and have fun with his children, to just be together, to tell his grandchildren stories—stories his children never heard from their grandparents.

► GETTING TESTED AHEAD OF THE SYMPTOMS

Some experts recommend that everyone be tested for Alzheimer's in late adulthood. But not everyone agrees. No proven treatment exists to reverse Alzheimer's. No perfect test exists to predict or diagnose Alzheimer's before memory loss reveals itself in people's daily lives. We do not, therefore, recommend screening on the basis of age alone but rather on the basis of risk factors and/or symptoms of memory loss.

If you do go for early screening and the tests detect some changes, get a thorough evaluation to make sure those initial results are accurate. This also applies for do-it-yourself tests touted in advertisements. How you do on a few memory tests may not represent how well your brain is really functioning day to day.

In addition, people with a strong family history of early-onset Alzheimer's often ask if they should go for memory testing. Doctors don't agree on what to do, so maintain a lifestyle that is good for your brain and stay informed about new developments in the Alzheimer's field. Some research studies offer free testing for people with a family history, and that is often the best option for getting a baseline of your memory and free monitoring over the years.

▶ POST-OP TESTING

If you are in your fifties or older and having surgery that requires general anesthesia, be aware that heart or lung surgery may leave people's cognitive abilities a bit wobbly. Surgery may cause clots that block blood flow to the brain. Also, animal studies show that some types of anesthesia increase the buildup of brain-clogging amyloid plaque. A neurologist, neuropsychologist, or psychiatrist should check out memory problems that persist for more than a few days after surgery. Don't ignore it or put it off. But here's the good news: Most thinking and memory problems that begin immediately after anesthesia gradually clear within six months.

BEFORE YOU REALIZE YOUR RELATIVE HAS ALZHEIMER'S, YOU MAY FIND YOURSELF THINKING:

- He's just getting a little eccentric as he ages.
- If I'm nicer, she won't be so belligerent.
- I have to make him shape up.

(continued)

- Does anyone else notice?
- Why am I running to her rescue so often now?
- Where is the rest of my family?
- Gosh, something is really wrong.

▶ DEAR FAMILY: GET IT TOGETHER

Families have a choice: They can stand in the way of their relative getting a proper diagnosis or be the force behind the decision.

What Turns Families into Roadblocks

- Rivalry among family members surfaces when it is time to take control of a volatile situation and destroys any will to compromise.
- The family gets along well, but members simply disagree on what's best for the individual.
- Family members listen to well-meaning friends or a doctor who says that their relative's problems are just normal signs of aging.
- Family members can't afford the high costs of medical care and don't know where to turn or don't have access to less expensive options, such as joining a clinical study or filing the many forms for insurance coverage.

Social workers and psychologists have developed a number of strategies to help families work together to solve such problems, starting with the recommendation to begin with ideas you can all agree on. Knowing you agree on something, no matter how simple, can move the family toward consensus or compromise. Such starting points are as individual as the families themselves, but here are a few examples:

- "She is a great mom and deserves the best that medicine has to offer."

- "We are a family and we want to make this decision together."
- "Dad is not safe."

When presenting your ideas, it can help keep others from feeling defensive if you begin your sentences with "I." So try "I could never live with myself if Mom got hurt because she forgot to turn off the stove," or "I read an article that there are medicines that really work if you start them early."

This is not the time to share how you really feel about your relatives or to remind them of their shortcomings. If you want people to agree with you, skip the accusations. Give everyone equal time to express worries, fears, and desires concerning the diagnosis. Don't make assumptions about why someone is for or against an early or thorough assessment.

It's not just agreeing on what to do that can be difficult; sometimes it's putting the plan in motion. The solution is to enlist each family member to take on at least one specific responsibility. For example, your brother may be good at collecting information about diagnostic or treatment options, while you offer to accompany your mom to the doctor and your aunt figures out what the insurance will cover.

If you happen to have some experience in, say, health care or finance, don't automatically expect family members to accept your advice without question. In these circumstances, the emotions may be too complex for family members to be able to see your opinions, no matter how expert, as objective.

At the same time, realize that any health-care "expert" in the family may be too close emotionally to recognize and admit obvious symptoms of decline in your parent. Mental decline, more so than other ailments, is particularly difficult for spouses or close family members to recognize.

The relative who is trying to get the parent with probable Alzheimer's diagnosed or into a special living facility may face accusations of trying to seize the parent's money or to take over the family home. This is a double tragedy, for while the relatives are squabbling, the person with Alzheimer's is going without a proper evaluation or treatment.

If at all possible, include the person with the suspected memory problem in the conversations. In addition to helping to ensure her trust and cooperation, she may offer valuable insights. Try to respect the person's preferences for a physician or for whom she wishes to accompany her to a doctor's visit.

► CONVINCING A RELATIVE TO SEEK A DIAGNOSIS

Convincing a reluctant relative to get help requires tact and strategies, not anger or ultimatums. It requires getting the family member to buy into the value of a thorough evaluation. It may even require releasing your inner storyteller.

Try to see the world through your relative's eyes. Imagine getting up and not being sure where to go or what to do that day. Then, seemingly out of nowhere, your family wants you to go to a memory doctor. The prospect can be scary, so try to reduce the fear by explaining fully what a memory assessment will involve and the benefits of going.

Sometimes playing to their preferences and pride can help persuade reluctant family members to agree to an appointment:

- One older woman was willing to see a specialist who had a "Christian" medical practice.
- Snob appeal may hold the key, as in, "All the [movie stars, classy people in town, former World Cup soccer champions] go to this clinic!"
- Show a reluctant academic a news article quoting the specialist or doctor.
- Remind your relative that a nearby university medical center provided excellent care to a particular friend or relative. One man agreed to an evaluation at an Alzheimer's research center because he remembered that the same institution had "saved his father's life" many years earlier.

Now is not the time to expect anyone to overcome prejudices—even recent ones born of dementia. If Dad never went to female physicians, if he recently expressed uncharacteristic bigotry toward some racial group, try to find a familiar-looking doctor he feels comfortable with.

Emotional pleas often succeed where rational arguments fail. Try saying, "If I had a memory problem, I know that you would leave no stone unturned. I just want the same quality treatment for you."

Here are some other possible approaches:

- Maybe your father would agree to get his hearing checked by a neurologist, or your sister would say yes to an appointment to see why she is tired. Hearing and fatigue are frequent early complaints of people with memory loss, and getting them checked may just open the door to a memory assessment.

- If you and your spouse are both older, suggest a "tune-up and oil change" for both of you at a geriatrics clinic or a doctor who sees a lot of older patients.

- If the person trusts only his or her physician, ask the doctor to write a prescription to see a neurologist or other specialist who does memory assessments.

Tom, a seventy-year-old businessman, began to lose interest in his company, forgot important meetings, and was tactless and irritable with customers and his own family. Tom's daughter and his wife suspected a memory problem, because some of Tom's relatives had developed similar symptoms at the same age and were eventually diagnosed with Alzheimer's. Tom insisted there was nothing wrong with his memory, that he was just tired from a lifetime of work and from supporting his "unsupportive" family. Terribly hurt by his remarks, his wife sought help from a knowledgeable social worker.

The social worker asked if there was anyone Tom especially admired or trusted at work or elsewhere. Although Tom had become increasingly distrustful of his colleagues, he always listened to his attorney, a childhood friend. With the social worker's coaching, his wife and children talked privately with the attorney about the potential benefits for Tom of a thorough medical evaluation and early treatment. The attorney was able to encourage Tom to go to a clinic for his fatigue and loss of interest in activities. The clinic, which specialized in memory disorders, was out of town and offered the privacy Tom sought from "small-town people."

The staff diagnosed Tom with early-stage Alzheimer's, as well as previously undiagnosed heart disease. He immediately began treatment for both, and it took a month or so for all of the medications to kick in. At a follow-up visit, when his anger had subsided, the memory clinic staff encouraged Tom and his wife to join an Alzheimer's support group for couples in their hometown. Over time, Tom's wife was able to credit that group of four very different couples with preserving their social life and their identity as a twosome, which they had both always valued.

CHAPTER FOUR

WHERE TO GO—AND HOW TO PAY FOR IT

A hospital should have a recovery room adjoining the cashier's office.

—FRANCIS O'WALSH

Amid all the mixed-up emotions of deciding to seek a diagnosis, you may now find yourself asking, "Where should I go?" Obviously, you're not going to one of the McClinics that are popping up at drugstores for flu shots and strep tests, but would your regular doctor be much better? It's hard to say. It depends on the doctor's interests and areas of expertise. Read on to learn about your options for getting a memory checkup. (Note: The prep work for the appointment usually falls to the family, so this chapter is for you: spouse, sibling, offspring, friend.)

▶ WHERE TO START?

Although many family physicians provide excellent diagnosis and treatment, specialists are more up-to-date on the latest developments and have more experience. So we recommend that everyone with suspected dementia see a specialist at least once, particularly people with very mild, early-stage, or atypical memory complaints. Our first choice is a superspecialist, such as a geriatric psychiatrist, a geriatrician with a special interest in dementia, or a behavioral neurologist. If you cannot get an appointment or don't have insurance coverage for a superspecialist, then our second choice is a specialist such as a geriatrician, psychiatrist, or neurologist who has been recommended by your primary-care doctor. If your insurance allows you to see only a primary-care doctor, then take the checklist of tests we provide (page 98) with you to your appointment.

Kinds of Specialists

- *Geriatricians*, primary-care internists or family practitioners who specialize in complex conditions of older people, can provide a one-stop service for all of an older person's medical needs, including regular monitoring of chronic conditions. These doctors do the most thorough examination of a person's health status, but they do not specialize in brain or memory problems.

- *Geriatric psychiatrists* specialize in the mental and emotional problems of people over age sixty. They provide very thorough memory, mood, sleep, and thinking evaluations. They are particularly good at assessing memory problems associated with life stress, depression, anxiety, excess drinking, or family conflicts.

- *General neurologists* and *psychiatrists* perform memory evaluations but don't specialize in Alzheimer's and may treat few people with dementia.

- *Behavioral neurologists* specialize in cognitive problems such as memory loss. Often they are the best at detecting subtle brain injuries such as small strokes or infections that may be causing memory problems. They also perform very thorough neurological and cognitive exams.

- There are other doctors who do specialized tests but usually will not see patients without a referral. These include *neuropsychologists*, who do detailed memory testing; *radiologists* and *nuclear medicine doctors*, who do special brain scans; and *consultant pharmacists*, who check for harmful drug interactions. (Other specialists will review medications for interactions as well.)

► START WITH YOUR FAMILY DOCTOR?

Insurance companies sometimes require patients to see their regular doctor (primary-care physician, internist, or family doctor—they go by many titles) for a referral to a specialist, and some people just prefer to start with their regular doctor before seeing a specialist.

Advantages of Starting with Your Family Doc

- The doctor may know your relative well enough to pick up on memory shortfalls and recommend a specialist whom you will like.

- You trust the doctor and, therefore, can trust the specialist he or she recommends.

- If you and your family like the doctor, everyone may be more open with him or her and be honest about what is really going on. No one likes to admit that a beloved father or aunt can no longer play bridge or drive to the grocery store or host a family reunion.

- Primary-care physicians often have good referral sources and can speed up a referral to a specialist covered by insurance.

- The doctor should already have a complete history of your relative's medications and medical conditions. Knowing, for example, that your relative had borderline low thyroid, he or she will test the thyroid level right away. He or she may remember that your family has other relatives who developed Alzheimer's and so be particularly sensitive to memory complaints.

- It may be easier to get a family member to agree to see the family doctor than to go to an unfamiliar memory expert.

What to Watch for if You Start with Your Family Doctor

- The doctor may be familiar with the two most common memory tests and consider them adequate for assessing memory. However, those tests pick up only very obvious signs of Alzheimer's and not subtle or early memory changes.

- The doctor may be unfamiliar with the wide range of conditions that can affect a person's brain and the best possible treatments for memory disorders.

- If the doctor attributes memory problems or confused thinking to another plausible cause besides Alzheimer's, you may be falsely reassured and less likely to pursue another opinion. This is most often a problem for people in the early stage of dementia or who are able to take themselves to the doctor. They should, if possible, bring along a family member or friend, although the impaired person may be very reluctant to admit the problem to others.

- Because the doctor sees the patient fairly often, he or she may miss changes that are small or gradual but warrant a visit to a memory specialist.

▶ TRY A MEMORY CENTER

There are different facilities that provide memory testing and diagnoses. The quality of these places depends on the skills and attitude of the doctor at the helm. However, some types of facilities are more likely to offer you great care.

- Memory disorder clinics are just what they sound like—offices or entire centers that specialize in the treatment of

Alzheimer's and other diseases that affect memory. Such clinics are likely to offer the latest tests, as well as the option to participate in research studies. They are usually staffed by doctors from different specialties and affiliated with a university or community hospital. Some are also independent.

- At university-based clinics, you'll find doctors who focus just on memory problems and do extensive research on the topic, so they may be very well informed about the latest treatments. Also, a group of doctors may review and discuss your case.

- Doctors staffing memory clinics that are affiliated with a hospital will probably be involved in general practice as well. The reputation of any of these clinics depends heavily on the doctors who lead the practice. Hospital-based clinics have fewer checks and balances compared to a university practice, but that doesn't mean you won't get equally good care.

- A private memory center can be any office that has decided to call itself a memory center; the staff and facility don't have to meet any sort of qualifications. So these centers can vary greatly in staffing, services, and, most important, quality. You may find one doctor who has an interest in memory, or a staff of neurologists, psychiatrists, social workers, and nurses trained in memory disorders. Some memory centers have sophisticated memory assessment tools; others don't. Many of these centers are headed by reputable doctors. Compared with university-based centers, they tend to offer greater convenience in terms of parking and scheduling. If you find one near you that has a qualified staff and a good reputation, check it out. Don't expect the full range of experts that you would find at a university center, however.

- Most memory centers also conduct clinical trials of new drugs and diagnostic tests and will readily give you information about studies seeking participants. Some universities have an Alzheimer's Disease Research Center near you. There are thirty-two of these government-supported centers in the country and they offer study participants many useful opportunities. (To learn more about participating in clinical research studies and where to find one, see Chapter 9; also see the list of Alzheimer's Disease Research Centers in the Resources section.)

Advantages of Going to a Memory Center

- The staff at a memory center work together and share their different perspectives with the lead physician. They do all the tests at the center and one person coordinates the whole evaluation, from blood tests to billing.

- Centers at universities train specialists and primary-care doctors, and trainees are usually willing and able to spend extra time evaluating patients and answering their questions.

- Center doctors usually have access to a large network of social workers, therapists, and others who can help with the non-medical aspects of care.

The Disadvantages

- University memory centers are part of large organizations that may be bureaucratic and less than efficient. Thus, the wait can be a month or longer to get an appointment, and everything from parking to paperwork can be more cumbersome and time-consuming.

- Having trainees and students involved may mean telling your story twice or more in the same visit. Some people expect to see the head doctor immediately and are reluctant to talk openly or be examined by fellows, residents, trainees, or even allied health professionals like clinical nurse specialists, social workers, and psychometricians (people who administer neuropsychological tests for neuropsychologists to interpret).

Where You Go Matters

The accuracy of the testing and—in particular—of the interpretation of the test results varies among centers and practitioners. Studies show that memory specialists at research centers have a higher accuracy rate than internists or other primary-care doctors; the latter are more likely than specialists to either under- or overdiagnose Alzheimer's. Nonspecialists are likely to miss Alzheimer's when the patient comes in alone (without a family member) for symptoms unrelated to memory. On the other hand, nonspecialists have a tendency to assume that a hospital patient has Alzheimer's, when the person actually is suffering from confusion or delirium as a result of being ill or hospitalized.

Before choosing a doctor or center, check out the information in Chapters 5 and 6 about the elements of a thorough evaluation and diagnostic testing. Then ask the doctors what their memory assessment involves and see if it comes close to what you, as an informed consumer, know to be important.

TIPS FOR FINDING A MEMORY SPECIALIST OR MEMORY CENTER

- Ask your relative's regular doctor, who may be able to get him or her an appointment with a specialist quickly.
- Ask for suggestions from the local chapter of the Alzheimer's Association or another memory support group.
- If there's a medical school in your area, see if it has doctors who specialize in memory disorders.
- If you have friends who are doctors or whose families have dealt with memory problems, ask them for suggestions.
- Check www.alz.org/carefinder for health professionals who diagnose and treat Alzheimer's in your area.
- Do your homework and don't feel you have to settle for the first name you get. Most large to midsized cities often have a dozen or more excellent memory specialists. Even if you live in a small town, it may be worth driving a few hours to see a top specialist.

▶ DIFFERENT PEOPLE/DIFFERENT NEEDS

The right doctor is the doctor who is right for *your* family member. To start, you will need to consider the availability of the doctor and your insurance coverage. Then look at your relative's particular needs. A person who has early-onset Alzheimer's and is still only in his early fifties can go to a geriatric clinic that is equipped to handle Alzheimer's. If, however, he is uncomfortable going to a center for people who are much older, he can see a behavioral neurologist or a psychiatrist who specializes in Alzheimer's. An older person whose memory problems are fairly obvious does not need the same level of workup as someone with subtle memory loss. Someone with mild memory problems and other complex neurological conditions is trickier to diagnose and needs more sophisticated testing and resources than a primary-care doctor can provide.

▶ WHEN AND WHERE TO GET A SECOND OPINION

Any family should feel totally secure telling their doctor they want a second opinion. Just as many patients (including many doctors, for that matter) get a second opinion after being told that they or their loved ones have cancer, so should you seek confirmation of a serious diagnosis like Alzheimer's. If you have any doubts about the diagnosis or simply happen to be someone who likes to double-check, get a second opinion.

Where to go for that opinion depends on your needs. If something was lacking in the first evaluation—say, the neurological exam was incomplete or nonexistent—see a neurologist. If you just feel better having two opinions, get the name of another doctor from your first doctor, or go back to the person who referred you to that initial doctor. A university memory clinic or a well-respected behavioral neurologist or geriatric psychiatrist can also be a good source for a second opinion.

▶ THE MATTER OF MONEY

The cost of memory testing depends on how much Medicare or the patient's private insurance company is willing to reimburse for the expenses and, of course, how much the doctor charges. Several factors determine how much you have to pay (other than the type of test):

- The type of insurance plan the patient has
- Whether she qualifies for Medicare or Medicaid
- Whether the doctor participates in his insurance plan or with Medicare or Medicaid
- The state she lives in
- His diagnosis
- The billing codes the doctor uses
- The type of practice, such as family practice, specialist, research clinic, that she goes to

Different Specialists, Different Charges, Different Reimbursement

Universities are often more expensive than private centers, but they are also more likely to have clinics run by trainees who accept lower fees based on income. Dementia specialists charge more than general practitioners. They are also likely to order more tests and prescribe more drugs and support services, all of which add up-front charges. Those add-ons may or may not turn out to be expensive in the long run, as having the right treatment and care from the start may prevent costly problems later. Plus, not all "value" is financial; an early and accurate diagnosis can bring intangible benefits like peace of mind and an improved quality of life.

Health-care providers differ in the kinds of insurance they accept. For example, the doctor may

- not work with insurance companies at all
- accept private insurance but not Medicare or Medicaid. This type of provider usually requires you to sign a document saying

you accept responsibility for all charges not covered by the insurance company.

- accept whatever your insurance, Medicare, or Medicaid is willing to pay and not expect additional payment

For patients over age sixty-five who use Medicare, check out the search tool at the Medicare Web site (www.medicare.gov) for finding doctors in your area who accept Medicare. Under specialty/subspecialty, type in neurology/neuropsychiatry or psychiatry/geriatric psychiatry. Note the site disclaimer that some of these doctors may no longer accept Medicare or treat certain conditions. Some doctors accept Medicare only from longtime patients.

That said, although neuropsychological tests are key to making an accurate diagnosis of Alzheimer's in the early stage, Medicare pays a very small portion of what neuropsychologists charge. These tests can run to a thousand dollars or more, and your relative or his or her insurance company would need to pay the amount that Medicare doesn't cover.

The doctor needs to be savvy about what tests to order and for what purpose. For example, insurance companies or Medicare may not dispute paying for the standard tests for diagnosing memory disorders, such as an MRI and blood tests. But other tests may be trickier to get covered. Medicare reimburses for the use of a PET scan to distinguish Alzheimer's and a type of memory disorder called frontotemporal lobar dementia, but not to assess routine memory loss. Doctors need to be prepared to explain to insurance companies their reasons for ordering the tests.

CHAPTER FIVE

MAKING THE MOST OF THE DOCTOR'S APPOINTMENT

So many topics, so little time . . . An average of six topics surface in a typical primary-care office visit with elderly patients, leaving a limited amount of time to discuss all of the issues fully.
—A HEADLINE IN *FAMILY PRACTICE MANAGEMENT* MAGAZINE DISCUSSING THE DILEMMA OF A TYPICAL FIFTEEN-MINUTE SLOT

What to Do in Advance

Going to an appointment where you or your family member may get a diagnosis of Alzheimer's is not easy, yet it may be one of the most important things you've done in a long time. Now that you're taking this important first step, some simple preparations can help make it count.

- Try to schedule the appointment for the person's best time of day, when he is most awake, alert, and agreeable. Avoid appointments that are close to other traumatic or very stimulating events, such as a retirement party or memorial service (you'd be surprised what people try to do in one day). Still, it is more important not to delay seeking help than to wait months for the ideal appointment time.

- If possible, collect information on your relative's medications and medical conditions from his other doctors. They can mail the information directly to the doctor or you can bring it to the appointment. If you fax anything, alert the office that it's coming and then check that it was received.

- Ask the doctor's office if your relative should stop taking any of her regular medications prior to the appointment. Some drugs, such as some sleeping pills, antihistamines, and narcotic painkillers, can artificially slow people's thinking.

- Prepare yourself emotionally. Most clinics don't let the family watch the memory testing, but individual neurologists and others may. If you are with your relative as he takes a memory test, don't show your dismay even if he does poorly. Family members are sometimes shocked by what they see, because people with memory loss often conceal their shortcomings until they take tests designed to uncover them.

- Bring a list of questions. For example, you might be wondering whether her memory problems are related to a concussion she had or whether eating everything in sight is part of Alzheimer's.

- Fill out the Memory Inventory at the end of this chapter to give to the doctor. The more information you have, the better chances you have of getting an accurate diagnosis for your relative.

▶ HOW TO PREPARE YOUR RELATIVE EMOTIONALLY

Fear of the A-word (Alzheimer's) is the most common reason people don't get tested for a brain disorder. You can help prepare your relative by being honest and reassuring from the start.

If your mother knows she's going for a memory check, answer her questions as they arise about why she is going and what will happen. Remind her that she hasn't been feeling like herself or that she seems more frustrated, and it would be better to know what it is and what can be done. Say you have confidence in her and in the doctor you chose.

The goal is to normalize the test, for example by saying, "After a certain age, we get our hearts and blood pressure checked, and most people now get memory checks as well." Encourage her to be honest with the doctor about her memory complaints. Remind her that memory tests are supposed to be hard and no one does perfectly. Be sure to tell her that whatever the outcome is, you will deal with it together.

What to Bring

- Yourself! When we ask patients how long they've had memory problems or what medicines they are taking, many joke: "How should I know? I'm the one with the memory problem!" Which brings up a good point: To diagnose a patient correctly, doctors need collateral information from a family member or good friend. It's okay for two friends or family members to come along, such as the spouse to provide comfort and a son or daughter to take notes and remind everyone of questions they want answered.

- Bring all of your relative's medication bottles, as long as they have the accurate dosage on them. Include over-the-counter drugs, such as aspirin or antihistamines, and supplements, such as fish oil or vitamins, that your relative takes regularly.

- The appointment may take a few hours, so bring a snack, a bottle of water or juice, and reading material, plus a sweater in case the office is chilly. (It's not unusual for older people and particularly people with Alzheimer's to get cold easily.)

► AT THE DOCTOR'S: THE MUNDANE MATTERS

The appointment will begin with the doctor or nurse taking your relative's medical history, which, at a memory specialist's office, takes forty-five minutes or longer. Some of the questions may seem odd. You may wonder, for example, why they need to know the date of your father's gallbladder surgery or what kind of work he did. But experiences and medical conditions from a person's past can come back and haunt the brain. For example, having a stroke increases the likelihood of developing Alzheimer's or vascular dementia. If your father has recently worked with pesticides, he should be tested for residues that can harm the brain. Incomplete histories can lead to a delayed or inaccurate diagnosis.

► THE IMPORTANCE OF A DOCTOR-FAMILY CHAT

The doctor should talk to you in private about your relative and not rely completely on her account of her condition. The doctor will want to know when the memory problems began and how serious you think they are. You can make sure you get private time with the doctor by either calling ahead and letting the doctor know of your concerns or, at the appointment, slipping the nurse or receptionist a note for the doctor. There are many reasons for a doctor-family chat. Your relative

- may be in denial about her memory loss
- may be too embarrassed to admit to the doctor (or to you) the full extent of her impairment
- may be so anxious that she is exaggerating her problem
- may have lost insight into how well she is or is not doing
- may be unable to make decisions regarding her health and need you to help her make decisions (eventually you may need medical power of attorney—more on this later)

You should tell the doctor not only about your relative's memory but also about her

- mood
- daily functioning, such as her hygiene, cooking, and bill paying
- general behavior
- understanding of her location, the time, and what's going on around her

- ability to find words, follow conversations, and understand what's being said to her
- tendency to repeat herself

▶ HOW MUCH TESTING IS ENOUGH?

The types of tests and the number of tests a doctor administers depend on the severity of the memory problem, the doctor's particular preferences, the patient's medical conditions and family history, and the results of initial tests. If they uncover the source of the problem, no more testing is needed. If the results are abnormal yet inconclusive, a good doctor keeps testing.

While we are big supporters of thorough testing, some doctors can overdo it.

An elderly man had been acting oddly for about a year, but when he could no longer follow a football game, his wife and daughter took him to a neuropsychologist who specializes in memory disorders. The doctor saw obvious signs of memory loss and said she would like to schedule an appointment for further testing—an appointment that would last six hours, with a break for lunch.

The family members just looked at one another and laughed. "Six hours?!" The daughter knew her dad would never last that long, and the dad said it would just be a waste of time. Sadly, they never pursued any other testing.

Such an ambitious testing schedule can be the norm at some memory centers. But a typical assessment should last no more than three hours. If the results suggest that further testing would help clarify the treatment, the patient can come back another day.

Disadvantages of More Tests

- Added inconvenience. Even a normal amount of testing can require two or three appointments: one for the initial consult with the doctor, another for the actual tests, and a third visit to discuss the results.

- Greater risk of false positives. If your relative is tired from taking tests or if he's just having a bad day, he may not do as well on the cognitive portions of the test. Plus, the results of any test, whether a blood test or a scan of a person's brain, can be mistaken.

- Added expense.

To avoid unnecessary tests, ask the following questions. (See Chapter 6 for the tests that we consider routine and important.)

- What are the different tests for?
- What are the risks and benefits of the tests?
- Are the test results likely to call for a change of treatment?
- What are the chances the test will get a false positive result that leads to more testing?
- What are the chances that the tests will find something that isn't actually related to the memory problem?

If the tests are part of a clinical trial, make sure you have read Chapter 9 on being in a clinical study.

► PROTECTING PRIVACY

All test results become part of the patient's medical record. Patients concerned about having an Alzheimer's diagnosis in their record have a couple of options:

- Some doctors may code the diagnosis as "memory impairment" or "cognitive disorder" instead of as Alzheimer's.
- Patients can pay out of pocket. However, the tests may still become part of the patient's medical record. Also, "paying out of pocket" is just another way of saying "paying through the nose." Diagnostic tests can cost thousands of dollars.

Doctors must protect their patients' medical information from curious family members as well. But when a person develops serious memory problems, the rules must change slightly. It's standard when caring for people with Alzheimer's to include the spouse or other designated care provider in the treatment plan. In the early stage of the disease, the doctor will ask the person with Alzheimer's directly for permission to share information with the care provider. However, as the disease progresses and the person with Alzheimer's needs considerably more help with all medical decisions, the care provider needs to have a durable medical power of attorney in place that allows her to make all medical decisions, in accordance with what she knows her relative would want. Check out www.caringinfo.org/index?page=472; go to the bottom of the page and click on a state for information on how to put a durable power of attorney in place. (The rules vary from state to state.) You may also get information about medical power of attorney from local hospitals.

A word of comfort: A good doctor will still protect the privacy of the person with Alzheimer's by disclosing to the care provider only as much information as is needed. There are some things that a doctor might know about his or her patient that no one else really needs to know. Alzheimer's doesn't mean an end to privacy.

▶ WHAT HAPPENS AT A MEMORY CHECKUP

It depends on your age, how worried you are, and how impaired you are. But, in general, a thorough doctor does the following:

- Assesses how well the brain is working through formal testing and general questions. He asks if you still find the right words to say what you mean, understand and follow what you read, get your work done, and balance your checkbook.
- Looks for treatable conditions, such as infections, thyroid conditions, depression, vitamin deficiencies, and sleep apnea, which cause or worsen memory problems or in other ways mimic Alzheimer's.
- Treats conditions such as diabetes and hypertension, which increase the risk of dementia.

- Reviews the patient's list of medications to screen for drugs that contribute to poor mental functioning or that interact negatively with Alzheimer's drugs.

- Determines the patient's stage of Alzheimer's. Is it early, middle, or late stage? (Don't wait until it's late!)

- Looks at any factors in the person's environment (demanding job, unsafe housing) or diet that may be contributing to memory problems by exacerbating anxiety, sleeplessness, depression, or confusion.

- Gives the family an idea of what activities and responsibilities the person can still enjoy and manage, based on how well he or she scored on different tests of mental functioning.

You can expect to learn specific information from a memory assessment:

- Whether the memory loss is truly Alzheimer's or some other more treatable or unrelated condition. You want a specific diagnosis (which may include more than one condition, such as early-stage Alzheimer's and clinical depression).

- Whether a medical or emotional problem is making matters worse. Even if the person has Alzheimer's, your doctor still needs to find out if another medical condition or even a medication is exacerbating symptoms.

- A baseline assessment of the person's condition, so the patient, family, and doctor can monitor whether treatments are helping or not.

- What the person can still do—which skills or mental functions are still quite intact and which are not. Knowing this will help him or her pursue activities that are still good choices and drop those that are frustrating or even dangerous.

Memory and Brain Health Questionnaire

We recommend that you complete the following questionnaire on behalf of your relative so you can be ready either to answer the questions at the appointment or to actually give the doctor this completed form. The "you" in the questionnaire refers to the person with memory problems.

Forgetfulness   Yes No

1. Are you more forgetful now than ten years ago?   ❑   ❑

2. Did your forgetfulness come on gradually or did it start abruptly?

    _____ gradually

    _____ abruptly

3. Approximately when did your forgetfulness begin?

    _____

4. Has it worsened over the past six to twelve months?   ❑   ❑

5. What type of forgetfulness do you have trouble with?

    _____ recent or short-term memory

    _____ past or long-term memory (e.g., childhood events)

    _____ recalling words

    _____ remembering names

    _____ remembering appointments

    _____ balancing your checkbook

    _____ remembering time or date

    _____ directions

    _____ using new appliances

6. Have you changed any aspect of your life due to your memory (e.g., stopped going to church or parties)?   ❑   ❑

7. Do you have any difficulty with any of your day-to-day tasks at home?   ❑   ❑

8. Does your spouse, friend, or coworker think your memory is worse now than it was before?   ❑   ❑

9. Has your spouse, friend, or coworker ever asked you to get your memory checked by a doctor?   ❑   ❑

Medical History   Yes   No

1. Have you ever had a stroke?   ❏   ❏

2. Have you ever had a serious head injury
    (e.g., concussion) where you experienced
    loss of consciousness or lost some abilities
    temporarily?   ❏   ❏

3. Have you ever experienced transient weakness or
    paralyses of the muscles of your face, throat,
    eyes, arms, or legs?   ❏   ❏

4. Have you ever had a heart attack or heart blockage?   ❏   ❏

5. Do you have high blood pressure?   ❏   ❏

6. Do you have high cholesterol levels?

7. Has anyone in your family ever had dementia,
    Alzheimer's, Parkinson's, or Huntington's disease?   ❏   ❏

    If yes, at what age and how was the person
    related to you? _____

8. Have you ever been told you had a problem with
    your thyroid gland?   ❏   ❏

9. Have you ever been prescribed thyroid hormone
    supplements?   ❏   ❏

10. When was the last time your thyroid level was tested?

    _____

11. Have you ever been told you have low blood counts
    or that you are anemic?   ❏   ❏

12. Have you ever been told you are low in vitamin B_{12}
    or folic acid?   ❏   ❏

13. Do you have persistent tingling or numbness of
    your lower legs?   ❏   ❏

14. Do you have a leaky bladder or lose control?   ❏   ❏

15. Do you have trouble with your balance or gait?   ❏   ❏

16. Have you ever sought professional help for an
    emotional, psychiatric, or substance abuse problem?   ❏   ❏

    If yes, please explain: _____

    _____

17. Have you ever been diagnosed with clinical
    depression or been treated with a medication for
    your nerves or depression?   ❏   ❏

Medical History (cont.)   Yes No

18. Are you having fun in life?   ❏   ❏
19. Are you sleeping well?   ❏   ❏
20. Is everything going well in your family and social life?   ❏   ❏
21. Have you ever taken antidepressants?   ❏   ❏
22. Do you consume alcohol (beer, wine, liquor)?   ❏   ❏

    Approximately how many drinks do you consume
    per week? _____

23. Have you ever been treated for excessive drinking?   ❏   ❏
24. When was your last physical exam?

    _____

    Where was it done? _____

    Name of the doctor. _____

    Was anything abnormal detected?

    _____

25. When was your last EKG? _____

26. When was the last time you had your prostate
    checked?_____

    What was the result? _____

27. When was the last time you had a mammogram
    and pelvic exam? _____

    What were the results? _____

28. Have you ever had an MRI scan before?   ❏   ❏

    What were the results? _____

    Was there anything abnormal? _____

29. Do you have any metal (e.g., implants, pacemakers)
    in your body?   ❏   ❏

30. Are you under a lot of stress now?   ❏   ❏

31. Please list all the medicines you are taking now.

    _____

    _____

    _____

▶ GETTING THE NEWS

Rule 1: *The patient should have a friend or family member with her when getting the diagnosis.* Even people without mental impairments find medical diagnoses difficult to understand and process. Plus, learning you have Alzheimer's can be emotionally devastating. You may need to ask the doctor questions to help your relative understand what the doctor is saying.

Rule 2: *On the other hand, don't assume your relative will be or should be shocked or devastated by an Alzheimer's diagnosis.* He knows he has a memory problem and may not be surprised to hear it is Alzheimer's. He may even be relieved to know the cause of his problem, that millions of others have the same condition, and that lots of help and expertise are available to him. He may not even react, because he doesn't understand or can't keep in mind what the diagnosis means or its implications for his future.

Rule 3: *Get the precise diagnosis.* Some doctors avoid telling patients or their families that the patient has Alzheimer's. They dance around the diagnosis by using terms such as "memory disorder," "dementia," "cognitive disorder," or "organic brain syndrome." Other doctors embrace the Alzheimer's diagnosis too aggressively—before they have ruled out other possible causes of the memory failure. At the same time, realize that your relative's symptoms may be atypical and difficult to diagnose.

Memory disorder, dementia, cognitive disorder, or organic brain syndrome is acceptable only as working diagnoses. If your doctor uses one of those labels, ask if further testing is needed to establish a specific cause or diagnosis. You don't want to find out years later that it was indeed Alzheimer's. However, appreciate that a diagnosis is only as good as the information available to make the diagnosis, and so diagnoses may change over time as more information comes to light.

Rule 4: *Ask questions.* How did the doctor reach this diagnosis, and how certain is he or she about it? You are entitled to that information. If more questions pop into your head after you've left the office, call and leave a message for the doctor to call you back.

Difficult Diagnoses

Many people with memory problems and their family members leave the doctor's office feeling bewildered about their diagnosis. There are two reasons for this:

The patient didn't meet the criteria for any one distinct disorder. The line between Alzheimer's and vascular dementia in particular is blurry, and studies now suggest that many people probably have features of both.

Diagnosing memory disorders is a subjective decision and a difficult one, even for specialists. Two equally qualified, equally thorough doctors can look at the same patient, do the same tests, and come up with different diagnoses. So a doctor may be unsure about the diagnosis and, therefore, unwilling to be definitive until he or she sees how the symptoms get worse over time. Don't be surprised to leave the first evaluation with a diagnosis of "possible" or "probable" Alzheimer's.

► THE APPOINTMENT ISN'T OVER UNTIL THE DOCTOR . . .

- completes a thorough neurological or physical exam
- gives the appropriate memory and neuropsychological tests
- orders the essential laboratory tests and a brain scan
- considers how daily life, family issues, medications, or other medical and psychological conditions may be interfering with the patient's ability to think, learn, or remember
- tells the patient or the family the test results and diagnosis
- refers the patient or family to other specialists and to sources of support, such as a social worker, if appropriate

CHAPTER SIX

THE BEST MEMORY TESTS

Early diagnosis offers the best chance to treat the symptoms of the disease. . . . At specialized centers doctors can diagnose Alzheimer's correctly up to 90 percent of the time.
—NATIONAL INSTITUTE OF AGING

While no single test (other than a brain biopsy, which is a very invasive and risky procedure) can conclusively prove that a person has Alzheimer's, many tests can give us a good idea. A list of all the tests that help us assess memory and thinking problems appears at the end of this chapter. Meanwhile, let's take a good look at the whys and hows of a thorough memory assessment.

► WHAT A DIFFERENCE AN EXTRA TEST CAN MAKE

To understand why getting tested (and retested as symptoms change and the disease progresses) is important, check out the experience of Katherine, who went to the doctor complaining of a memory

BUT FIRST, PAYING FOR THE DIAGNOSIS

Ignorance can be costly, yet so is information. At the first visit, ask the doctor to spell out which tests he or she wants to run, then check that your insurance covers those tests and whether there are any conditions that are not covered. At the end of this chapter you will find the approximate costs of different tests.

slowdown. She took five of the most important neuropsychological tests, which assess brain function without actually physically looking at the brain. Then she underwent brain scans, a cardiovascular workup, and blood tests to see what else was going on that might be undermining her mental function.

Was it all worth it? Well, if she had stopped at just the two most common tests, she could have walked away with a very inaccurate diagnosis.

First, the doctor wanted to know if she had a family history of Alzheimer's and, if so, at what age the relative developed Alzheimer's. The doctor also needed to know her age. That's not surprising—seems the older you get, the more people ask. But for an Alzheimer's diagnosis, age really matters, because after age sixty-five the risk of Alzheimer's doubles every five years, and below age fifty the disease is relatively rare. Your education level is important, too. People who didn't complete high school have a greater risk of developing Alzheimer's than people with a higher level of education. Finally, women are more likely to get Alzheimer's than men.

Katherine was seventy-two, a college grad, and had no family history that she knew of. Her parents both died before their seventy-fifth birthdays, but they certainly didn't have early-onset Alzheimer's.

► THE STANDARD OF MEMORY TESTS

The test that all doctors should give at the first memory assessment, which Katherine's doctor did, and at every follow-up visit is the

Mini-Mental State Exam (MMSE), a short but very useful test that assesses a lot of different abilities.

What the MMSE Asks and Why

- To demonstrate orientation: The patient tries to answer, "What is today's date?" and "What county are we in?"
- To demonstrate memory skills: The patient tries to repeat the names of three objects immediately and again after five minutes.
- To demonstrate concentration: The patient tries to count backward or to spell backward.
- To demonstrate language abilities: The patient tries to name objects in the room, repeat a tongue twister, or follow simple directions such as to take, fold, and put a piece of paper on the desk.
- To demonstrate motor skills: The patient tries to copy a picture that includes intersecting shapes.

What the MMSE Does

- Serves as a quick screen for dementia of any kind
- Provides a general measure of brain function
- Helps determine if the patient is in the early, middle, or late stage of Alzheimer's
- Monitors changes in mental functioning over time, including the effects of treatment
- Provides a common language. Everyone from a general practitioner to a memory specialist understands the test results, so they serve as a common language spoken across different specialties.

What the MMSE Doesn't Do

The MMSE doesn't do subtle. It was developed thirty years ago to help doctors screen hospital patients for problems with their mental functioning. Now people are driving themselves to the doctor for a memory test, and the MMSE is not sensitive enough to pick up on subtle problems in thinking and memory. Nor does it probe any one aspect of mental functioning in depth or distinguish among memory disorders.

Some individuals with a very high IQ or those who are really good test takers appear merely "normal" on the MMSE when in fact they have an Alzheimer's-induced memory slowdown. Doctors should, though not all do, consider IQ, gender, occupation, education level, and an individual's age when scoring the MMSE. An assessment may not include a formal IQ test, but the doctor should find out about the person's personality, capabilities, and occupation prior to developing memory problems, because Alzheimer's is about a *decline* or *change* in memory and thinking. For example, the MMSE score of 26 is normal for a man in his early sixties who has an eighth-grade education, but it would be below normal if he had gone to college. (A chart showing what MMSE score is normal for a person's age and education is available at www.tuftsnemc.org/psych/mmse.asp.)

Katherine did okay on her MMSE. She scored a respectable 26 out of a possible 30. No big red flag there for most doctors, who don't worry until they see a total score below 24. But the score actually concerned her doctor, who happened to know that for her years of education and age, normal for Katherine would be closer to a 28.

Doctors sometimes neglect to home in on how the test taker did on each set of questions. For example, forgetting today's date is less important than missing other assessment questions. Before leaving the doctor's office, find out your (or your relative's) total MMSE score and what items were missed.

Katherine ended up taking the MMSE many times over the years. Her scores declined slowly because, as the tests revealed, she had MCI (mild cognitive impairment). But after three years, she, too, was diagnosed with Alzheimer's and her decline accelerated.

It's Time . . .

Probably the second most popular test to screen for dementia is the clock-drawing test, which requires patients to draw a clock showing a specific time. The test is a good way to screen for overall mental abilities, and it can reveal problems that the patient has been able to hide during day-to-day activities. Katherine did great on the test, which was lucky for her daughter, whose own little girl was just mastering the skill of telling time. It's upsetting for family members to see a parent or spouse fail at a task most kids master in grade school.

Most general practitioners consider talking with the patient, ordering some blood tests and a brain scan, and giving the MMSE and clock-drawing test sufficient for diagnosing dementia. It might be sufficient for someone with obvious signs of Alzheimer's. But it could miss the early-stage Alzheimer's or MCI. Fortunately for Katherine and her family, her doctor did more.

► ASSESSING LANGUAGE SKILLS

A diagnosis of Alzheimer's requires being impaired in memory and one other mental function, such as language or attention. Language problems usually indicate that Alzheimer's is somewhat progressed or that the problem is another type of dementia that strikes the language centers of the brain first.

To assess language, beyond just listening to how the person formulates and understands words, a doctor will ask the patient to name common objects, such as chair, shoe, or elbow. More sensitive tests of language skills involve asking the patient to name, for example, all the four-legged animals he or she can think of as quickly as possible, or to repeat complex phrases, such as "Nelson Rockefeller had a Lincoln Continental." Katherine took one section of a language test called the Boston Naming Test that required her to name uncommon objects depicted in line drawings. She got only twenty-six out of thirty right, which is slightly worrisome.

The Delayed Recall Test

One of the most sensitive tests to distinguish normal aging from Alzheimer's is the delayed recall test, which tests a person's memory for a story or list of ten to sixteen words heard thirty minutes earlier. It's usually given as part of a larger memory test that also assesses immediate recall. Katherine's MCI came out of the shadows here. She was in the bottom nineteenth percentile on these recall tests.

One delayed recall test, called the Buscke Selective Reminding test, helps distinguish Alzheimer's from normal aging, because the tester is allowed to give clues to jog the test taker's memory. A prompt usually does not help if Alzheimer's is at the wheel, but it does help if the memory malfunction is due to depression or attention grabbers.

There are other tests, too. To assess attention, doctors see how well the patient can follow directions. They also ask the patient to spell words forward and backward or to subtract numbers forward and backward (for example, subtract by 7s starting at 100). There are computerized tests of attention as well, which are becoming increasingly popular in private practices and research centers.

Daily Living

The activities once taken for granted, from using the phone to fixing dinner, go from routine to frustrating to impossible as Alzheimer's storms the brain. Katherine's doctor used a Functional Activities Questionnaire (FAQ) to rate her ability to perform several common daily activities. The questionnaire assigns one point if a person has trouble with the activity but can do it alone, two points if he or she needs assistance, and three points if he or she is dependent on someone else to do it. The highest score, 30, indicates impairment in all activities; a score below 9 is normal. Katherine scored a 5, because she needs some help balancing her checkbook and assembling tax records.

► DEPRESSION, DEMENTIA, OR BOTH?

Depression is a must-check condition for every person complaining of impaired thinking. Depression and Alzheimer's have an insidious relationship: Depression masks Alzheimer's, is mistaken for Alzheimer's, worsens Alzheimer's, may precede the onset of Alzheimer's, and can be caused by Alzheimer's. To screen for depression, the doctor may start by just asking a few important questions:

1. Are you able to have fun or experience pleasure during a normal day?
2. Are you sleeping well?
3. Are you in pain?
4. Is everything okay with home and family life?
5. Have you lost weight unintentionally? Are you overeating?

Katherine's answers were: 1. not really; 2. not really; 3. not really; 4. I don't have much of a home life; 5. I wish.

Her doctor decided to give her the Geriatric Depression Scale— Short Form, which asks fifteen questions to probe for depression. A score greater than 5 warrants further assessment and a score greater than 10 indicates clinical depression. Katherine scored 11. After asking a few more questions and reviewing her medical record, the doctor prescribed an antidepressant. He also recommended that her family get her more involved in physical and social activities, including walking. Three months later, her depression eased. Her memory problems persisted, but she was thinking more clearly and her attention and concentration improved. Also, she regained a good portion of her former desire to see her friends.

Doctors often give the relative of the person with Alzheimer's the brief Neuropsychiatric Inventory (NPI) to assess changes in the patient's sleeping and eating habits, appetite, depression, euphoria, irritability, hallucinations, paranoia, impulsivity, and nighttime behaviors. The family member also describes how much each of these behaviors is disrupting the family. To fill out the survey, family members can rely on their memory or keep a weekly diary of changes they notice in the person with Alzheimer's. The NPI can help a doctor:

- Be more thorough. Unusual symptoms, such as extreme euphoria or impulsivity, may point to frontal lobe dementia, for example.
- Determine if the person needs psychiatric drugs, such as antidepressants
- Identify the stage of Alzheimer's—more severe behavior problems usually indicate more advanced dementia
- Monitor improvements following the start of new medications (such as Aricept or Namenda)

This scale is particularly useful if one is being treated by a nonspecialist, since most general practitioners often lack the time or experience to assess behavioral problems in detail. Doctors use the NPI when first assessing a patient and again at subsequent appointments to monitor change. Roughly one-third of people with MCI and two-thirds of people with mild to moderate Alzheimer's have a behavioral change.

Computerized Neuropsychological Tests

For people with mild memory loss, computerized tests of all aspects of mental functioning, including memory, are particularly useful though not widely used. Unlike paper-and-pencil tests, computerized assessments can easily be made more difficult to challenge patients who are only slightly impaired or who are highly able test takers. Computerized tests are becoming very feasible to administer, as more patients (though not all) are becoming more technology-savvy and comfortable with a keyboard. You probably have to go to a specialist to take them, however, as they are not readily available elsewhere.

At-Home Tests

There are dozens of tests that you can use at home to self-diagnose Alzheimer's or measure memory loss. No test stands out at this time. Many of these tests are based on sound principles and were developed by respected researchers. But whether you are at home or in the doctor's office, diagnosing Alzheimer's and ruling out conditions that worsen Alzheimer's require a sophisticated battery of tests, test givers, and interpreters. If you or a family member does take an at-home test, bring the results to your doctor and let him or her interpret them. Online, at-home memory testing may someday become the norm, but we're not there yet.

▶ THE PHYSICAL EXAM

When Katherine first went to her doctor complaining of memory loss, she learned that she would be getting a complete physical exam as part of the effort to determine the cause of her memory problems. Of course, "complete" means different things to different doctors. Her doctor gave a very wide battery of tests, but others take a more moderate view—using a set of about six tests and then adding others as needed. The results from any test, including those offered during a complete physical exam, may or may not change a person's diagnosis, Katherine's doctor told her and her family, but they will shed light on her condition and how she could feel better.

Physical illnesses can both trigger memory problems and make existing problems much worse. When fighting an infection or even suffering from heart disease, a person with Alzheimer's can go from being mellow though memory impaired to oddly mean or depressed.

As part of the physical exam, it is standard to obtain blood and urine samples to be tested for

- urinary infection
- thyroid deficiency
- vitamin deficiencies, including anemia
- liver, kidney, or electrolyte problems
- diabetes
- blood infections such as syphilis

Katherine scored "slightly elevated" on everything—blood pressure, blood sugars, and cholesterol, and, not surprisingly, her weight was higher than desired. Together, these problems increased her risk of having a stroke and developing Alzheimer's. So she saw a dietician, who put her on a low-fat diet and helped her find a walking group that met three times a week. She felt a little better, thanks to her efforts.

People with memory problems can turn out to have all sorts of treatable conditions that show up in a thorough physical. But sometimes a doctor may chase a few false leads before finding the real problem. Katherine's doctor had another patient, Stephan, in the early stage of Alzheimer's who had mild tremors in his hands, joint stiffness, and trouble sleeping. His blood work looked fine, and he didn't have vascular disease (clogged arteries). The doctor was concerned about the tremors, because combined with the memory problems they are a possible sign of two tricky-to-diagnose conditions: Parkinson's disease or Lewy Body Dementia. Fortunately for Stephan, a neurological exam revealed that his tremors were benign and not indicative of either condition.

Stephan's sleeping problems needed to be addressed also. Early Alzheimer's can sometimes change the brain in ways that cause sleep problems, and being sleep deprived makes any brain more sluggish. However, discussions with his family revealed that the patient's coffee and napping habits were causing the sleepless nights. (See Chapter 13 for more information on sleep problems.) After he improved his sleep habits, his family reported he was more alert during the day and less moody.

► LOOKING FOR PHYSICAL PROBLEMS THAT COULD AFFECT MEMORY

Some of the tests doctors give when looking for causes of memory problems might surprise or even insult you—"Why do *I* have to be checked for syphilis or HIV?" Depending on your doctor, you may not, but HIV and syphilis can cause dementia and you don't have to be sexually promiscuous to get these conditions. A woman may wonder why she is being checked for anemia when she hasn't had a period in years. Well, severe anemia can cause a type of memory loss. Plus, lots of conditions, from severe hemorrhoids to a poor diet to cancer, can cause anemia. Here are some other conditions doctors look for when tracking down the cause of a downturn in memory or thinking:

The Less-Than-Trusty Thyroid

Get your thyroid tested. Nearly one in five people over age sixty has some degree of hypothyroidism, meaning a sluggish thyroid. The symptoms include forgetfulness, weight gain, depression, dry skin, intolerance to cold, joint or muscle aches, and fatigue. People who are hypothyroid feel as though they have mild Alzheimer's and depression all mixed into one bad day. It's particularly important to catch thyroid deficiencies because there are effective medications to treat them—but you won't know that you need treatment unless you get tested. Patients with hypothyroidism should get their thyroid levels checked regularly, as the amount of thyroid hormone replacement they need may change over time.

Liver and Kidney Tests

It's a good idea to get blood and urine tests that look for liver and kidney diseases, since they can impair mental functioning if left untreated. In addition to standard tests, the doctor may run a liver enzyme test called gamma-glutamyl transpeptidase (GGT) or a urine test called ethyl glucuronide (EtG) to help detect surreptitious alcohol abuse, which can also cause memory problems. However, diseases other than alcohol abuse can affect levels of GGT and some experts question its use.

Getting to the Heart

If your memory is suffering, your heart may be, too. People with memory problems need a cardiovascular workup and, as part of that, their blood sugar checked for diabetes, which increases the risk of heart disease. Having heart disease or diabetes increases the risk of having a stroke and of developing vascular dementia and Alzheimer's. Having had a stroke also increases the risk of developing Alzheimer's and makes any brain problem worse.

Homocysteine and C-Reactive Proteins

Talk to your doctor about getting tested for both of these potential troublemakers. When elevated, they may increase the risk of developing heart disease and Alzheimer's, but the research is mixed on that. High homocysteine levels are an indicator light for vitamin B_{12} and folic acid deficiencies. Vitamin B supplements normalize homocysteine levels, studies show. However, in two recent studies, B vitamins did not help slow down Alzheimer's memory loss. Routine homocysteine testing is controversial and may be most useful in individuals suspected of having inherited disorders that lead to heart attacks or strokes at a very young age.

Having a high concentration in the blood of C-reactive protein is an indicator of heart disease or vasculitis, a potentially serious but rare inflammation of the blood vessels. Its cause is not known, but some believe that it occurs when the body's immune system goes slightly crazy and attacks the blood vessels, including those in the brain.

EKG

An electrocardiogram (EKG) is very simple and painless. The technician tapes electrodes to your chest and a few spots on your body, and a machine records your heart's electrical activity. An EKG can detect problems with the heart's blood supply. It also detects an irregular heartbeat called atrial fibrillation, among other heart conditions that increase the risk of developing Alzheimer's or that exacerbate an existing memory problem. An EKG is particularly important for people who take Alzheimer's medications, because people with a condition called sick sinus, which shows up on EKGs, can't use three of the four FDA-approved drugs.

Carotid Check and Ultrasound

Now for your neck. There may be a few vampires in the Alzheimer's assessment business, but most are interested in your neck for one reason: to monitor the blood flowing through your carotid arteries, which run up your neck and feed oxygen and nutrition to your brain. Doctors can hear the blood flow by simply putting their stethoscope to your neck, which they should do annually. Plaque that comes, in part, from having high cholesterol can clog those valuable arteries. In addition to limiting blood supply to the brain, the plaque can break loose from the lining of the artery, travel through blood vessels to the brain and, in the worst case, cause a stroke.

If the doctor hears the telltale sounds of a blockage or if your relative is at a high risk of having a stroke because of high blood pressure or high cholesterol, be sure he or she undergoes a carotid ultrasound test or an MRI of the carotid. An ultrasound is a painless examination that uses high-frequency sound waves to create images of blood flow through the major blood vessels. Both MRI and ultrasound are equally acceptable, but an MRI might be easier to get. Most people with memory problems undergo an MRI anyway, so the doctor just needs to make sure it also includes images of the neck. Some experts believe that routine screening for carotid ultrasounds could reduce stroke-related deaths by half. Blockages of 70 percent and above may require carotid surgery, and less severe blockages may require medication.

▶ **Check This Out:** Many cognitive abilities (memory, attention, information-processing speed) were much more impaired among 189 older people with blocked carotids, compared with 201 individuals of the same age bracket whose carotids were clear. These individuals had not yet had a stroke, so the study demonstrates that blockages alone may lead to mild memory problems.

Lessons learned:

- Anyone who has a memory problem needs to have his or her carotid arteries checked.
- Routine physical exams may not detect subtle or even severe carotid blockages.
- Routine brain MRI scans do not image the neck unless the doctor orders it.
- Carotid blockages are frequently missed, and the results can be fatal.

It's not just the carotids that get blocked; other vessels that carry blood to the brain can become blocked as well. In fact, such blockages are more common in people with memory impairment than in those without memory problems. A recent study comparing the two groups showed that 30 to 40 percent of memory-impaired individuals had small clots traveling daily in the blood vessels going to their brain, compared with only 15 percent of the nonimpaired individuals.

▶ IS IT VASCULAR OR ALZHEIMER'S?

Vascular dementia and Alzheimer's often overlap, and distinctions between them are somewhat arbitrary. But in some cases they require different treatments, so it's worth trying to separate the two conditions. To this end, doctors fill out the Rosen-Hachinski Ischemia Rating Scale, a questionnaire about the patient's physical complaints, emotional changes, and various vascular risk factors, such as whether the person has had hypertension or a stroke. The scale also asks whether memory problems came on abruptly or gradually. A high score (above 8) points to a vascular dementia; a lower score points to Alzheimer's or a mixed diagnosis of both disorders. Asking your doctor if he uses this scale is a good test of his expertise in vascular dementia. The regular physical exam and history done by any doctor should provide all the information needed to fill out the questionnaire and interpret the results. No extra testing is needed.

▶ NO-NONSENSE NEUROLOGICAL

As part of a standard neurological exam (which can be done by any doctor, not just a neurologist), the doctor will check your relative's vision, reflexes, and the sensitivity of his arms and legs to touch or a pinprick. The doctor may also ask him to smile, grimace, raise his brows, touch his finger to his nose, or walk down the hall. (It has an uncomfortable resemblance to a tough sobriety check.) The doctor is looking for neurological problems that cause or contribute to memory loss. Your relative's walk alone may tell the doctor whether he has Parkinson's disease, which causes dementia in some patients.

If his facial movements are abnormal, that may mean his cranial nerves, which connect the face and brain, are malfunctioning. However, problems with the cranial nerves are a sign that the person probably *does not* have Alzheimer's, because Alzheimer's doesn't harm the cranial nerves. Tumors, vitamin B_1 deficiencies, stroke, and other serious conditions can cause the combination of malfunctioning cranial nerves and a poor memory. The doctor is checking the cranial nerves when she shines a light into the eyes; cranial nerves deliver electrical impulses to move muscles controlling the pupil.

Next Level of Neurological

If the basic neurological test results aren't definitive or if a patient needs a very thorough assessment for whatever reason, these are the tests.

For Finding Infection

Spinal taps, which involve extracting spinal fluid under local anesthesia, are becoming more common. Studying the spinal fluid is important for detecting chemical changes in the brain that suggest a person may have or be at risk of developing Alzheimer's. Spinal fluid tests are also important for ruling out other serious conditions, including multiple sclerosis, tumors, and prion diseases, such as mad cow disease.

Spinal taps carry a small risk of serious complications, including infections or a debilitating headache that results from the injection site hole not sealing and spinal fluid leaking inside the spinal membranes.

To minimize complications, doctors can do spinal taps using an X-ray machine to guide where they place the needle. Using a small-bore (24-gauge) needle also helps, as does experience at doing the procedure. A severe headache is usually cured by either lying flat or, if that doesn't work, getting an injection of your own blood, called a blood patch, at the needle site.

Detecting Electrical Difficulties

Quantitative electroencephalography, a version of the standard EEG, measures electrical activity in the brain using painless electrodes on the patient's scalp. The test can detect seizures and rare abnormalities, yet it poses no serious risks. People with Alzheimer's have slightly slower than normal electrical activity in the brain.

When the Problem Is (Not) Sleeping

As you may have already found out, people with dementia often can't sleep well—and can sometimes wake up everyone in the family or even the neighbors. Family members can usually reveal enough about a person's sleep habits for a doctor to diagnose and treat what's going on. Other times, the doctor will order (or the family will request) a formal sleep test, called a polysomnogram (PSO). The patient spends the night at a sleep center, hooked up via an electrode to a device that records brain waves, eye movements, breathing rate, and other bodily functions. Once the doctor figures out the cause of the sleeplessness, he or she will probably recommend medications and better sleep hygiene (such as no daytime napping).

UNDER CONSTRUCTION

Researchers are developing new tests for diagnosing Alzheimer's and assessing brain function. (By participating in clinical trials, you can be part of the testing process—see Chapter 9 for more information on joining such trials.) Here are some of the possible and more interesting tests that we might see in the future.

Look into My Eyes

A new eye test still being developed may help to diagnose Alzheimer's in its earliest stages. The doctor shines an infrared laser into the patient's eye to look for a type of cataract caused by amyloid plaque, the same protein that is thought to cause Alzheimer's. If there is plaque in the eye, that's a sign that there is also plaque building up in the brain.

Name That Smell

You may have heard that when people get Alzheimer's, their sense of smell weakens. It's true in some people; early on in the course of the disease, Alzheimer's often harms the part of

(continued)

the brain that processes and identifies odors. So researchers have developed a standardized smell test that requires patients to identify a series of odors. The test is simple and less stressful than a memory test but is not yet perfected. It can't control for conditions not related to Alzheimer's, such as having a cold or being a smoker, which also distort a person's sense of smell.

Testing Your Diet

As mentioned earlier in this section, nutritional deficiencies can affect memory, so make sure that your family member's memory assessment includes a good nutritional assessment as well. The B vitamins are particularly important to memory function. People may run low on B_{12} because of a very poor or strictly vegetarian diet. Absorption problems, which can occur with chronic illness, bowel surgery, and age, also lead to a B vitamin deficiency.

Anemia is dangerous for brain cells, as it means the brain may not be getting a good supply of oxygen. Anemia signals that the body is low on hemoglobin, the protein in red blood cells that carries oxygen from the lungs to the body's tissues, including the brain. Some types of anemia may signal a B vitamin deficiency. Among older people, anemia is usually the result of an iron-deficient diet; blood loss, such as from severe hemorrhoids, colon polyps, or cancer; or absorption problems.

The brain also requires a healthy balance of electrolytes, such as sodium and potassium. Cells communicate electronically, by transferring electrical impulses to other cells, but that process breaks down if the brain is running low or high on electrolytes.

Metals on Our Minds

A pervasive myth is that cooking with aluminum pans causes Alzheimer's. We wish the problem of what causes Alzheimer's were that simple. Lead, mercury, aluminum, copper, or zinc can cause memory loss but only in people who are exposed to high levels, such as through a very contaminated water supply, diet, or work or home environment. They should have their urine tested to detect metal residues and any imbalance that may have resulted in the proteins and enzymes involved in the transport and absorption of metals.

► DO YOU HAVE THE ALZHEIMER'S GENE?

Some families have a lot of members who develop Alzheimer's. They have probably inherited a faulty gene or genes that predispose them to developing the disease. Scientists are developing tests that can give us some clues about our own genetic profile.

About twenty thousand of the human body's thirty thousand genes have a role in how our brain functions, and scientists have identified several hundred that may be related to memory. One of these is apolipoprotein E4 (ApoE4), which gives carriers a three- to eightfold higher risk of developing Alzheimer's than people without the gene. Blood tests and cheek swab tests that can determine if someone is carrying ApoE4 are already available. Whether a person inherits one or two copies of the faulty gene also affects the risk of developing Alzheimer's.

ApoE4 may influence how well the body metabolizes certain lipids and nerve cells repair themselves after injury. Preliminary studies suggest that ApoE4 carriers are particularly sensitive to the effects of a head injury, sleeping pills, and heart bypass surgery, and face an increased risk of having a stroke or heart attack. Some studies also suggest that people with the gene will start losing their memory, have abnormal brain scans, and develop Alzheimer's at an earlier age than people without the gene.

Should You Get Tested?

Experts disagree on the answer. Here's what you need to know before you decide:

- The test is widely available but not always covered by insurance.

- About 25 percent of people in the United States test positive for having one copy of the ApoE4 gene.
- Half of all people with Alzheimer's do not test positive. So not having the ApoE4 gene does not mean you won't get Alzheimer's.
- At least 20 percent of people with ApoE4 won't develop Alzheimer's.
- If you have memory loss and ApoE4, the odds are you probably have Alzheimer's or will be diagnosed with it in a few years.
- Whether or how quickly a person with ApoE4 will get Alzheimer's, or how severe his illness becomes, depends on many factors, including what other diseases he has and whether he lives a "brain-healthy" lifestyle.
- Inheriting one copy of the ApoE4 gene poses the same risk as having a parent who has Alzheimer's. In one study of MCI, the ApoE4 gene was a major predictor of who would get diagnosed with Alzheimer's over the next three years.

Because the ApoE4 genetic test is not a perfect predictor, many Alzheimer's experts don't recommend getting tested if you don't already have memory loss. They do not want people to become despondent because they have this susceptibility gene. However, a recent research study of 196 families suggests that getting tested in the context of proper counseling may not have negative effects, and many of those who found they were indeed ApoE4 carriers increased such efforts to protect themselves against Alzheimer's as controlling their cholesterol levels.

▶ **Our Take:** Genetic testing will become part of a package of routine Alzheimer's tests in the near future. Based on their comfort level, people can get tested for ApoE4 only if they have memory loss and/or are under the care of an expert who can counsel them appropriately. At-home genetic testing for ApoE4 will likely become available soon.

About two hundred very rare but very devastating genetic mutations can cause early-onset Alzheimer's. If many members of your family have developed Alzheimer's symptoms at an early age (in their forties and fifties), you could (should, in our opinion) consider signing up for a research study that offers genetic testing, counseling, and cognitive or imaging tests.

PROTECTING YOUR INSURANCE AND YOUR PRIVACY

Are you at risk of losing your insurance if you test positive for ApoE4? Probably not, but read on. Federal laws prohibit companies from canceling a policy. However, if the insurance company thinks you have a high risk of getting Alzheimer's in the near future, they may turn you down if you apply for insurance on your own (not through a group), or may raise your rates.

What to do: Ask your doctor if you can get the test done anonymously, or request in writing that you don't want the results to go on your medical record. If you get tested as part of a research study, get it in writing from your doctor that the results will be stored in a locked cabinet that only the doctor and nurse can access.

► **Consider:** Despite the value of tests, doctors learn the most from talking with the patient and the family. Doctors use their judgment, not just test scores, to make a final diagnosis and treatment plan.

► STOP IMAGINING, START IMAGING

Doctors and patients alike can think up all sorts of explanations for why someone feels poorly. Doctors must occasionally make educated guesses for problems that lie in our favorite little black box (the brain). But researchers are making progress toward turning on a small light in that black box, in the form of imaging devices or scanners for the brain.

The existing scanners can't detect the plaques and tangles that define Alzheimer's. What they look for is damage to the regions of the brain that are harmed by Alzheimer's. Researchers are also using imaging techniques to assess the brain's synapses, where cells connect to relay their chemical messages, because this is where Alzheimer's strikes first.

Because brain scans are far from perfect and humans far from uniform, a person with fairly bad cognitive problems can have a fairly normal-looking brain scan, and people whose brain scans look as though they should be impaired actually feel and behave quite normally. So imaging devices are most helpful when used along with a regular exam with the doctor and neuropsychological tests.

Where to Start: Magnetic Resonance Imaging (MRI)

Anyone complaining of or suffering from a memory problem should get an MRI scan, which provides the best view possible of the brain's memory tissues. MRI machines, long tubes that patients lie in, use very strong magnetic fields and radio waves to create pictures of the size and shape of different tissue in the brain. They can image blood flow, tumors, infections, aneurysms, nerve injury, and much more.

There are different types of MRIs. Any basic thirty-minute MRI will assess the brain for strokes, tumors, and inflammatory conditions and assess the degree of shrinkage in the memory and other regions of the brain. However, an MRI with *diffusion-weighted imaging* (DWI) is being increasingly used at top research centers. A doctor will request a DWI if he or she suspects the patient has had a recent stroke. But to be safe, some experts feel a DWI should be routine for all patients; many strokes are silent and produce no obvious symptoms. If you have any risk factors for stroke, such as high blood pressure or diabetes or high cholesterol, a DWI scan may be useful. If you go to a special memory clinic, such as at a university, the MRI will include additional images to get a better look at the brain.

When a diagnosis is still unclear or a patient has signs of cancer, infections, inflammation, or meningitis, the doctor may order a *contrast MRI*. The patient gets an injection of a dye called gadolinium, which shows up on the MRI as it flows through the brain. Patients who have kidney disease, certain allergies, or anemia can't take this test. Some memory centers routinely order a contrast MRI, because it provides a better picture of the health of the brain than a regular MRI does.

MRI angiography, which also uses a contrast dye, shows the blood flow through vessels in the neck and brain. Doctors use it when they suspect aneurysms, narrowing of vessels, and carotid blockages.

MRI Downsides

There can be false positives. The scanner may reveal something such as a cyst that looks significant but doesn't actually need to be treated. The patient may have to undergo further testing if it is unclear whether or not the cyst is benign. The routine MRI may also detect signs of a stroke but not discern if it happened recently or long ago.

Our advice is to get a second opinion if in doubt. Also, agree to a treatment plan or further testing only when you feel that there's sufficient evidence it will help.

The MRI has been in use for more than twenty years. Because of the strong magnets, MRIs are not suitable for people who have any metal in their body, and people with pacemakers, eye shrapnel, or certain types of stents may need to have a brain CAT scan instead of an MRI.

Claustrophobic individuals may not be able to use a traditional MRI machine. MRI is very sensitive to motion, and the picture quality will be poor if the patient cannot lie still. Some doctors allow patients to take a sedative before the procedure. Another option is to use an open MRI, which, as you may have guessed, is not completely enclosed. Another possibility is a CAT scan (see below).

Alternatives to MRI

Although MRIs are very common, many other good alternative imaging devices are being used everywhere from primary-care offices to special memory clinics.

Positron Emission Tomography (PET)

Used routinely to detect cancer, PET scans have become widely available in the last few years. PET scans involve getting an injection of a radioactive glucose that shows up on the PET scanner as it travels through the brain. This is useful for detecting Alzheimer's, because the disease causes cells in the brain's hippocampus and parietal and temporal lobes to take up less glucose than normal. If the brain's frontal lobes take up less sugar, that may indicate a frontal lobe dementia.

Some research suggests that PET scans may be among the most sensitive tests for detecting early signs of Alzheimer's. The actor Charlton Heston announced that PET scans helped in his early diagnosis. In some people with mild memory loss, a PET scan may show Alzheimer's-like changes even before a regular MRI can.

Studies suggest that using PET to assess whether a person has Alzheimer's would cut the number of false diagnoses (and unnecessary drug treatment) by half. But critics say that PET's diagnostic or predictive value has yet to be fully tested and PET should be reserved only for special cases, such as when frontotemporal dementia is suspected.

New PET scans under development (called FDDNP and PIB) map plaques in the brain, and FDDNP also maps tangles, the two hallmarks of Alzheimer's. Preliminary studies suggest these experimental scans may be able to differentiate between healthy brains and Alzheimer's. In the future, PET will probably be used to assess a person's risk for developing Alzheimer's long before symptoms appear and to monitor a person's response to therapy.

Computed Axial Tomography (CAT)

Faster and more comfortable than an MRI, CAT scans transform X-ray images of the brain into a 3-D image. Using a CAT scan, doctors can spot a tumor, damage from a stroke, or hydrocephalus (the fluid pressure in the brain increases and compresses tissue). Although they are still not preferable to an MRI, CAT scans are a fine alternative when an MRI is unavailable. Their shortcomings: CAT scans are less useful than MRIs for imaging the brain's memory regions and nerve fibers that connect the regions. CAT scans also expose patients to a low dose of radiation.

After five months of being forgetful, confused, and headachy, sixty-nine-year-old Peter went to the doctor. A CAT scan revealed that he had a large blood clot, called a subdural hematoma, compressing the tissue on the left side of his brain. After a surgeon drained the clot, all of Peter's symptoms went away. These kinds of clots can result from taking blood thinners, drinking heavily, or, as was the case for Peter, suffering a head injury. He had not connected his head injury, which had happened a year earlier, with his more recent forgetfulness. Subdural hematomas, which can be deadly if untreated, occur in about 5 percent of all serious head injuries.

Single-Photon Emission Computed Tomography (SPECT)

Some medical practices are more likely to offer a SPECT, which is fast, comfortable, and one-third the cost of a PET scan. However, the resolution of SPECT is lower than that of PET and, like PET, it also involves being injected with a radioactive compound.

Very popular before MRI and PET scans became common, SPECT creates a 3-D model of blood flow using gamma rays, rather than X-rays. An injected radioactive compound emits the rays as it moves through the brain. Areas of the brain stricken by Alzheimer's produce a weaker signal.

▶ BRAIN BIOPSIES

A surefire diagnosis of Alzheimer's requires proof of a high density of plaques and tangles in the brain tissue. Yet the only way to get this level of evidence is to biopsy brain tissue, an invasive, risky procedure, done only if a definitive diagnosis is important for the family, for providing treatment, or to rule out a possibly contagious disease. The procedure makes sense only for younger patients with unusual forms of dementia or for people who may have a serious infection, such as HIV or CJD. Even though brain biopsies today are safer than decades ago, they still pose serious risks.

► AUTOPSY: THE ULTIMATE ALZHEIMER'S DIAGNOSIS?

For Alzheimer's and other diseases of the brain, autopsies provide an accurate diagnosis—at least most of the time. To do an autopsy, a pathologist removes samples of tissue from different parts of the dead person's brain, then examines these tissues under a microscope. If the number of plaques and tangles in these samples meets the criteria for Alzheimer's, then the pathologist will say the patient had the disease. However, determining what is plaque and what is normal tissue is a bit of a judgment call, and so not all pathologists would come to the same diagnosis for a patient.

That's not the only opportunity for confusion. Some doctors see signs of vascular disease and immediately say the patient had vascular dementia, while others might call it a "mixed dementia"—Alzheimer's and vascular dementia. Also, although damage from a stroke can be quite apparent, how long ago the damage occurred is not. So it's very difficult to determine if a stroke occurred many years before the patient's memory faded, or if the stroke and memory problems went hand in hand. Some brain tissue appears to have suffered a stroke, yet the owner of that brain never officially had a stroke.

Despite their shortcomings, autopsies can be very valuable to families. Alzheimer's has its roots in our genes, so family members can benefit from knowing their relatives' cause of death.

Autopsies are important to medical science as well, by allowing researchers to peer into the brain's tiniest wheels, the structure and chemistry of its molecules. Without autopsies, our current drugs to treat Alzheimer's wouldn't exist. Many people who develop Alzheimer's choose to join a clinical study that includes donating their brain tissue to Alzheimer's research after their death.

► THE TEST OF TIME

No matter how much expertise goes into a diagnosis, doctors frequently need to follow a patient over time to get an accurate diagnosis. Doctors would like everyone to believe that they are right the first time out, but as one eighty-year-old liked to remind her frustrated family members as they watched the doctor's multiple mistakes, "Dears, they don't call it 'practicing medicine' for nothing." It's up to family members and patients to go to their doctors whenever symptoms change and to understand that this diagnosis business is an ongoing process.

WHAT TESTS COST

Tests that each cost $25–$250, which insurance usually covers: physical exam; X-ray; urine analyses; blood tests for homocysteine, thyroid, vitamins, ApoE4; MMSE; depression assessment; EKG

Tests that each cost $250 to $750, and insurance covers if patient gets precertification, meaning approval from the insurance company before undergoing the tests: hearing analyses; carotid ultrasound; spinal tap with analyses for plaque and tangle proteins; second opinion with an Alzheimer specialist

Tests that cost $750 to $2,500 and insurance covers if patient gets precertification: MRI, MRI angiography or MRI diffusion imaging, CAT scan, neuropsychological testing

Test that costs $1,500 or more and has Medicare coverage if the patient's diagnosis is uncertain or if the patient is in a clinical trial: PET scan

These costs are approximate, and actual costs can vary widely. While insurance companies usually set rates, doctors who don't accept insurance can charge whatever they feel is appropriate. For example, the cost of neuropsychological testing can vary from $250 to $3,000, depending on how many tests are given and the type of practice.

▶ **The List.** Take a copy of this list of tests and assessment tools to your doctor. Ask which of the tests he or she does, and later, be sure to see the test results.

▶ ESSENTIAL TESTS

Tests 1 through 16 are considered the standard tests to give to someone who is suspected of having Alzheimer's. In some cases, these tests alone will reveal that the patient's memory is normal. If not, then doctors order additional tests.

Core Essential Tests

1. Interview with family
2. Check for inappropriate drugs
3. Memory and medical history
4. MMSE
5. Clock test
6. Depression screen, such as the Beck scale, Geriatric Depression Scale
7. Delayed recall memory test
8. Physical, neurological exam, hearing, vision, smell, weight, blood pressure, waist measurement
9. Vascular risk assessment
10. Brain MRI or CT scan (MRI is better)
11. Urine analysis
12. Blood cell counts (to look for infection or anemia)
13. Thyroid function with ultrasensitive TSH
14. Blood tests for liver function, kidney function, electrolytes, glucose
15. Fasting cholesterol and lipids (blood test)
16. Vitamin B_{12} and folic acid (blood test)

Considered Essential at Some Centers

17. Syphilis test (blood test)

18. Neuropsychological testing (paper-and-pencil test)

19. Brain MRI FLAIR and oblique thin slice

20. Brain MRI diffusion-weighted imaging

21. Carotid ultrasound

22. EKG

Other Essential Assessments
Done at Most Centers

23. Activities of daily living to assess day-to-day functioning

24. Assessment of behavioral problems using a test or interview

25. Determining the stage of the disease using a test or interview

26. Caregiver/home needs assessment (usually done by social worker)

27. Assessing the person's legal needs, driving ability, and home safety

Optional Steps

28. Referral to specialist

29. Chest X-ray

30. Brain FDG PET scan

31. Brain SPECT scan (if PET not possible)

32. Homocysteine, thiamine, and vitamin C levels

33. C-reactive protein, lipoprotein A, ESR

34. Routine lumbar puncture (spinal tap)

35. CSF beta-amyloid, tau, and phosphorylated tau

36. CSF viral or 14-3-3 prion protein markers

37. Genetic testing: ApoE4, APP, presenilins, CJD, MTFR

38. Rosen-Hachinski Ischemia Rating Scale, stroke risk scale
39. Polysomnogram
40. Test for metals: iron, lead, ferritin, transferrin, zinc, copper
41. Brain MRI with contrast or MRI angiography
42. Transcranial Doppler
43. Gait tests, cisternogram
44. EEG, muscle biopsy
45. Urine neural thread protein (NTP)
46. Computerized neuropsychological tests
47. Simulated driving test
48. Erythrocyte cholinesterase
49. Serum anticholinergicity
50. Expanded smell tests

Research Tests
(usually done only after you give written consent)

51. Blood amyloid test
52. Amyloid PET
53. Functional MRI
54. MRI spectroscopy
55. Lens amyloid test
56. MRI volumetry
57. MRI tensor imaging
58. Other genetic tests

PART TWO

► STATE-OF-THE-ART TREATMENT

CHAPTER SEVEN

THE TRUTH ABOUT ALZHEIMER'S TREATMENT

Few Alzheimer's patients get state-of-the-art care.
—HEADLINE, *PSYCHIATRIC NEWS,* 2001

In the past decade, we have made tremendous progress in developing treatments for the symptoms of Alzheimer's disease. Researchers have completed more than a hundred clinical trials testing various treatments for Alzheimer's, which have taught us a great deal. Just as in cancer or heart disease, Alzheimer's treatments are based on the latest science and are tested rigorously using standards set by the U.S. Food and Drug Administration, as well as by worldwide government agencies. Older treatments are being replaced with newer and better ones.

Despite all these advances, many people still see Alzheimer's as a part of normal aging. People say a relative or friend is "senile" or that he or she has "old-timer's disease." Even doctors (trained prior to the advances in treatment) and insurance companies can share this fatalistic view. That may be one of the reasons why about half of the people with mild-stage or moderate-stage Alzheimer's are *not taking any* of the FDA-approved medications.

We want to correct misperceptions about Alzheimer's in a way that helps people with the disease and their families the most. The two most important points about Alzheimer's treatment:

1. Early treatment is important.
2. Treatment can help people at all stages of Alzheimer's.

► THE TEN BIGGEST MYTHS ABOUT ALZHEIMER'S TREATMENT

Here are ten of the most common fallacies and their antidotes (the true story).

Myth 1: Dementia is just old age, so it is best to leave the person alone.

Truth: Because dementia, especially Alzheimer's, was traditionally viewed as "senility" or normal aging, physicians and families long held that dementia was untreatable or not worth treating. As we discussed in the beginning of the book, we now know there are numerous dementia copycats, including depression, vitamin deficiencies, and thyroid problems, that can be improved or even halted through treatment.

Myth 2: Alzheimer's is untreatable.

Truth: Alzheimer's is incurable, but it is not untreatable.

Myth 3: There is no need to start treatment early—it's all downhill anyway.

Truth: Studies suggest that people who start treatment early usually remain better off than those who start treatment months later (more on this topic below). That is why most expert doctors begin treatment right after a person is diagnosed.

Myth 4: Treatment will stop the course of the disease or bring someone back to normal.

Truth: Unfortunately, the available medicines cannot do this, but they can help people with Alzheimer's to think more clearly and function better and longer than they would have without the medication.

Myth 5: Memory pills should be stopped after a few weeks if there aren't any clear benefits.

Truth: It may take from several months to a year or longer to tell if a memory drug is working.

Myth 6: Drugs for Alzheimer's work only in the early stages, so there is no use treating people in the moderate or severe stages.

Truth: These drugs are effective for treating moderate and severe Alzheimer's. They may help people in the moderate stage even more than those in the early stage. People at every stage should have access to any treatment that helps.

Myth 7: Vaccines and stem cells to cure Alzheimer's will soon be on the market, so let's just wait until they're available.

Truth: It will be years, if ever, before vaccines and stem cell therapy are available. To date, researchers have found no experimental treatment that improved thinking and memory better than the four drugs already in use: Aricept, Exelon, Razadyne, and Namenda. (All of these drugs are discussed in detail in the following chapter.)

Myth 8: It is worth trying a memory supplement or herbal pill before trying these drugs.

Truth: It's best to make a choice such as this after you discuss it with your doctor. Supplements or herbal treatments vary widely in their benefits and risks, and none are as well studied for Alzheimer's as are the four prescription drugs.

Myth 9: Not seeing any change after treatment means the drug is not working.

Truth: The course of untreated Alzheimer's is a progressive decline. So not seeing a change is usually a good sign that the disease has stabilized, at least for the time being.

Myth 10: The side effects of the current drugs are too strong to justify taking them.

Truth: Most beneficial drugs have side effects, and most people generally tolerate Aricept and Namenda quite well.

▶ WHAT YOU CAN EXPECT FROM THE MEDICATIONS

In general, the drugs allow people with Alzheimer's to function at a higher level for a longer period. Depending on the stage of the disease, you may see one or more of the following:

- Actual improvements and stabilization in the person's mental functioning are more likely in the earlier stages of the disease. In one study of people with mild and moderate Alzheimer's, 82 percent of patients on medication improved or stayed stable for six months, compared to 59 percent on placebo. Of participants on medication, 58 percent showed a meaningful improvement after six months, as did 28 percent of the placebo recipients.

- Among people who are in the moderate to severe stages, the chance for actual improvement is lower than for people in the mild stages, but symptoms may stabilize or get worse more slowly. In one study, about 40 percent of people on medication improved or stayed the same for six months in their cognitive abilities compared to about 22 percent on placebo.

- People who take medications are less likely to develop behavioral problems than those who don't.
- Care providers may find that the person with Alzheimer's requires less time to care for.
- The brain's memory center shrinks less quickly, though researchers have yet to prove that.

(Side effects vary among the various drugs; see the detailed discussion in Chapter 8.)

Finally, as much as we wish you could, you *cannot* expect the following from the medications:

- A complete reversal of the disease, that is, "getting back to normal"
- No further decline
- Dramatic or overnight benefits. This is possible but not likely, and if it happens, it won't last more than a few months

FAMILIES KNOW BEST

Family members see benefits in their relatives taking Alzheimer's medications. The reported benefits include:

- More alert and motivated
- Less forgetful, less frustrated
- "Holding her own"
- In a better mood, less depressed
- Worrying less, is less pessimistic
- More interested in life and derives more pleasure from it
- Easier to get going, gets ready more quickly
- Not as repetitive
- More able to chat on the phone and carry on conversations
- Not hallucinating or imagining things
- Less suspicious

(continued)

- More likely to remember to flush the toilet
- More likely to rely on memory aids
- Better able to handle themselves at a restaurant or a friend's house

People who developed Alzheimer's at an unusually young age and took Alzheimer's medication said that they could continue to do the following (especially if they could do these things before treatment):

- Engage in hobbies such as painting or knitting
- Play musical instruments
- Appreciate art, music, and humor
- Read books, watch television and films
- Give speeches
- Work part- or full-time
- Send e-mails and use the computer
- Use most devices around the house
- Socialize with family and friends
- Go to church, pray

▶ THE IMPORTANCE OF STAGING

When your doctor starts talking about staging, she's probably not digressing to discuss her interest in theater. She's talking about how to determine if the disease is in the mild, moderate, or late stage of Alzheimer's. It requires evaluating day-to-day functioning, memory ability, and general behavior. Rating scales developed for this purpose take between fifteen and forty-five minutes.

Unfortunately, staging still hasn't caught on with many doctors, though it's becoming more common because insurance companies ask the doctors for this information. When done correctly, staging has several benefits:

- Gives doctors and families a good baseline for tracking progress or treatment benefits over time
- Helps the doctor choose the best initial drug, since different drugs are approved for different stages
- Allows doctors to better predict what benefits or risks to expect from treatment. For example, for a person in the very early stage of Alzheimer's, a doctor may choose to use a slightly lower dose of a drug to minimize nausea or diarrhea.
- Gives doctors and families a better sense of what to expect over the next few months or years. We know that for some, thinking abilities and test scores on the Mini-Mental State Exam (MMSE), for example, decline slowly at first, then more quickly in the moderate stage, then slow down again in the later stage. (Behavioral and speech problems don't follow this same pattern of decline.)

At a minimum, most doctors will perform the Mini-Mental State Exam, which provides a good clue about the stage of the disease. Here is how MMSE scores translate in terms of stages:

Very mild: 27–30
Mild: 21–26
Moderate: 11–20
Severe: 1–10

MMSE cannot be used actually to diagnose Alzheimer's. People with MCI and mild Alzheimer's have very similar scores, so doctors who rely solely on the MMSE may mistake MCI for mild Alzheimer's. In addition, the MMSE is not a perfect staging tool because it doesn't assess behavioral problems or a person's functioning in daily life, and a person's education level can affect scores.

▶ **Check It Out:** See Appendix A for a more detailed description of the early through moderate stages of Alzheimer's.

► SHOULD YOU START TREATMENT IN THE EARLIEST STAGES?

Truthfully, there are pros and cons to starting early. Most experts agree that the pros strongly outweigh the negatives, but below we give you both sides of the issue so you can judge for yourself. Note that our "pro" list is a lot longer than the "con" list!

Understanding how Alzheimer's spreads in the brain reveals the importance of early treatment: It starts in very small regions and then spreads over a period of years to damage more and more of the tissue. Although it has not been proven that current drugs stop this deadly march, doctors hope that starting treatment early gives patients their best chance of preserving their independence.

The Pros

- Alzheimer's relentlessly damages nerve cells and mental abilities and causes brain tissue to begin shrinking even in the early stages.

- Mental decline is slow in the early stage and then speeds up dramatically in the moderate stage, when the ability to function independently decreases and wandering, suspiciousness, and other serious problems emerge. Starting treatment early offers the best chance to keep people in the early stage for as long as possible.

- Medications have shown modest but consistent benefits on mental and functional abilities in early Alzheimer's. Some studies suggest that people who start treatment early retain better mental ability longer than those who start treatment months later.

- We hope the drugs may protect against Alzheimer's-related harmful effects, such as neurochemical imbalances and possibly even against brain shrinkage.

- Alzheimer's treatment may delay the emergence of behavioral problems and possibly reduce caregiving time by protecting people's ability to care for themselves.

- In people with moderate Alzheimer's, treatment offers added hope to keep them functioning better (and possibly longer) in the community.

- Last but not least: The available drugs are not miracle drugs and they don't cure the disease. But they are the best we have, and from the vantage point of a scientist who sees the broad trends in Alzheimer's studies, there is no better treatment on the horizon for the next several years. So at this point, no one can afford to wait for the perfect pill.

Henry is a fifty-four-year-old doctor who was diagnosed early in the course of the disease. He had to stop practicing after a colleague discovered he was forgetting important details that could have hurt his patients. Once diagnosed, Henry began taking Aricept. He also took up new activities he'd always wanted to do, such as singing in a rock band, and he became an active advocate for Alzheimer's charities. He attended lectures and managed most of his daily activities for a couple of years after treatment began. He even delivered four lectures to large groups about his memory-loss experience. The disease eventually progressed and gradually reduced his independence, but he had several good years.

Ample scientific evidence illustrates the value of starting treatment early, as these studies of Aricept, Exelon, and Namenda show.

- When researchers gave either a placebo or Aricept to people with mild or very mild Alzheimer's, the thinking of 20 percent of the placebo recipients and 40 percent of the Aricept recipients improved by about 15 percent over the course of the six-month study.

- In a one-year study of people with mild- to moderate-stage Alzheimer's, the people taking the placebo declined steadily right away. However, it took almost nine months on average for the people who took Aricept to decline below their baseline. Such results underscore the value of starting treatment early and staying on it for at least one year.

- Another study showed that by about twelve months, approximately half of the people who received Aricept had not declined in their ability to manage day-to-day tasks, compared to about 35 percent of people on the placebo.

- Researchers gave Exelon to one group of Alzheimer's patients, then gave it to another similar group six months later. Those who started Exelon earlier performed at a much higher level mentally for two years longer than the late starters.

▶ **Good to Know:** In our experience, it is wise to stay on an Alzheimer's medication for at least one year. Most of our patients stay on them for years.

The Negatives

- There is no definite proof that early treatment extends life, keeps nerve cells alive longer, or slows the buildup of plaques and tangles in the brain.

- Not all studies have been positive. For example, long-term studies of the effects of Aricept, Exelon, and Razadyne on people with MCI have yielded mixed or negative results. Likewise, studies of giving Namenda to people with mild Alzheimer's were not positive enough to meet the FDA-approval standard.

- There is no strong proof that the drugs' effects last beyond two or three years.

- The drugs can have side effects in some people.

- Critics feel the benefits may be too small to justify their cost to society.

▶ UP AND RUNNING: PUTTING A TREATMENT PLAN IN PLACE AND KEEPING IT USEFUL

In the previous chapters, you read about how doctors diagnose Alzheimer's. After the diagnosis, you should expect more than a pat on the back and a prescription.

First, let's talk about where to find the best doctor for long-term treatment and care. Most of our recommenation in Chapter 4 about how to find the best doctor to make your diagnosis also apply to choosing a doctor for your ongoing care. You may be able to stay with the doctor who made the diagnosis. Some doctors, however, specialize in diagnosis and want you to see your general practitioner for ongoing care. (Doctors get reimbursed less for ongoing care and treatment.)

In general, for ongoing memory care in the early stage, your best bet is to go to a neurologist, a geriatric psychiatrist, or a specialized memory clinic. In the later stages, more health and behavioral problems emerge. Then it's wise to find a geriatrician or primary-care physician who will treat the physical health problems, and you may also need a psychiatrist to help you handle the emotional and behavioral issues. What's most important is that you find a doctor who will spend time with you and really focus on your needs and concerns.

An important factor to consider in choosing a doctor for long-term care is the doctor's approach to medications. In general, we see three types of approaches:

1. *More is better.* These doctors like to prescribe the newest medication, regardless of the cost. They favor combining medications for maximum effect and using drugs for purposes not yet approved by the FDA if some evidence exists to support such use. For example, they may recommend an imported drug from Europe to treat mild Alzheimer's, even though it's not approved by the FDA to do that. They also usually are more likely to recommend that patients stay on medications for longer periods of time.

2. *Less is more.* These doctors avoid medications that don't meet their own criteria for success, wean you off any that aren't absolutely necessary, and give medications for the shortest time possible. They declare failure quickly. They may work in a managed-care system where doctors benefit by keeping prescription numbers down and the HMO's profits up.

3. *Follow the rules.* These doctors adhere to the formal evidence. If a study showed that a drug worked for six months, these doctors will use the drug for six months. They live and die by the clinical studies. However, the studies they live by may include some innovative or alternative approaches.

Our advice? Find a doctor who suits your philosophy of care, recognizing that you need innovative approaches when dealing with Alzheimer's.

_____

How to Recognize a Good Doctor

- *Establishes treatment targets.* Documenting the MMSE, as well as any specific problems you have now, will help the doctor gauge the effectiveness of treatment later on. For instance, you may have trouble remembering names, repeat yourself, misplace objects, or have difficulty keeping your finances in order. On subsequent visits, the doctor will assess how treatment is affecting these behaviors.

- *Reviews all medications.* The doctor should ask about psychological problems, such as anxiety, or other medical conditions, such as heart disease, and how these are being treated. It is important for the doctor to have a complete list of medications, because some drugs, including those for incontinence and depression, can nullify Alzheimer's medications.

- *Thoroughly explains the treatment options.* You are entitled to a complete explanation of the diagnosis and prognosis, along with the overall treatment plan, available medications, and possible side effects of drug treatment. This is the time when you should expect the doctor to discuss the possible usefulness of taking at least one of the four FDA-approved medicines for Alzheimer's disease that are described in the next chapter.

- *Helps you choose a friend or relative who will serve as your official assistant.* Your assistant may be a family member who will be able to keep an eye on you, observe any changes, and fill the doctor in as needed. Ideally, your helper lives with you or close by. An adult child who lives two hours away and visits you once a month, for example, wouldn't be a good helper for your doctor visits. Your spouse, who knows you the best, would be.

- *Helps your family set up an integrative treatment plan.* More than just helping to pick a helper, a doctor should discuss ways that you and your family can monitor medication use and keep track of changes and responses to medication. The best doctors will help you enhance the positive effects of drugs, such as by getting family support, educating yourself on the disease, and trying nonpharmacologic strategies. They will also help keep your family's expectations of treatment realistic. None of these drugs is a magic bullet, so a doctor should help you appreciate any small improvements.

When to Wait

Most doctors will recommend that you start treatment immediately after diagnosis. However, on occasion, a doctor isn't sure of the diagnosis. If that's the case, it's better to err on the side of caution. She may have you come in again and undergo a few more tests, or even watch you for a few more months to be certain of what she's seeing. If you trust and like your doctor, go with her judgment.

Joe, fifty-five, was labeled with possible Alzheimer's, and his family urged his doctor to start him on Razadyne and Namenda as soon as possible. Joe started taking the drugs, but in the next two years, he got so much worse that the doctor decided to order a special spinal fluid test to make sure the diagnosis was correct. The test showed that Joe didn't have Alzheimer's after all, but Creutzfeldt-Jakob disease (a rare infection) that these drugs are unable to help.

What Your Doctor Should Do at Follow-up Appointments

- Review your medication and any other health issues that may need monitoring. Drugs affect people differently, and both primary and secondary effects must be monitored regularly.
- Weigh the risks and benefits of your medication in relation to the stage of Alzheimer's and health status.
- Consider combining or switching drugs, based on the latest data concerning the risks and benefits.
- Discuss any changes in your condition (or that of a loved one), including safety-related concerns such as driving skills and wandering.

- Periodically administer tests to see how the disease is progressing over time. At the minimum, he should perform the Mini-Mental State Exam (MMSE), a quick measure of brain function. If he isn't doing this, ask him to.
- Discuss whether you need to consult with other specialists.

In general, it takes at least six months and several visits to judge whether a medication is working well or not. For instance, people's memory may fluctuate a lot in a short period of time for reasons ranging from getting a poor night's sleep to battling a flu bug. For this reason, expert doctors rely more on patterns they see over several visits than on a single visit.

► TREATMENT MISTAKES AND WHAT TO DO ABOUT THEM

Not all doctor's visits to treat Alzheimer's are optimal.

"The doctor saw my mother for thirty minutes and gave her some pills. Since I live so far away from her, I can't check on her daily. She took the pills he gave her for four weeks, but we didn't see any improvements. When I called the doctor, he said we could stop the pills since they didn't seem to be helping, but then my mom's memory got a lot worse when she did stop."

This scenario is all too typical when a doctor is not well versed in Alzheimer's or is simply not doing a good job. The doctor tried unsuccessfully to assess over the phone how the mother was doing and whether her medication was working. He didn't counsel the family about what they should expect from treatment. (In this case, counseling the mother wouldn't have been very useful because she was too forgetful.) He should have taken the time to call and speak to the daughter herself and warn her that it usually takes several months to determine how a medication is working.

The mother's memory got worse when she stopped the medication, probably because the drug was actually helping. Remaining stable may well indicate that the medication is doing its job.

Unfortunately, she lost the benefits she could have seen from the drug.

The Top Ten Mistakes and How to Avoid Them

1. *Delaying treatment.* As mentioned, starting treatment early may preserve mental skills longer.

2. *Documenting the person's baseline status and stage incorrectly or incompletely.* If the doctor doesn't fill out the forms correctly, patients and their families will have difficulty assessing how the treatment is working (and the family is likely to have problems with insurance). Ask the doctor how he or she is documenting the baseline status.

3. *Not counseling families about side effects or evaluating the person for drug interactions.* If families and patients don't know about possible side effects, they may respond inappropriately when side effects occur—either too alarmed or not alarmed enough. Make sure you ask for this information if the doctor doesn't volunteer it. (As with all drugs, the list of possible side effects is long, so the best doctors focus on the most common and dangerous ones.)

4. *Having unrealistic expectations.* This can lead families to stop their relative's medications when they don't see dramatic improvements.

5. *Increasing the dose too fast.* Drug companies' recommended dosages are based on the average amounts used in studies. Doctors should sometimes deviate from the package inserts if newer research has come out on how much to prescribe, or if they need to modify the dosage to fit the patient's unique needs.

6. *Stopping a drug too soon.* This can lead to loss of future benefits and exacerbate symptoms for a few days to a couple of weeks. Restarting the drug after a few months may not make up for lost time.

7. *Not fully assessing symptoms at follow-up visits.* Seeing a patient only briefly or not assessing all of the different aspects

of the person's mental and functional status can lead to poor decisions such as stopping a drug or giving a person the wrong dose. If you encounter this, speak up and ask for more time or a follow-up visit if necessary.

8. *Sticking with the tried-but-not-so-true.* If a drug doesn't appear to be working as well as it should, a doctor should switch to another one or add a second medication. Likewise, being too aggressive and adding a second drug when it is not indicated can lead to unwanted, avoidable side effects.

9. *Mistaking disease symptoms for drug side effects, and vice versa.* For example, if a doctor or family member thinks agitation is a drug side effect when it is actually part of the progression of Alzheimer's, he or she may mistakenly stop the drug instead of trying to raise the dose or add a second medication to treat the agitation.

10. *Being too aggressive.* Some doctors combine two Alzheimer's medications for every single patient, while others routinely overshoot the recommended dose limits. Clearly one dose does not fit all, but such aggressive strategies must be well justified.

TAKE THIS LIST TO THE DOCTOR

Questions to Ask Before Starting Treatment

- What is the stage of Alzheimer's? What is the MMSE score?
- Why did you choose this specific drug instead of the others, and what are the expected benefits?
- What are the expected risks? Will treatment interfere with any current drugs or illnesses? Is there anything in the EKG (heart rhythm) that would suggest a problem with using one of these drugs?
- How much does treatment cost? If needed, can you sign us up for a Prescription Assistance Program, and do you provide free samples? (See more on what treatments cost and how to pay for them in Chapter 8.)

- How often do we need to come for follow-up visits? (At least every three months is ideal.)
- Will my insurance pay for the medications, and if so for how long?

Questions to Ask at Follow-up Visits

- What kinds of tests did you do? How does the MMSE score compare to her prior scores? What kinds of improvements or decline are you noticing?
- Is the diagnosis still Alzheimer's? Could it be vascular dementia or Lewy Body Dementia?
- Is treatment working? Is this the best dose? Would changing drugs or adding a second drug help?
- Can I continue to get free samples?
- Is there any suggestion that the drug is adversely affecting the liver or heart rhythm? What about weight loss?
- Has any new information come out about the risks or benefits of the drug(s) since the last visit?
- Has the FDA approved any new drugs that might be helpful? Have any new drugs become available in Europe but not here? If so, should we try them?
- Are there any worthwhile new clinical trials to consider?
- Should we get the second opinion of a specialist?

CHAPTER EIGHT

THE BEST DRUGS TO TREAT ALZHEIMER'S

Recent research results suggest that pharmacologic and psychosocial interventions may forestall cognitive decline among people with dementia, provided they are implemented early in the course of the disease.

—CHRONIC DISEASE PREVENTION, A JOURNAL OF THE
U.S. CENTERS FOR DISEASE CONTROL

Alzheimer's drugs evolve over time. In the 1980s, a drug called Hydergine (ergoloid mesylates) was used to treat dementia, but it fell out of favor in 1993 when Cognex (tacrine)—a drug more specifically targeted at Alzheimer's—came on the market. Cognex, too, lost its status when Aricept, a safer drug used widely today, was approved in 1996. Since then, the FDA has approved three other medications in addition to Aricept to treat Alzheimer's. The table on the following page shows which stage of Alzheimer's these newer drugs, Aricept, Exelon, Razadyne, and Namenda, treat most successfully.

	Mild	Moderate	Severe
Aricept (donepezil)	✓	✓	✓
Exelon (rivastigmine)	✓	✓	
Razadyne (galantamine)	✓	✓	
Namenda (memantine)		✓	✓

As you can see, there are drugs that are shown to help at every stage of Alzheimer's.

► WHAT THE ALZHEIMER'S DRUGS HAVE IN COMMON

Aricept, Exelon, Razadyne, and Namenda are all approved by the FDA to treat Alzheimer's symptoms. The FDA bestows its blessings only when two independent six-month-long studies have shown that the drug improves memory and thinking abilities and increases overall functioning.

Aricept, Razadyne, and Exelon are cholinesterase inhibitors (ChEIs). They block the brain enzyme cholinesterase that in healthy people automatically clears up excess acetylcholine, a major neurotransmitter in the brain. Acetylcholine is vital to learning, memory, and many other bodily functions. However, an excess of it can overstimulate the parts of the body that it supplies, causing side effects.

People with Alzheimer's have too little acetylcholine, because the disease hits the part of the brain that produces it. So people with Alzheimer's need the extra acetylcholine that cholinesterase normally removes. Scientists created ChEIs on the theory that blocking cholinesterase might be a good approach to alleviating Alzheimer's symptoms—and to a large extent, they were right.

All are "symptomatic drugs," meaning they are better than a placebo at treating symptoms but haven't yet been proved to change the pathology of the disease in people. For example, if you stop taking a ChEI, you stop getting its benefits and will soon be no better off than if you never took the drug. In other words, these drugs don't appear to provide a permanent fix.

Aricept, Exelon, and Razadyne differ slightly in their chemical makeup, so they stay in the body for varying lengths of time and have their own unique side effects. The body also harbors many types of cholinesterase enzymes, and the three drugs differ in how they affect them. As a result, people who cannot tolerate one drug sometimes do well on another. So don't give up if the first medicine you try causes side effects.

> Roger, sixty-nine, was diagnosed with mild Alzheimer's. When he took Aricept, he developed muscle cramps and had nightmares, even at the lowest dose. The doctor halted the drug and put him on Exelon instead. While the new drug didn't cause cramps or nightmares, it did make Roger feel nauseated. The doctor suggested that Roger take his pills with a full breakfast and a glass of whole milk, which slowed his absorption of the drug. Over the next two weeks, Roger's nausea gradually subsided. He has continued to benefit from Exelon.

A Word of Caution: All ChEIs carry some common warnings and precautions. Acetylcholine is involved in regulating heart rhythm, stomach acid secretion, and lung function. Hence, ChEIs may worsen stomach ulcers or bleeding, especially in those taking anti-inflammatory pain medicines, may increase the risk for seizures or breathing problems, and may also lead to abnormally slow or blocked heart rhythms. ChEIs can also interfere with muscle relaxants used during general anesthesia. Common side effects of individual drugs are described under each drug profile below. Consult the product labels for complete descriptions of all possible side effects and discuss side effects with your doctor before starting treatment.

We don't have good studies testing efficacy beyond two to three years, but many patients have been treated with these drugs for more than five years. The benefits of ChEIs disappear three to six weeks after you stop taking them and may not come back in full if you start them up again.

WEB SITES WORTH KNOWING

When you type "Alzheimer's" into Google, your top hits may be for Web sites sponsored by the maker of an Alzheimer's drug. To find the official site for any drug, just use its name in the Web

address—for example, www.Aricept.com or www.Namenda
.com. These Web sites contain up-to-date information that you
should definitely check out about the drug itself, patient-
assistance programs, study results, and the latest safety
warnings. However, these sites shy away from controversy and
focus only on information approved by the FDA. For more
cutting-edge information, breaking news, or debates on
Alzheimer's—particularly controversies surrounding drugs—go
to the Alzheimer Research Forum (www.alzforum.org), which
has a discussion board where doctors freely exchange their
opinions. For the latest information on clinical trial results,
especially negative studies that have not been published, go to
www.clinicalstudyresults.org.

► MEET THE MEDS

These are the four newer FDA-approved drugs for treating
Alzheimer's disease. (For lifestyle and alternative approaches to treating the symptoms of Alzheimer's, check out Chapters 16 and 17.)

Aricept (donepezil)

Pluses: Aricept has been studied longer and in more people than the
other two ChEIs, is the easiest to use, and is the best tolerated. Aricept clears more slowly than the other drugs from the body, which
has both pros and cons: If you miss taking a dose, there is still some
drug in your body; if you are having side effects, it will take longer
for them to stop. Only one dose a day is needed. It is the most widely
prescribed Alzheimer's drug, accounting for 70 percent of doctors'
written prescriptions of the four drugs. *It is a great first choice for people in the mild stages.* Aricept may offer benefits for at least a year.

   Common Side Effects: Possible nausea, vomiting, diarrhea, bruising, fainting, not sleeping well, loss of appetite, feeling tired, and muscle cramps. Most of these are mild and tend to subside as the body
adjusts to the medication over a few days. Aricept may be more likely
than Exelon or Razadyne to cause mild sleep problems such as vivid

dreams and nocturnal illusions. Urinary problems are also occasionally seen with Aricept.

Who Is Aricept Best For? People at any stage of Alzheimer's.

Best Dosage: Ten milligrams a day provide the most consistent benefits and is the optimal amount. Doctors start Aricept at 5 milligrams once daily, and after four to six weeks, they raise the dose to 10 milligrams. Both 5 milligrams and 10 milligrams daily are effective, and so people who cannot tolerate 10 milligrams can remain on 5 milligrams. In very frail people or those with concerns about side effects, it can be started at an even lower dose (5 milligrams every other day). Usually taken with dinner or breakfast, Aricept is also available as an Orally Disintegrating Tablet (ODT), which dissolves in the mouth and does not need to be swallowed.

Latest Studies of Aricept

- Aricept was approved by the FDA for treating severe Alzheimer's, making it the only drug indicated for all three stages.

- Three preliminary studies report that people who take Aricept may have slightly less Alzheimer's-related loss in brain volume than those not taking it.

- A major three-year study by the National Institutes of Health found that Aricept helped delay dementia for about eighteen months in people with MCI. At thirty-six months, only a subset of participants maintained the benefits: those with the ApoE4 gene, which increases a person's risk of developing Alzheimer's. Aricept is not approved by the FDA for treating MCI, however.

- Aricept is the only ChEI studied exclusively in elderly African Americans with Alzheimer's, who had a similar response to others. But because ethnic groups metabolize some drugs differently, scientists view drugs tested in diverse ethnic groups more favorably. All of the four FDA-approved drugs have been studied in Asians and in Latin Americans.

- When used for people with vascular dementia, Aricept improves thinking. During one study, one concern was that more people taking the drug died than those on placebo. The reasons are not known and the pattern was not seen in other Aricept studies. Aricept is not approved for treating vascular dementia.

- A recent one-year study found that 5 milligrams a day of Aricept plus weekly mental-stimulation therapy helped people more than Aricept alone.

- Another small study found that people could safely take doses of Aricept as high as 20 milligrams a day. However, the information is considered too limited to judge whether it provides greater benefits at that dose. People with inadequate response to recommended doses sometimes may require bigger doses in general, so this study provides us with important safety information about the effects of larger doses.

- Several studies (some lasting five years) following up on the original ChEI trials found that people with Alzheimer's who remained on the drugs declined at a slower rate than previously predicted. These studies were not well controlled and the numbers of people staying on treatment were small after two to three years.

Razadyne (galantamine)

Razadyne was originally made from daffodils, using the same extract that soldiers in ancient Greece purportedly used to stay alert on the battlefield. The drug now uses a synthetic version of the compound.

Razadyne not only blocks cholinesterase in the way that Aricept does but also stimulates the brain's nicotine receptors, which are involved in attention and learning. Researchers originally hoped this double action would double the drug's benefits as well, but unfortunately, that theory was not borne out in clinical trials. Razadyne is just as effective as the other two ChEIs.

Razadyne's original name was Reminyl, and American manufacturers changed its name in June 2005 because it overlapped with other drug names in this country.

Pluses: Razadyne may not disturb sleep and dreaming as much as Aricept.

Common Side Effects: Possible nausea, vomiting, diarrhea, fainting, loss of appetite, and weight loss. Most of these are mild and tend to subside as the body adjusts to the medication over time. In MCI trials, thirteen Razadyne recipients died, compared to only one death among placebo recipients—a finding that not many doctors are aware of. The FDA has not approved the use of Razadyne in MCI patients. Because more deaths occurred in the Razadyne group than in the placebo group, doctors can't rule out that the deaths were somehow due to Razadyne. At this time, we wouldn't use Razadyne in people with MCI.

Who Is Razadyne Best For? People with mild to moderate Alzheimer's.

Best Dosage: Razadyne comes in regular and extended release, or ER, capsules. You take Razadyne ER once a day and regular Razadyne twice a day. The regular and ER verisons should not be taken together.

The effective dose of both Razadyne ER and regular Razadyne is 16 to 24 milligrams per day. Doctors usually recommend starting with 8 milligrams a day and then increasing it to 16 milligrams a day after a period of at least four weeks. Once you've been taking 16 milligrams for at least four weeks, your doctor may increase it again to 24 milligrams a day. Take ER in the morning with breakfast.

Latest Studies of Razadyne

- Taking Razadyne ER once a day is as effective as taking regular Razadyne twice a day.

- Two studies of Razadyne in people with mild cognitive impairment showed it did not delay the onset of dementia. But paradoxically, one of these studies suggested that Razadyne might help protect against shrinkage of brain tissue.

- A study comparing Razadyne with Aricept found that they improved thinking and memory about the same.

- Razadyne might help improve cognitive abilities in people with vascular dementia, two studies find. As with other ChEIs, it is not approved by the FDA for this condition.

- An Australian study showed that 70 percent of people with mild Alzheimer's who started on Razadyne and kept taking it for six months had a 10 percent improvement on their tests of thinking.

- In animal models, Razadyne protects against the buildup of amyloid plaques.

Exelon (rivastigmine)

Unlike Aricept, Exelon is not a selective cholinesterase inhibitor. Instead, it blocks two related enzymes: acetylcholinesterase and butyrylcholinesterase. Scientists think the latter enzyme may also play a role in Alzheimer's and inflammation.

Pluses: Unlike most drugs, Exelon is not metabolized by the liver so it is unlikely to interact with other drugs. The drug is also available in a patch form, which provides the drug throughout the day. The patch may be better for people who find that the drug makes them feel nauseous, because the drug bypasses the stomach.

Common Side Effects: In clinical trials, Exelon capsules caused much higher rates of nausea and vomiting, and higher rates of weight and appetite loss, than Aricept did. Vomiting can sometimes be so severe as to lead to throat injury. That said, the reason for these effects is probably that researchers used an aggressive dose aimed at having the biggest impact. Other possible common side effects include diarrhea, headache, stomach pain, dizziness, fainting, feeling tired, sweating, and tremors. It is recommended that Exelon capsules be taken with meals to reduce the severity of nausea and vomiting. If treatment is temporarily interrupted for more than a few days, it should be restarted at the lowest daily dose to reduce the risk for nausea and vomiting.

The Exelon patch was designed to release the drug more slowly over a twenty-four-hour period and so has much lower rates of nausea and vomiting. It is as effective as the capsule. As with any patch, it can cause local irritation. Make sure to apply it properly. Also, it may come off accidentally.

Who Is Exelon Best For? People with mild to moderate Alzheimer's. People with Lewy Body or Parkinson's dementia.

Best Dosage: Doctors start Exelon at 1.5 milligrams a day and increase it gradually over several weeks to 6 milligrams twice a day in sequential steps. Three to 6 milligrams twice a day taken with food is considered the optimal dose. If the lower dose does not work, the goal is to get people to the highest dose in this range if they can tolerate the drug. The Exelon patch is usually applied daily, to a person's back. People taking oral capsules can easily be switched to the patch.

Latest Studies of Exelon

- A large Canadian study of 2,633 people with Alzheimer's found that Exelon might help people who do not benefit from or can't tolerate Aricept or Razadyne. Switching to Exelon improved their thinking, and care providers felt less burdened. However, this was an uncontrolled study, so participants' hopes may have influenced ratings.

- A study comparing Aricept and Exelon found that Aricept caused less nausea, though the two drugs were about equally effective.

- A study of Exelon in people with MCI found it did not delay dementia.

- Exelon is the first ChEI shown to improve thinking and functioning in people with Parkinson's dementia. It has received FDA approval for this.

- Exelon is also the first ChEI found effective for improving thinking, memory, behavior, and attention in people with Lewy Body Dementia. It is not yet FDA approved for this purpose.

The Bottom Line: To date, no independent studies have compared Aricept, Exelon, and Razadyne to one another. But all three drugs have been compared two at a time. All three ChEI drugs appear to be equally effective, but people seem to find Aricept the easiest to use. Aricept also has been studied the most, is the only ChEI approved for severe Alzheimer's, and is covered most fully in most insurance plans. It's worth asking why your doctor chose a

HITTING THE RIGHT DOSE

Doctors have discovered that nausea and vomiting occur if the ChEI drugs are increased too quickly. So now we start patients at a low dose, increase it gradually, and recommend taking the medications with a meal. That way fewer patients stop the medications before hitting an effective dose. Both extended Razadyne and the Exelon patch were developed to reduce nausea.

particular drug, as the reasons may include the stage of the disease, insurance coverage, risks of side effects in light of a specific medical history, as well as the doctor's own comfort level with the various drugs.

Huperzine A: Herbal ChEI?

Huperizine is an herbal ChEI currently undergoing testing. (For more details, see Chapter 16.) We do not yet recommend it routinely because Aricept, Exelon, and Razadyne are better studied. If you are on a prescription ChEI, do not combine it with Huperzine A unless your doctor has recommended it.

Namenda (memantine)

Namenda is the second most widely prescribed of the four major Alzheimer's drugs and was available for about twenty years in Europe before it came to the United States in 2003.

Namenda has been studied widely in many kinds of patients. Millions of people worldwide have taken it for a variety of conditions, including various dementias. It has also been studied in Parkinson's disease, neuropathic pain, depression, HIV, and glaucoma.

Chemically speaking, Namenda is in a class of its own. It gets its name from a glutamate nerve receptor, NMDA (N-methyl-D-aspartate), that Namenda blocks. Glutamate is a brain neurotransmitter that is critical in helping us form long-term memories. However, surges of excess glutamate acting via the NMDA receptor may contribute to the risk factors for many brain diseases, including strokes and Alzheimer's. Namenda is thought to serve as a surge protector, shutting down the excess glutamate action but allowing normal memory formation.

Pluses: Namenda has a good safety track record and is usually well tolerated. It was the first drug approved for moderate to severe Alzheimer's. In studies, people given Namenda and Aricept did better than people given Aricept alone. For this reason and because it has a unique mechanism of action, doctors frequently use it in combination with all of the ChEIs.

Common Side Effects: It may sometimes cause dizziness or confusion if it's given too quickly at too high a dose. Less commonly, it causes constipation, fatigue, pain, headache, or sleepiness. Side effects tend to be mild.

Caution: Namenda should not be combined with a Parkinson's drug called amantadine, or with Ketamine or dextromethorphan, as they are similar drugs and combining them can be toxic. Moreover, it shouldn't usually be used in people with seizures. If you have epilepsy, alert your doctor.

Who Is Namenda Best For? People with moderate or severe Alzheimer's.

Best Dosage: Start at 5 milligrams a day for seven days, then increase to 5 milligrams twice a day. After another seven days, raise the dose by another 5 milligrams, and seven days after that, by another 5 milligrams until you reach the optimal dose of 10 milligrams twice a day. Namenda comes in a "starter pack" that makes it easy to follow these dosing steps. If a person develops side effects, doctors will increase the dose more slowly or keep it at 5 milligrams twice a day. In one study of severe Alzheimer's and vascular dementia patients, 10 milligrams a day was effective.

Latest Studies of Namenda

- People tolerate a combination of Namenda and Exelon or Razadyne well.

- Studies of Namenda's effects on people with mild Alzheimer's weren't consistent enough to receive FDA approval for this group. Two studies were negative, one was positive, and the results of these studies combined showed that the drug had only a small benefit. However, the drug was safe, and no new risks emerged from these studies.

- A group of experts recently recommended Namenda to treat mild Alzheimer's if the disease is progressing rapidly or the patient can't tolerate ChEIs. Many clinicians are already using this drug for people in the mild stages, usually along with a ChEI.

- Animal studies show that Namenda blocks plaque accumulation and toxicity, although this has not been proved in humans. Researchers are now testing this possibility in people using brain scans.

- Although Namenda is now given twice a day, a study found that it is well tolerated when given once a day.
- An analysis of several clinical studies suggests that Namenda may ward off certain behavioral problems such as agitation.
- Namenda may help thinking processes in people with vascular dementia, two studies find. But many doctors disagree and it is not FDA approved for people with vascular dementia.

A CONTRARIAN VIEW FROM THE UNITED KINGDOM

Not everyone agrees that drugs approved for Alzheimer's should be widely used. In 2004, a regulatory arm of the United Kingdom's National Health Service—the National Institute of Clinical Excellence, or NICE—provoked controversy when it issued a statement saying it was withdrawing Aricept, Exelon, and Razadyne from the British formulary (the list of drugs that the public health system will pay for). Why? Lack of effectiveness. (To read the full review, go to www.nice.org.uk.)

NICE based its recommendations in part on an independent study of Aricept done in the United Kingdom, called the AD2000 trial. Researchers treated 565 people with mild to moderate Alzheimer's with Aricept or a placebo, and followed them for up to three years. While Aricept users were doing better at the second year on measures of thinking and memory, by year three, the two groups were faring about the same in their ability to function on a daily basis.

Critics point out that the study enrolled fewer subjects than originally planned and the medication was temporarily interrupted during the study. Thus, stopping the medicine may have led to a loss of benefits. So it's unknown whether a bigger study would have produced different results.

Several organizations, including drug companies and the independently run Alzheimer Society, protested the removal of the drugs. NICE then relaxed its original statement, saying it

(continued)

would allow the three drugs for people with moderate Alzheimer's but not those in the mild stage. NICE felt that the effects for mild-stage patients were simply too small to justify payment by the government. The Alzheimer Society criticized the decision as "blatant cost-cutting." NICE said Namenda can be used only in clinical studies.

Other groups of physicians weighed in on the controversy. The British Association for Psychopharmacology supported the use of the drugs by saying, "There is ample evidence that there are effective treatments for people with dementia, and Alzheimer's disease in particular. Patients, their caregivers, and clinicians deserve to be optimistic in a field which often attracts therapeutic nihilism."

► FREQUENTLY ASKED QUESTIONS ABOUT MEDICATIONS

Q: How long should I stay on ChEIs or Namenda?

A: There is still debate over this. Doctors cannot precisely determine how someone would have fared if he or she never went on the drug. So the decision tends to be subjective, based on the drug's benefits and side effects for each individual. However, try a medication for at least six months, the length of FDA trials showing a drug's effectiveness and safety. See your doctor at least twice during those six months for a quick progess inspection.

If you are declining rapidly on a drug before the six months are up, the doctor needs to reassess the situation and perhaps stop the drug, switch to another drug, or add a second drug. If you are doing well, the doctor will probably want you to continue it. Many of our patients have taken these drugs for five years or more.

Studies also show that you will lose the benefits of ChEIs if they are withdrawn for three to six weeks. Restarting them may not get you back to the same level as prior to stopping the drug.

Q: When should the drugs be stopped?

A: This is a difficult issue without a clear answer. Certainly when a person is having serious or intolerable side effects, the drug should be stopped. The question then is, should one of the other drugs be started?

Many experts feel that treatment with a ChEI or Namenda should continue long-term even when there is evidence the person is deteriorating. That's because withdrawing these drugs often leads to a worsening of the condition. Other doctors feel that the drugs are not cost-effective, should be used for the shortest period of time, and should be stopped as early as six weeks if there's no dramatic evidence a person is improving. So the average length of treatment with Alzheimer's drugs is still only about five or six months.

Q: Should ChEIs be used to prevent Alzheimer's?

A: None of the ChEIs is recommended for prevention, and long-term studies with all three ChEIs have been disappointing. Because Razadyne was linked to more deaths (see the section on Razadyne for details), it is our least favorite choice for treating MCI. However, some doctors use Aricept to treat MCI. As noted before, Aricept appeared to improve some mental abilities in MCI patients and reduce the risk for developing dementia in people with MCI who have the ApoE4 gene that increases their risk for Alzheimer's.

Q: Do you recommend combination therapy?

A: It's unlikely that any single drug could correct all of the conditions that contribute to Alzheimer's. Hence, combination therapies may soon become the norm in Alzheimer's, much as they are in cancer, HIV, and high blood pressure.

Already we are using combinations, such as Aricept and, as the disease progresses, Namenda. A survey indicated that nearly 60 percent of physicians would use a combination of therapies (such as Aricept and Namenda) to treat their family members with Alzheimer's. A 2006 report recommended that a combination of ChEIs and Namenda is the best practice for people with moderate Alzheimer's.

Q: What about alternative therapies, such as ginkgo biloba, that are reported to show as good a success rate as ChEI?

A: A small study suggested that ginkgo may be as effective as Aricept, but study results have been too mixed on the effects of their being taken together. No alternative therapy has been as rigorously studied as any ChEI for mild Alzheimer's. However, studies have shown that ginkgo may be useful for people who have both Alzheimer's and vascular disease. (See Chapter 16 for more details on alternative treatments.) But we may learn more soon: A report of a large trial of the effectiveness of ginkgo at preventing Alzheimer's is scheduled for release in 2009.

Q. Is it okay to take two ChEIs at once?

A: Not usually, since it may double the chances of serious side effects and no study has shown added benefits of this type of combination. Some aggressive doctors do combine two of these drugs because they found it helped certain patients. If you are on two ChEIs, make sure you call your doctor right away to confirm that this wasn't a mistake and to talk about side effects.

Q: Can Namenda be used by itself, or must it always be used in combination?

A: Namenda can be used by itself. It is effective on its own for moderate to severe AD. Your doctor needs to make this determination. Also, check whether your insurance coverage will pay for two drugs for your disease stage.

Q: Should a person with moderate Alzheimer's start with Namenda or a ChEI?

A: People in the moderate stage of Alzheimer's can start with either a ChEI or Namenda or their combination because all of these drugs are indicated for this stage. But people in the mild stage generally are started on a ChEI.

Q: Can Namenda be used for mild Alzheimer's?

A: The FDA has not approved Namenda for mild Alzheimer's because its positive benefits for this stage of the disease haven't been consistent. However, doctors can choose to use it off-label as long as they counsel patients on their reasons and the possible risks. Many doctors use it this way for people who cannot tolerate ChEIs or if the disease is progressing rapidly despite ChEI use; in some cases it does help.

Q: Can you start someone on Namenda and a ChEI at the same time?

A: There is a lot of debate among researchers about this issue. Proponents of starting two drugs at once argue that doing so may produce bigger benefits early on. More cautious doctors start one drug at a time to lower the risk for side effects and because it will be harder to tell which drug is causing what if there is a side effect. To get the right answer, we'd need a study comparing these two strategies. Regardless of whether the drugs are started one at a time or at the same time, many people with Alzheimer's end up taking a combination of the two drugs.

Q: Can a ChEI be safely added if a person is already taking Namenda?

A: Yes.

Q: Are ChEIs better than Namenda?

A: There are no studies comparing Namenda with Aricept, so we don't know.

Q: What should I do if I develop confusion while taking Namenda?

A: Consult with your doctor about a smaller dose or taking a short break from it. Also ask your doctor to check on whether the confusion might be the result of some other cause, such as natural worsening of the disease or urinary infection.

Q: Can everyone tolerate these medications?

A: Most people can if they are dosed correctly. We listed the side effects under each drug in a previous section. People usually need to stop taking ChEIs before surgery that requires general anesthesia, but ask your doctor about what you should do.

► PAYING FOR THE PRESCRIPTIONS

Everyone these days must consider, and often worry about, the high cost of medications. However, most private prescription drug benefit programs cover the cost of one or more Alzheimer's drugs, usually with a co-pay. Without insurance, they cost about $150 a month, and most doctors can give free samples of the newer Alzheimer's drugs, such as Razadyne ER or Namenda. For anyone age sixty-five or older, Medicare pays for prescription medications if you have purchased a supplemental-payment plan called the Prescription Drug Plan, or PDP. Check the following Web sites for details.

- Medicare offers assistance to consumers at www.medicare.gov and by phone, 1-800-MEDICARE.

- More online help is available through the Medicare Rights Center, a national nonprofit consumer group, which provides tools at www.medicarerights.org. Counselors also answer questions for consumers who call its toll-free hotline, 1-800-333-4114, ext. 1. If you are denied coverage, call its appeals hotline (1-888-466-9050). All are free services.

- Good sources of information on finding help with the costs of prescription medications in general include benefitscheck-upRX.org and Senior Health Insurance Information Program (SHIIP), www.shiip.state.ia.us/. Some states, such as North Carolina, also have prescription assistance programs.

PDPs have a three-tiered structure where the co-pay is lowest for Tier 1 (generic drugs); higher for Tier 2 (preferred-brand drugs); and highest for Tier 3 (nonpreferred-brand drugs). The drug plans determine which drug is preferred or nonpreferred, based on evidence of the drug's success and other business considerations. Hydergine, which most experts no longer recommend, is Tier 1 in many plans since it is generic. At least one ChEI is Tier 2 in most plans, as is Namenda.

The co-pays on PDPs range from $0 to $22 per month for generic drugs and $15 to $100 per month for brand-name drugs.

Preauthorization

Some PDPs require preauthorization, meaning that doctors or patients have to call the insurance company to get approval for the drug before they use it, or the insurance company may not pay its share of the costs. In addition, the doctor also must document what stage of the disease the patient is in, using the MMSE.

If the patient is younger than sixty-five and doesn't have insurance coverage, medication can get pricey. Aricept, Exelon, Razadyne, and Namenda cost about $150 to $200 per month. The only generic (read: cheaper) option for Alzheimer's, Hydergine, is less well studied than the four brand-name drugs and we don't usually recommend it. So question your doctor if he or she prescribes it instead of the others.

How to Get Free Alzheimer's Drugs

Although some doctors have chosen not to, your doctor may be able to provide a week's to several months' supply of free samples. All of the brand-name drugs are also available at much lower costs in other countries, so if you or a relative is planning a trip to Canada, it might be worth looking into. But be aware that drugs in other countries may carry different names, so check with your doctor before making the purchase. As discusssed in Chapter 9, research studies may also offer free samples of already-approved drugs and monitor your relative while he or she is taking them.

In addition, all drug manufacturers have patient-assistance programs that allow you to get free drugs if you qualify, and you should feel quite comfortable asking the doctor about them. Patients have received free drugs for years through these programs. The companies don't always have strict standards for deciding who qualifies for free drugs, but if wealthy people take advantage of this, they may deprive people in need.

> Judy, a seventy-two-year-old grandmother, was mixing up the names of her friends, repeating herself, and having trouble finding words. Not surprisingly, she was also becoming withdrawn. Her husband, Paul, was afraid to leave her by herself for extended periods.
>
> Paul took her to the doctor, who diagnosed her as being in the

early stage of Alzheimer's. He started her on 5 milligrams a day of Aricept, which she took at supper. After six weeks, the doctor increased her dose to 10 milligrams, the optimal dose for most people. Fortunately, the drug had no bothersome side effects.

Three months after her diagnosis, Paul realized that Judy was slightly more social and eager to go out, including to church, and she wasn't repeating herself as often. She said she was finding it easier to talk on the phone to friends. Memory testing showed that her overall mental abilities had improved by about 15 percent.

Over the next year, Judy continued on Aricept, and her memory stayed about the same—but it didn't get worse, which it would have without treatment. Her only side effects were occasional vivid dreams. But Aricept isn't a cure. Over the next two years her memory got worse, she became frustrated and agitated more easily, and she took longer to do simple tasks, such as dressing herself or getting ready to go to an appointment. She also became confused when she and Paul took a trip to the beach; she kept asking where they were. Also, her appetite was plummeting. Her illness was progressing to the moderate stage, although somewhat slower than it might have without treatment.

Paul asked the doctor if they could stop the Aricept because he was worried about Judy's eating. But when she stopped the medication she seemed to get more confused, so they put her back on and the doctor added a second drug, Namenda. She took 5 milligrams of Namenda each morning, and eventually 5 milligrams at supper also. It made her feel a little dizzy for a few days, enough of a side effect that the doctor decided not to increase the dose. He also recommended a nutrional drink once a day. It worked: Paul said that she handled her daily activities more easily, got going more quickly, and was less frustrated. After three more months Judy's memory test scores seemed stable, and she seemed less frustrated and agitated.

Nothing stays the same in the land of Alzheimer's. Six months later Paul said Judy's memory and behavior had slipped again, noting that she was mixing up her grandchildren. She also was more afraid of being alone, more confused in new surroundings, and less able to help with chores. Her doctor increased Judy's dose of Namenda to 10 milligrams twice a day, which Judy tolerated well except for two days of constipation. The dose increase seemed to slow (not stop) her decline. With this drug regimen, she was able to live at home with Paul for three more years and manage most of her dressing and bathing on her own.

CHAPTER NINE

CLINICAL TRIALS: CAN YOU (SAFELY) GET TOMORROW'S TREATMENTS TODAY?

If we knew what we were doing, it would not be called research, would it?

—ALBERT EINSTEIN

You have probably seen an ad like this in a newspaper or heard it on the radio:

ALZHEIMER'S RESEARCH DRUG TRIAL NOW RECRUITING!

Are you 55 to 90 years of age and interested in MEMORY LOSS DISORDERS? You or your family member may be eligible for participation in an investigational drug study for

(continued)

Alzheimer's disease. Qualified participants will receive free medical evaluations and tests, free MRI scan, and free experimental medication or a placebo. Qualified participants will also receive up to $300 for their time and travel expenses. For more information, call the Memory Research Institute at (800) xxx-xxxx.

This is an invitation to join a clinical drug trial. Similar advertisements appear in newspapers throughout the country seeking volunteers for clinical trials of experimental drugs. Should you sign up?

Consider these statistics: The average time from an Alzheimer's diagnosis to death is about eight years. The average drug takes from eight to twenty years to reach the market. So a valuable drug could be invented when, say, a man in his late sixties is first diagnosed and not become available until his Alzheimer's is no longer treatable. The only exception would be if he took part in a clinical trial—or a research study—in which he received the drug.

In this chapter, we'll help you decide if you might want to enter a clinical trial and how to use trials to your advantage. We start with some important questions to ask about any clinical trial that you are considering participating in. The more yes answers you receive to the questions, the more patient-friendly the trial is likely to be.

- Is it a Phase 3 or 4 study? (What this means is explained below.)
- May I take FDA-approved Alzheimer's treatments while participating in the trial?
- Will you avoid invasive procedures and take less than 20 milligrams of blood per visit?
- Does the trial pay for my time and travel costs?
- Are all the procedures free?
- Will I be able to learn about the treatment I was on within a few months after the end of the study?
- Does the consent form describe all of the drug's side effects?

- Do I have a choice to get into an "open label" drug trial after this study ends? (Open label simply means that all participants get the drug and not a placebo.)
- Does the trial follow participants for a few months after the study ends?
- Will the trial report all of my test results to my personal doctor?

▶ CLINICAL TRIALS 101

Clinical trials are studies designed to assess the safety and effectiveness of potential medical treatments or diagnostic tools when they are used on people. Some clinical trials compare a new treatment with the best existing treatment or with a placebo (sugar pill); others test new diagnostic tools against existing ones. Some clinical trials also study possible measures to prevent memory loss in people with mild forgetfulness or in family members of people with Alzheimer's.

Generally, either pharmaceutical companies or the federal government sponsors the trials. Private or university clinics run them.

Clinical trials give us hope for improving our understanding of Alzheimer's and discovering potential new treatments. They also offer you or your family member free, often high-quality medical care and monitoring, as well as access to nurses, doctors, or social workers who specialize in Alzheimer's to answer your questions and provide emotional support.

Each year, thousands of people sign up for Alzheimer's clinical trials, including savvy medical consumers such as doctors and nurses who are in varying stages of the disease or are interested in preventing it. You can get into a trial whether you are already diagnosed with the disease or still need to be evaluated.

But the other side of this shiny coin is the reality that most experimental treatments fail, so your chance of actually getting early access to the next breakthrough drug for Alzheimer's is as small as it is for any other serious disease, such as cancer. Also, all clinical trials pose potential risks to participants.

► WHAT ARE THEY STUDYING?

Dozens of clinical trials are devoted to Alzheimer's. Of these, most are pursuing treatments that rely on medications. A couple dozen are testing nondrug strategies to help ease the symptoms of Alzheimer's, including short-term memory lapses, difficulty finding words, disorientation, and personality changes. Scientists are also looking into treatments that may help protect healthy people at high risk of developing Alzheimer's. Researchers are investigating exercise, diet, herbs, memory training, lifestyle changes, yoga, music therapy, and more. Future trials will also test combinations of drug and nondrug strategies.

In addition, scientists are comparing the value of new and existing tests for diagnosing Alzheimer's, including new memory assessments, blood and urine tests, and brain scans. (Studies examining the biology of the disease, and how the disease affects family and society, are research studies rather than clinical trials.)

Most clinical trials take place at private clinics that run such trials for pharmaceutical companies. Some of these clinics' sole function is to run trials, but most also see regular patients. University research clinics also conduct trials for both drug companies and government agencies. A large university clinic is likely to run ten to fifty research studies each year.

► WHAT'S IN IT FOR YOU?

If you enroll in a clinical drug trial, you are usually agreeing to take either a placebo that looks and tastes similar to the real pill but has no active ingredients, or a drug that has undergone little or no human testing. Does that make you a (a) two-legged guinea pig, (b) do-gooder, or (c) well-informed patient?

It's all of the above, but let's take a closer look at the pros and cons. Many, but not all, trials provide

- Free diagnostic tests and memory monitoring
- Free medical care unrelated to the Alzheimer's tests and treatment, including more tests than patients get in routine annual physicals

- Payment for participants' travel costs or time
- Access to caring, supportive Alzheimer's experts, including specialists who would be hard to see outside of a trial
- Access to a doctor who may have particular expertise in your area of concern, such as sleep problems or depression

When Ed, an older man in the early stage of Alzheimer's, was beginning to worry about his memory, he read in the newspaper about a drug trial for mild cognitive impairment. Since most internists don't know much about mild cognitive impairment, Ed decided that a university hospital might be the place to go for some expertise. He found it gratifying to talk to people who were interested in the problem. To most doctors, he said, "I fall into the category of old guy complaining."

Some people join clinical trials partly to double-check their diagnosis with an Alzheimer's expert. The husband of a trial participant explains: "The main reason we thought she should join the trial was to see if her doctor's diagnosis and treatment plan were correct and to see what else could be done for her."

▶ **Good to Know:** Many of the nation's top Alzheimer's experts run clinical trials and maintain a separate appointment book with short waiting times for study participants.

The support and advice that care providers receive when their family member joins a clinical trial varies from study to study but can make a big difference in a person's life. As one wife explains, "His Alzheimer's disease progressed despite being on the study medication, so I don't know if the drug helped him or not. But I know that having him in the study helped me! The support I got from the staff means so much—they really care and they also know what's going on with you. When I had questions, I always had someone to answer them."

Is everyone's experience so good? No. It depends on the trial staff and on the efforts of the care provider.

Clinical trials can involve lengthy testing and unanticipated risks or delays. But in many research clinics you are also pampered and appreciated, particularly compared to what you might be used to at a regular, busy doctor's office.

A Dose of Hope

Trials give participants and their family members hope, which in the incurable-disease business is quite a commodity. Available Alzheimer's medications can only stall or limit symptoms, so participating in a trial that just might lead to a cure now or in the future can be rewarding. As one participant explained, "I look forward to my visits to the university, because they are doing objective scientific measurements, and if there is any help for my particular problem, it would be in a place like that."

Last but (we hope) not least: Being in a trial makes people feel good about doing good. Clinic staff say that even people who have fairly advanced Alzheimer's still know that they are a parent or grandparent, and they understand that they are helping their loved ones. In the quest for an Alzheimer's cure, the key players are the study participants—no study participants, no research. No research, no treatments. Laboratory animals do their part, but then it's up to us humans. Clinical trials are vital, even when they produce negative results or advance our understanding of Alzheimer's only slightly. Many small steps may add up to a cure, or at least better treatment options for future generations.

How do you measure success as a clinical-trial participant? You can't use "cured!" as the gauge, since we just aren't that close to finding the magic potion. But if participants and their families feel supported and hopeful, and if they receive an expert second opinion, high-quality information about their disease, and some symptom relief, that's success. The thousands of families who took part in the trials that resulted in the four Alzheimer's medications on the market today enjoyed early access to what is now accepted treatment. That's success.

Still, while we have four successful drugs, several dozen others have been tested without positive results over the past ten years, including some that had serious side effects. The many families that took part in these trials were not so lucky. The key to maximizing your luck is to talk regularly to the doctor about updates on the test results of not only your drug but of others being developed.

▶ **Consider:** Study participants may choose to quit their current study if emerging results are discouraging and join one that

appears more promising. You must wait at least one month between experimental drug trials and in some cases longer, depending on the drug. However, most patients stay with a trial once
they've joined.

▶ PROS AND CONS

"You don't join a trial just because you have a free afternoon," explained one participant with early-stage Alzheimer's. "I did it because I have a real need and was willing to put up with the
downsides of participating."

Exactly. People join trials because they are willing to accept
some risk to get better medical care, to find a reason to feel optimistic, or maybe just to get the good feeling that comes from helping others. But how do you know if the benefits outweigh the risks?
For Alzheimer's trials this is a particularly important question,
since the likelihood of a trial proving hugely beneficial to a participant (as in curing or halting memory loss) is very small.

Why You Might Want to Take Part in a Clinical Trial

- Not participating means missing out on the chance to take a
  promising drug.
- If no one participated, researchers couldn't develop new
  drugs.
- Doctors who run Alzheimer's trials don't work alone. Ethics
  committees oversee the trials, government offices will inter-
  vene if problems arise, and the clinic staff and participants
  can report wrongdoing directly to the FDA if necessary.
- Many drugs in clinical trials are already used for other conditions and are being tested for a secondary use.

*"At first I was a bit uneasy about my husband joining a trial because
I thought that he needed help and I didn't want him to be taking sugar
water. But then I thought, It's a trial, so he has a fifty–fifty chance of*

getting the drug and maybe he'll get on the drug once he's completed the study."

                                               —The wife of a participant

---

Why You Might Not Want to Participate

- Inconvenience. Trials last from a few months to a few years and may require that you take hours off from work or other activities. They involve testing, including less-than-pleasant ones such as blood tests and MRI scans, and frequent memory testing. The appointments can be tedious and tiring.

- Family members and participants may resent having to answer personal questions.

- Participants in a Phase 2 or 3 trial usually have a chance of getting the placebo.

- Side effects can be worrisome. Common side effects of medications in general include having a metallic taste, feeling dizzy, fluctuating heart rate or blood pressure, diarrhea, constipation, or a rash. Study participants have died or suffered serious complications such as liver injury, cardiac arrest, brain swelling, strokes, stomach bleeding, and allergic reactions from drugs used in Alzheimer's clinical trials.

A highly touted trial of a vaccine that cleared plaque from the brains of mice with Alzheimer's illustrates what can go wrong with an experimental treatment. When no major side effects showed up in preliminary human trials, the vaccine manufacturer tested it on people with Alzheimer's in a larger trial. The vaccine appeared so promising that practically every noted Alzheimer's doctor wanted to be an investigator in the trial. But, tragically, about 6 percent of people injected with the vaccine developed a serious swelling of membranes covering the brain. At least one person died and the trial was halted. The lessons learned from this study led the company to develop other, hopefully safer versions of the vaccine, which are now undergoing clinical trials.

While such seriously negative outcomes are rare, they remind us:

- Animal studies can't tell us everything. For example, mice don't complain of headaches that may signal brain swelling.

- The more promising the drug, the bigger the pressure to test it quickly in people with Alzheimer's.

- Drugs need to be widely tested before they can be declared safe. Some side effects may not emerge until thousands of people take the drug.

- Quickly halting a trial after initial reports of serious side effects can save lives, so it is essential that independent safety experts monitor trials.

Since drugs can linger in your body for weeks, sometimes side effects may emerge days or weeks after you stop the trial. But most trials don't schedule any follow-up visits after the trial ends, so it is up to you to report any new side effects. Some trial doctors may not ask you to report the side effects, but you should.

When the trial ends, always ask if you were getting the drug or sugar pill. Unfortunately, it can take months or years for a company to release this information. However, if the drug comes to market, you will want to know if you have already tried it and how you reacted to it. Further, by staying in touch with your trial doctor, you will be able to get timely updates on any new findings related to the drug you were exposed to.

A Personal Choice

In the end it comes down to your preferences and those of your loved ones. Some people participate in two to three trials; others have never been in a trial and never will be.

> *"My wife works full time and she cannot help me participate in studies that involve too much time. Also, unless I was sure of what I was getting and that it was efficacious, I don't think I'd be interested. Plus, I really don't want to go through those stressful memory tests multiple times."*
> *—A man in his sixties who has mild Alzheimer's*

We often hear both positive and negative reactions to trials, and clearly, clinical trials aren't for everyone. All patients should have access to a trial and the right to make an informed choice for themselves about whether they wish to participate. If you are leery but curious, talk to other families who have participated in trials. You may decide to avoid all trials, or you may decide to join a low-risk, low-stress trial, such as a study that requires that you take only a brief survey.

► HOW CLINICAL TRIALS WORK

How do you find a good trial and get the most from it? Learning the ins and outs of these studies will help.

The first item for consideration is the "phase" of the trial. Just as you'd check the depth of a pool before diving in, it's vital to know the phase of the trial before signing up. Phase 1 is the most preliminary and most risky, and Phase 4 is the least.

Phase 1 trials are the first set of human trials that researchers do on a product, drug, or diagnostic test. In most cases, drugs are tested in humans only after being tested on animals. We may not look alike, but humans and rodents have a lot in common on the inside. The goal of most Phase 1 Alzheimer's trials is to determine whether or not the product is safe enough to warrant continued study. Researchers are looking primarily for information on:

- The most frequently occurring or acute side effects
- How the body metabolizes the drug
- The safest doses to give

Compared to other trials, Phase 1 trials offer the greatest risks and inconveniences, as well as the greatest monetary rewards. Some Phase 1 participants receive thousands of dollars in compensation if, for example, they have to stay at a hospital or undergo invasive procedures.

Most Phase 1 trials enroll only between twenty to eighty participants. Those who sign up at the end of the enrollment period can take comfort in knowing that others have taken the drug or undergone the procedure before them. Before signing up, you can always ask the clinic staff how many people are already enrolled. While you're at it, ask how many other Phase 1 trials the researchers have done. You may want to avoid a Phase 1 trial that is headed by a novice.

Most trials you will come across are in Phase 2, 3, or 4. The safety inspection continues in Phase 2, but on a larger group of one hundred to one thousand participants. Researchers are now asking another important question: Will the product work? Regarding safety, if you join a Phase 2 trial at its beginning, the only people who will have tried the drug or undergone the procedure are the Phase 1 participants. If you join toward the end, more people will have tried it. Researchers use what they learned in a Phase 1 trial to make a Phase 2 trial safer.

Phase 3 Alzheimer's trials usually enroll between three hundred and one thousand participants. Researchers use what they learn in Phase 1 and 2 trials to make Phase 3 trials safer. The Phase 3 trials are designed to reveal short-term (six- to twelve-month) effects of the product, seal the case concerning its effectiveness and safety, and maximize the chances of FDA approval. In the United States, new Alzheimer's drugs are not required to show advantages over competing products already on the market, so most Phase 3 trials do not compare newer drugs with older ones.

Companies sponsor Phase 4 trials to get information that will make the drug more marketable, such as showing that it is more convenient to take or better tolerated than the competition. Phase 4 trials are your best bet in terms of safety and the possible efficacy of the product being tested, but they are more difficult to find in academic centers since most of these are done in private centers.

PREVENTION TRIALS

Sadly, we have not progressed very far in prevention research. Why?

- The drugs used must have an extremely strong safety record.
- The studies take three to seven years to complete.
- The studies require one thousand to five thousand participants and can cost millions of dollars. In terms of Alzheimer's, researchers don't know exactly when the disease first shows up in the brain, so we can't know when to begin prevention strategies. Plus, the onset and progression of the disease vary considerably among individuals.

► TURNING THE TABLE: INTERVIEW THE DOCTOR

To figure out if you feel comfortable participating or having your family member participate in a trial, ask the research coordinator or the doctor the following questions. Then discuss your plans with your personal physician.

Q: How do the possible risks, side effects, and benefits of the treatment being studied compare with my current treatment?

A: About one in five studies does not allow you to take or start the four FDA-approved medications to treat Alzheimer's (Aricept, Exelon, Razadyne, Namenda). So if the new drug isn't necessarily more promising than what you or your family member are already taking or could get from your regular doctor, you may choose to skip the trial.

Q: Will I have to change my daily routine?

A: The requirements of some clinical trials could indeed affect your day-to-day routines. Consider

- the number of clinic visits you may have to make
- the length of those visits
- annoying side effects, such as dry mouth, diarrhea, or dizziness, that would require you to plan your days a little differently

That said, most Phase 3 drug trials require no more than one to two days per month of your time.

Q: Will I be reimbursed for expenses?

A: Your gas and parking costs will most likely be paid. Most studies will pay for an overnight hotel stay if you drive from a long distance. You probably won't be compensated for missed workdays, but there's no harm in asking.

Q: How long will the trial last?

A: Phase 1 trials may last just a few days or weeks. Others can last several months to a few years.

Q: What is the purpose of the study?

A: Get a clear explanation of the study's primary goal, whether it's a treatment, prevention, or diagnostic trial, and of course what phase it is in.

Q: Has the product been tested before, including for conditions other than Alzheimer's?

A: "No" means that study participants have a greater chance of running into unexpected risks, as well as unknown benefits. "Yes" means that the product is not a complete unknown.

Q: The million-dollar question: What is the likelihood the drug will actually help and how?

A: Almost by definition, experimental drugs do not come with guarantees. If this is a Phase 2 trial, the clinic staff will not be able to answer this question. But if it is a Phase 3, the staff should clearly explain the results of prior studies.

Q: Once I start taking the drug, how will I know if it's working?

A: You can ask the trial staff to summarize the results of memory or other test scores over time, and ask family members if they see any changes.

Q: Who oversees participants' care during the trial?

A: A licensed doctor oversees drug studies. Studies that look at treatments other than drugs (such as exercise or music therapy) usually don't involve medical doctors. No detailed standards exist for who can conduct a trial, and experience and qualifications vary widely. So make sure that key staff members, including the research nurse, the social worker, and the doctor, are skilled at helping people with Alzheimer's. They will be asking participants (you or your family member) to go along with procedures that may be uncomfortable or novel, such as lengthy memory testing, multiple blood draws, shining a light in your eye, or even a spinal tap.

Q: What tests and experimental treatments are involved?

A: At the beginning and end of most drug trials, participants undergo a physical exam, including blood and urine tests and heart monitoring, as well as paper-and-pencil memory tests that last one to three hours. Most drug studies also require a brain scan as part of the diagnostic workup. Some studies also require spinal taps or genetic testing. If the study you are considering is a Phase 1 trial, ask if you will be hospitalized, whether you will undergo any invasive procedures, such as having a catheter inserted for blood draws, and how your safety will be monitored.

Q: Will I receive long-term follow-up care or monitoring after the study ends?

A: Not usually, as participants are expected to go back to their regular doctors for care. However, the clinic staff needs to know about any side effects that participants experience during the thirty days after the trial has ended.

▶ FINDING THE TRIAL YOU WANT

Outsourcing has hit the world of clinical trials: The goal of many drug companies is to have 30 to 40 percent of their Alzheimer's study participants residing in lower-cost places such as India, South Africa, and Eastern Europe. Unless you have the travel bug or locate a uniquely promising trial, apply only to trials near you and base your selection on the drug or device being tested and its potential benefits and risks to you.

About fifty centers nationwide are part of the Alzheimer's Disease Cooperative Study network. Some of these sites are at universities, some at private hospitals, and others at private clinics. These sites run a variety of trials of drugs and diagnostic tests. Go to http:// adcs.ucsd.edu for more information. Subsets of these sites, with the highest federal research funding ranking, are called Alzheimer Disease Centers. You can find a listing of such centers in the Resources section of this book or at www.nia.nih.gov/Alzheimers/ResearchInformation/ResearchCenters/#statelist.

You can also:

- Contact the local chapter of the Alzheimer's Association, as they maintain lists of local sites and ongoing trials.

- Ask your doctor for a recommendation of a trial that you or your family member might join.
- Call the Alzheimer's clinic at your local university to see if they are running or know of any trials.
- Look for advertisements of clinical trials in your local newspaper or the paper of a nearby city.
- Check out these databases of clinical trials:
  - www.centerwatch.com/
  - http://clinicaltrials.gov/
  - www.nia.nih.gov/Alzheimers/ResearchInformation/ClinicalTrials/

If you have a choice between a trial run by a university and one run by a private clinic, consider that university clinics are overseen by their own ethics committees and may offer slightly more safeguards, but they usually take much longer to make key decisions. Also, universities cannot match the convenience and compensation offered by private research clinics. Many of the doctors running private clinics are also highly respected researchers. If you live in a midsized to big city, it's not a bad idea to visit one or two different Alzheimer's research clinics and then make your choice.

► **Note:** Any clinic can call itself an Alzheimer's research center, so look into its affiliations.

Many families learn about Alzheimer's trials through advertisements or from other families. Few learn about them from their own doctor, even if that doctor has a colleague who is running a trial. Why? The doctor probably just didn't think of suggesting a trial, or he fears having other doctors second-guess his assessment of a patient or being blamed if something goes wrong during the trial. But once you ask your doctor for advice on finding a trial, he may be happy to help, including reviewing a list you have compiled of local psychiatrists, neurologists, or geriatricians who are running trials.

▶ WHAT THOSE ADS REALLY MEAN

Here's an example of an advertisement for a clinical trial, with our explanation of how to read between the lines. [Our comments are in brackets.]

Alzheimer's Drug Trial Now Recruiting!

Are you fifty-five to ninety years of age [researchers may be willing to let people join who are slightly older or younger than the designated age] and interested in MEMORY LOSS DISORDERS?

You or your family member may be eligible [only about one in five callers ends up being eligible for most trials] for participation in an investigational ["investigational" or "research" means that the FDA has not yet approved the drug] drug study of mild to moderate [determined by your score on a brief test] Alzheimer's disease if you

- Have been diagnosed with or are experiencing symptoms [meaning you don't need a formal diagnosis to inquire about the study] of Alzheimer's disease

- Have a care provider or family member who can accompany you to clinic visits [the researchers will most likely ask the care provider a lot of questions about the participant throughout the study]

You may continue taking Aricept (donepezil), Exelon (rivastigmine), Razadyne (galantamine), or Namenda (memantine). [But study participants must be on their medication for about three months before enrolling, so the researchers know the drug's effects. Some studies require participants to stop taking certain medications.]

Qualified participants will receive free, study-related assessments [applicants can get the results of their screening exams, even if they are found ineligible for the study], including

- MRI brain scans

- psychiatric evaluations and laboratory tests

Qualified participants will also receive free experimental medication or a placebo. [Find out the drug name or chemical number so you can ask your doctor about it or look it up on the Internet. Also ask about the odds of getting the drug versus the placebo, how many participants the study has enrolled, and how participants at other study sites have fared.]

For more information, call Sally Martin at Memory Research Institute, (800) xxx-xxxx. [Call the clinic only when you have time to talk, in case the study coordinator wants to interview you right then to see if you or your family member qualifies for the study. Ask for a copy of the informed consent form at this first interview.]

▶ HOW TO GET ACCEPTED INTO THE TRIAL YOU WANT

Unfortunately, it's sometimes a leap between finding a trial that's right for you and getting in. Trials really need study participants, but their specific requirements rule out a lot of applicants. These requirements are intended to exclude people who

- may be at significant risk for side effects
- have certain conditions, such as poor hearing, that may confuse the interpretation of the study results

A coordinator of an Alzheimer's clinical trial might have to talk to ten people to get three candidates to come for a screening interview, and of those only two may qualify.

▶ **Good to Know:** Most centers have ongoing Alzheimer's trials, so if you don't qualify for one trial, ask the staff about other ones. Sometimes the clinic staff will try to steer you to a trial that has attracted few participants, but you can always decline and ask about others.

One of the key criteria for entry in a study is the applicant's score on a very simple test of cognitive impairment called the MMSE. Ask your doctor for your, or your family member's, score. Most trials enroll participants who score in the mild to moderate range on this widely used test. Scoring in the 26–30 range and having MCI usually qualifies a person for a prevention trial. The zero–10 range qualifies a person for a study of severe Alzheimer's. Scores can fluctuate by two or three points, so many trials allow applicants to retake the test.

The following is a generic list of inclusion and exclusion criteria that apply to many (not all) drug trials for people with mild to moderate Alzheimer's. You must meet *all* the criteria on the inclusion list. Having just *one* of the conditions on the exclusion list can disqualify you.

Inclusion List: What You Need to Get into Most Trials

- A formal diagnosis of Alzheimer's, such as a brain scan taken in the last six months that suggests Alzheimer's
- A low score on a measure of vascular dementia
- Be able to take part in all aspects of the trial
- If you are taking any medications, you must have been on them for at least one month and, for Alzheimer's medications, at least three months
- A care provider with whom you have almost daily contact and who will participate in the study with you
- An IQ in the normal or above range
- No hearing or eyesight problems that would interfere with test performance
- Be between fifty and eighty-five years old

What May Exclude You from a Trial

- Having donated blood in the previous hundred days
- Suffering from a major physical or mental illness, including anemia or clogged arteries
- Having a history of strokes, seizures, certain cancers; having had a recent heart attack or infection; alcohol or drug dependence
- Taking Parkinson's medications
- Taking certain drugs to improve cognition, other than cholinesterase inhibitors and memantine (Namenda)
- Starting or stopping certain medications within the last couple of months, including psychiatric medications, herbal medications, sleeping aids, sedating anti-allergy medications, and large doses of certain vitamins

How to Improve Your Odds

- Bring a formal diagnosis of Alzheimer's to the first visit to the clinic, as well as the results of a recent physical.

- Inquire about a study only after being stable on all medications (including those for Alzheimer's, thyroid, and heart disease) for two to three months, so that the clinic will be better able to distinguish the effects of the test drug from those of normal medications.

- Correct any health problems before the interview. Treat thyroid problems, vitamin deficiencies, or mental health issues, for example, before inquiring about a trial.

- Correct any hearing and vision problems, since being impaired in either area may resemble cognitive impairment.

- Find out what the trial requires regarding care providers, and then make sure that person is available for your visits. The care provider must answer a lot of questions about how the participant is doing.

- Be sure to have already lined up a trusted family member to serve as legal representative or durable or medical power of attorney. This is usually the spouse or child (if the spouse is not alive).

- Have all contact information in order. Line up transportation for getting to the clinic for regular appointments. If you are concerned about the expense of getting to the clinic, ask about reimbursement even if it isn't routinely offered.

LEGAL REPRESENTATIVE

People with Alzheimer's may not have the capacity to make health-care decisions for themselves. Hence, most trials will not permit even a mild-stage Alzheimer's patient to sign up for a trial unless a spouse or next of kin (acting as a legal representative) also consents on his or her behalf.

► GETTING INFORMED BEFORE GIVING CONSENT

Before enrolling in a study, you will be asked to sign an Informed Consent Form (ICF). This eight- to ten-page document outlines all of the procedures you are agreeing to, the science behind those procedures, and most of the known risks and benefits of participating.

Given its length and technical information, the document can seem daunting. Here are a few hints:

- Give yourself at least half an hour to read the document before signing it or, better yet, ask that the form be sent to you before going to the clinic for your first appointment, so you have time to read it thoroughly.

- Mark anything you don't understand, so you can ask the staff about it.

- Don't sign it until you understand.

- If you are uncomfortable with a particular test or activity (spinal tap and genetic testing come to mind) that would prevent you from participating in the trial, ask if you can skip it. You won't always get a yes, but it's worth asking.

- *Check out the fully annotated sample of an ICF in Appendix B.*

Over the course of the trial, you will sign at least five to six versions of the form. The staff revises the forms when new information becomes available about the drug, when the study sponsor decides the study or the form needs tweaking, or for a host of other reasons. Ask why it was revised. Before you sign a new version, the staff should show you how it differs from the old one. Keep each version, so you have a record of what has happened over the course of the trial.

Signing the ICF does not bind you to stay in the study; you may change your mind and quit anytime.

► STICKING WITH THE TRIAL

People drop out of clinical trials all the time for a variety of reasons: They don't feel they are getting better, participating becomes inconvenient because of changes in their life, they don't like the doctors, or they are experiencing bothersome side effects.

The dropout rate for most Alzheimer's trials is 15 to 20 percent over six months, and 30 to 50 percent over a year. So we've prepared tips for finding happiness in a clinical trial. Family members, if you have a relative in a clinical trial, be his or her advocate.

- Tell the clinic staff before you take any new medication, including over-the-counter pills, drops, and supplements. A new medication could alter the test results, interact poorly with the study drug, or prove dangerous when used with the procedure being tested.

- Keep your personal doctor in the loop. Both during and after the trial he or she will continue to handle your routine care as well as any emergencies.

- Don't expect the nurses to tell the doctor all your concerns; tell the doctor yourself.

- Tell the doctor any and all side effects you are experiencing, even if you aren't sure they result from the trial drug or procedure.

- If you are the care provider, you may need to encourage your quiet relative to voice any problems or concerns to the doctor.

- If you know you will have to miss an appointment, tell the clinic as far in advance as possible. The staff should accommodate you by giving you extra medications and a new appointment time.

- If you have a medical emergency, the doctor running the trial must notify the doctors handling the emergency whether you are taking a placebo or the drug.

- If a procedure or test is really bothersome, the staff may be able to let you skip it.

- If you are experiencing medical, financial, or emotional problems, don't suffer in silence. Talk to the staff.

▶ GETTING RESULTS

After going through a trial, participants or their family members want to know if the drug or diagnostic procedure being tested actually worked. Did the drug improve cognition? Did the diagnostic tool tell the doctors anything useful about the participants' condition?

Unfortunately, it's not always easy to find out the answers, but here is some advice on how to get that information.

If it's a so-called double-blind trial, which all Phase 2 and Phase 3 Alzheimer's drug trials are, even the investigators don't know which participants are taking the drug until all of the data are in and analyzed. If the trial is taking place at multiple centers, none of the doctors running the trial know the full results until the trial is over.

When a drug or procedure has a positive effect—meaning it helps—trial results are reported rapidly at scientific meetings or in press releases. In some cases, negative results may take much longer to become public. After you complete the trial, every month or so call the doctor who ran the study you participated in to see if the results are available. The doctor is your best source.

Finally, as the trial is coming to an end, enlist the clinic staff to help you plan your transition if you plan to go back to your regular doctor. The clinic staff can write a summary of what happened in the study, including test results. Don't wait for the staff to offer these benefits to you—ask about them yourself.

Keeping a Good Thing Going

Some of the benefits of being in a study may continue after the trial is officially over. In about 50 percent of Phase 2 and Phase 3 trials, participants have the option of joining an open-label trial, which enables them to continue receiving the research drug for free. In some cases, participants may get a few months of free samples from the clinic if the study drug is already on the market.

▶ **Good to Know:** If you like the doctor overseeing the trial, you can ask to continue as a patient in his or her regular practice.

► WHAT FRAUD LOOKS LIKE IN A CLINICAL TRIAL

As with any enterprise, clinical trials have their share of unethical individuals. The fraud can take a variety of forms, including but not limited to

- using consent forms that minimize side effects and hype the promise of the drug or procedure
- deviating substantially from what is in the consent form
- using verbal instead of written informed consent
- reporting fudged test results or diagnoses to enroll more people
- not having licensed doctors on site
- offering large inducements to join or stay in a trial
- asking the participants to pay for research procedures

If you suspect fraud, always call the Institutional Review Board (IRB) overseeing the trial. A telephone number for IRB staff should be listed in the materials that you receive when you join the trial. If it's not, ask for it.

► THE FUNDERS AND THE WATCHDOGS

Curious about who is funding trials and who is looking over the researchers' shoulders? You've come to the right place.

The federal government is the biggest backer of Alzheimer's research studies, including human studies. Not surprisingly, the other big backers of Alzheimer's clinical drug trials are the pharmaceutical and biotechnology companies that produce most of the products being tested. Companies generally pay private clinics or universities directly to run trials.

However, companies take a very hands-on approach to the trials, as they have huge investments in them. The company's interest in a trial benefits patients because it may prevent the rogue or simply naive researcher from taking an action that harms the study or its participants. At the same time, most company-funded trials are designed to maximize the drug's chances of gaining government approval. Their priority is not necessarily to answer key public-health questions. Keep in mind that companies own the data that come out of the study and analyze the data themselves, although the FDA audits the data before they allow the drug to be sold. (Anyone can analyze the data from government-supported research.)

All trials must have some sort of oversight board. You should look for trials that have a data safety monitoring board (DSMB). Made up of doctors and other professionals, DSMBs analyze safety information on individual participants and may stop the trial if necessary. However, members of DSMBs, and other oversight boards, must rely on the researchers or companies to give them accurate data.

▶ LEARN THE LINGO

Be prepared for your screening interview and check out this vocabulary list of words that doctors and clinic staff might use, or that might appear in the informed consent document.

The Overseers

Food and Drug Administration (FDA). The federal agency required to protect human health by regulating drugs, biological products, medical devices, the nation's food supply, and cosmetics.

Good Clinical Practices (GCP). International guidelines of how clinical trials are to be conducted. All study doctors and staff members are required to follow GCP guidelines, which are published at www.fda.gov/cder/guidance/959fnl.pdf.

Institutional Review Board (IRB) or *Ethics Committee (EC).* The group of doctors, statisticians, researchers, community advocates, and others who together monitor a clinical trial. They make sure it adheres to FDA regulations and protects the rights of participants.

The Trials

Double-blind trial. A study that compares two or more drugs, but neither the researchers nor the participants know which drug the individual participants are taking during the study. This level of secrecy reduces researcher bias when interpreting the results. The staff breaks the seal if a study participant has a medical emergency and when the study is completed.

Randomized trial. A study in which participants are randomly assigned to receive either the treatment drug or a placebo. The goal of randomization is to minimize the impact of differences in age, gender, and disease severity between the treatment and placebo groups.

Who's Who

Principal investigator (PI). The lead researcher or doctor on a study. He or she is responsible for all aspects of the study, although a team of doctors, researchers, and support staff help the PI run the trial.

Subject or participant. The person who has volunteered to participate in the clinical trial.

Sponsor. The company, government agency, or private group that is covering the expenses of the trial.

The Forms

Inclusion or exclusion criteria. The criteria an individual must meet to be either included in or excluded from a trial.

Informed consent form (ICF). A document participants or their legal representative must sign that outlines how the study works, its goals, and its risks and benefits to participants. See Appendix B for a sample ICF, along with a full explanation of what it means.

CHAPTER TEN

HOW WILL WE TREAT ALZHEIMER'S IN THE FUTURE?

There is no medicine like hope, no incentive so great, and no tonic so powerful as the expectation of something better tomorrow.
—ORISON MARDEN, INSPIRATIONAL SPEAKER (1850–1924)

In Chapter 9 you learned about clinical trials: the pros and cons of participation, what to expect if you do participate, and how to make the most of a clinical trial. Here we'll walk through a number of actual drug treatments under study. Be aware that while some of these drugs and other strategies hold particular promise, none is proved (hence the term "experimental treatment"), and a medication that looked like a panacea one day could turn into a real problem pill the next.

▶ STARTING OUT

Before scientists test any treatment on people, they run safety tests on mice, and often these mice are genetically modified to include human Alzheimer's genes—so-called transgenic mice. When the mice mature, their brains begin to form human Alzheimer's amyloid plaques and tangles, the hallmarks of Alzheimer's. Then researchers can directly see the effects of drugs on the disease, although mice are clearly not perfect models for people.

Scientists can never be completely sure when the theories that guide their research may be faulty. For example, scientists believe that amyloid plaques are toxic to the brain, and that removing these plaques would help correct the symptoms of the disease. Based on animal research, they've been testing a number of strategies aimed at minimizing or destroying the plaque. But what if plaques are actually protecting the body from some other underlying problem? If that were true, removing them might actually worsen symptoms. So for better and sometimes worse, the best we can do is to keep testing and revising treatments based on new information until we reach a point where the right insights and treatments come together.

Scientists are developing more than sixty new drugs for Alzheimer's, including standard medications in use for other conditions, vaccines, and hormones. They are also testing an array of other treatments such as surgeries, meditation, and herbal treatments. Here is a look at some of the strategies.

▶ DRUGS (AND PROCEDURES) THAT TARGET ALZHEIMER'S

Alzhemed

Made from a form of natural amino acid, Alzhemed appears to block substances in the brain that help to create plaques. Small studies have shown that Alzhemed is safe, so scientists launched larger and more definitive trials here and in Europe to see if the good findings hold up. The first large U.S. trial failed to confirm its cognitive benefits, and its manufacturer terminated its second trial. Surprisingly, they decided to instead sell this over the counter as a nutraceutical.

Don't rush out and buy amino acids over the counter. There is no definitive evidence that they work, and until there is, save your money for an exercise class or a curry dinner (more on that in Chapter 16).

Ampakines

A class of drugs that may enhance people's attention span and memory, ampakines do their work via the brain chemical glutamate, known to assist people in forming long-term memories. So far results have not been too encouraging: In one large study of people with MCI, one ampakine had little impact on memory. A second study of another ampakine was halted for safety reasons. Nevertheless, researchers are continuing to investigate their potential usefulness.

Anti-inflammatories

Many diseases are marked by inflammation, and Alzheimer's is no exception. Researchers are looking into whether anti-inflammatory medications could reduce this inflammation, which appears to occur in brain cells, and thereby improve Alzheimer's symptoms. Trials have looked at a variety of medications, none of which proved useful so far, including ibuprofen. In the past, some animal studies have suggested that NSAIDs also appear to directly block the formation of amyloid plaques. (NSAIDs are aspirin substitutes, such as ibuprofen and Aleve.)

► **Caution!** Don't take NSAIDs to treat or prevent Alzheimer's.

Unfortunately, so far research has found that many of these medications appear to do more harm than good. Prednisone, for instance, seems to worsen mood problems in people with Alzheimer's, while Vioxx appears to increase the risk of strokes and the chance that people will develop dementia more quickly.

Based on these data, investigators are examining whether insulin taken via nasal spray could help to prevent or treat Alzheimer's. Since the nasal passage is connected to the brain, inhaled insulin goes directly to the brain's memory centers without having a big impact on blood sugar levels. Hence, scientists believe it may be safe even for people without diabetes.

Researchers looked at whether the diabetes drug Avandia (rosiglitazone), which makes the body more responsive to insulin, could help. In one large study, Avandia did not improve symptoms, but researchers are testing it further. The fate of this drug emerging as a treatment for Alzheimer's is in doubt given concerns over its heart risks. They're also testing the diabetes drugs Actos (pioglitazone) and Glucophage (metformin).

Dimebon

Researchers were recently very excited to discover that Dimebon, an old Russian allergy medication, operates like a blend of Aricept and Namenda, FDA-approved drugs for Alzheimer's. It may also have other mechanisms that could help Alzheimer's. In a Russian clinical trial, Dimebon substantially improved memory and day-to-day functioning in people with Alzheimer's, and the benefits seemed to last for at least one year. It was also well tolerated except for mild increases in depression. Researchers are now testing the drug in a much larger trial. If the results are positive, Dimebon could soon become widely available.

Dopamine Enhancers

Rasagiline (Azilect), a drug approved by the FDA to treat Parkinson's disease, is now being tried in people with Alzheimer's. It sustains and increases levels of dopamine in the brain, a neurotransmitter in short supply in some people with the disease.

Enzyme Inhibitors

Enzyme inhibitor drugs block the action of either gamma- or beta-secretase, two enzymes needed for plaque formation in the brain.

However, because these enzymes are also involved in other needed functions, scientists are treading carefully by conducting sufficient safety studies before they launch larger trials on people.

FK962

The drug FK962 works by encouraging the release of the brain chemical somatostatin into an area of the brain involved in learning and memory. Scientists studying it are hoping it benefits people with Alzheimer's.

Flurizan

Flurizan (Tarenflurbil) is a new drug that's a component of an old anti-inflammatory drug called flurbiprofen. Scientists discovered that flurbiprofen contains two parts: one that reduces inflammation and the other that blocks plaque formation. So they reasoned that if they created a drug that eliminated flurbiprofen's anti-inflammatory properties while retaining its plaque-fighting ability, they could side-step the potential ill effects of anti-inflammatories while creating a drug that tackles a main disease component of Alzheimer's.

In one recent study of this drug in people with mild- and moderate-stage Alzheimer's, the group as a whole did not benefit much on average. But a subgroup of patients with mild Alzheimer's did improve, both in memory and thinking. Researchers are conducting another study with mild-stage Alzheimer's patients to see if they experience the same gains.

Gene Therapy

You'd think that with all the talk about genes, gene therapy might be curing Alzheimer's *and* world hunger. But gene therapy is not far along in any field. Scientists are proceeding carefully to make sure they do not expose people to unnecessary risks.

The only gene therapy trial currently under way for Alzheimer's is with NGFs. Researchers are injecting a gene for NGF directly into the brain. At first, participants experienced bleeding into the brain, so the researchers redesigned the study to eliminate this risk and are continuing the study. The recent death of a participant in a trial of a gene therapy for arthritis has led to the suspension of most gene therapy trials across the country.

Metal-Removing Meds (Chelation Therapy)

So-called chelator drugs may remove the metals, including iron, copper, and zinc, in the brain that plaque binds to. The technique has been used for years to treat lead poisoning. Note that aluminum does *not* seem to be a culprit in Alzheimer's, as was previously suspected.

Nerve Growth Factors (NGFs)

Alzheimer's causes networks of nerve cells to break down more rapidly than in people without the disease. Scientists are therefore testing nerve growth factors that fertilize the brain. The hope is that NGFs will help the brain establish new connections between nerve cells and repair or trim old ones.

One drug that mimics the effects of an NGF, cerebrolysin, passes from the bloodstream into the brain. In a small pilot test, people with mild to moderate Alzheimer's who took it did better on tests of memory and thinking than people who received the placebo. In a larger follow-up study, those taking cerebrolysin improved too, but only in overall functioning. What's more, the effects lasted for two months after the most recent infusion. Researchers expect more results from this promising treatment soon.

▶ **Good to Know:** Some fun and pleasant ways to increase NGFs in your brain without drugs include getting more exercise, reducing your stress load, learning new things, and socializing. See Chapter 17 for information in these areas and more.

Neramexane (Glutamate Receptor Blocker)

Similar in makeup to the FDA-approved Alzheimer's drug Namenda, neramexane protects the brain against harmful surges in the neurotransmitter glutamate. It may also keep the brain from forming plaques. However, initial studies were somewhat disappointing.

ONO-2506 (Cereact, Proglia)

ONO-2506 is a chemical cousin of an old drug called valproic acid that is being developed to treat stroke, Alzheimer's, and Parkinson's disease. Researchers think it may stimulate NGFs and other brain chemicals to protect the brain, but because valproic acid itself doesn't improve memory in Alzheimer's, it remains to be seen if this version will help.

Stem Cells

These multitalented cells are found in the fetus, bone, and umbilical cord. Doctors hope that if they put them into brain areas attacked by Alzheimer's, they will grow into normal brain cells and replace lost ones. At present there are no stem-cell trials for Alzheimer's under way in the United States, though they are taking place in other countries.

Tumor Necrosis Factor (TNF) Alpha-Blocking Drugs (Enbrel and Remicade)

Tumor necrosis factor, or TNF, is a natural chemical that modifies the body's inflammatory response. Scientists have begun testing two drugs that block the effect of this chemical in hopes they will modify the brain's inflammatory response in people with Alzheimer's. One of these, Enbrel (etanercept), is currently used to treat arthritis; the other, Remicade (infliximab), is now used to treat Crohn's disease. The drugs work via different pathways: Enbrel is an antibody that binds to TNF and deactivates it, whereas Remicade blocks a receptor for TNF.

So far, results look quite good. In one small study where researchers put Enbrel into the spinal fluid of people with Alzheimer's, their memory and thinking improved dramatically. Some participants' communication and daily abilities improved as well. Unfortunately, one person died. It's too early to tell how safe and effective this drug will be for people with Alzheimer's. Investigators are now conducting larger clinical trials to test the drug in greater numbers of people.

Xaliproden

As with the drug cerebrolysin discussed above, xaliproden mimics the actions of NGFs. It was initially studied without success in Lou Gehrig's disease, a condition, like Alzheimer's, that involves progressive brain damage. Scientists tested it in people with Alzheimer's in hopes of better results, though results again were disappointing. The development of this drug will likely be stopped.

► GETTING A SHOT OF PROTECTION

Imagine going to the doctor's and getting an injection that would keep you from getting Alzheimer's. Well, scientists love the simplicity of that idea too. To this end, they have been developing several types of vaccines intended to break up or even prevent the formation of plaques and, more recently, tangles too.

They are working on two basic types of vaccines. One, an "active vaccine," is made from material taken directly from plaques or tangles. Theoretically, the body will mount an immune response to the material, and from there, it is tricked into mounting a response against existing or new plaques or tangles in the brain. So far, researchers have tested an active anti-plaque vaccine successfully in mice but, sad to say, unsuccessfully in humans.

Active vaccines for tangles in humans have yet to be tested. But some researchers believe that anti-tangle vaccines may be more promising than anti-plaque vaccines. Compared with plaques, tangles appear to be more directly linked to memory decline.

The other type of vaccine is called a "passive vaccine." It uses antibodies to plaques and tangles rather than the actual plaque or tangle material itself. Researchers are testing several forms of these vaccines to fend off plaques, and the final results aren't in yet. In addition, they're about to launch trials of passive vaccines against tangles.

For several reasons, researchers think passive vaccines may be a more promising approach than active vaccines. Passive vaccines don't force the body to react to a foreign entity as active vaccines do, so they may have fewer side effects. Moreover, passive vaccines already have been successfully used to treat other diseases, including cancer and arthritis. Also, passive vaccines might benefit people who cannot mount an immune response to active vaccines.

But passive vaccines could turn out to have their own risks as well. Some people taking antibodies have developed rare infections or fatal brain diseases, while some mice receiving passive anti-plaque vaccines developed bleeding in the brain. Researchers therefore plan to use brain MRI scans to monitor people. One such drug, Bapineuzumab, is completing a Phase 2 trial. Another, called IgG, or gammaglobulins, is also in Phase 2 testing.

▶ HELPFUL HORMONES

Hormones—those wonder chemicals that put a spring in our step— take a real nosedive as we age and take some youthful feelings and functions with them. So scientists are testing whether hormone therapy might help the brain function better, for longer.

Evista (raloxifene)

Low estrogen levels may cause brain changes and memory lapses, so scientists are testing estrogen-based drugs to see if they help women with Alzheimer's. The estrogen drug Premarin actually increased women's risk for memory problems, but Evista works differently in the brain. (Evista targets only one type of estrogen receptor, whereas Premarin acts on multiple receptors.) But don't get your hopes up: So far, Evista, now used to treat osteoporosis and to help prevent breast cancer, has not been shown to improve memory in older people with or without Alzheimer's.

Leuprolide

This naturally occurring hormone influences the release of testosterone and estrogen in the body. Again, researchers hope it might reverse the effects on the brain of age-related declines in hormone levels.

RU486

RU486, a drug that blocks the effects of reproductive hormones and cortisol, may also minimize the effects of stress on the brain, doctors hope. You may have heard of this drug in a much different context: It is commonly known as "the French abortion pill."

Testosterone

Guys, forget hair gel—think testosterone gel. Researchers are investigating whether a gel that contains the male hormone testosterone might help memory function in men with Alzheimer's. Testosterone levels decrease with age, and replacing it improves mood and quality of life in older men who have low levels of the hormone. However, so far testosterone injections have not improved memory and cognition in people with Alzheimer's.

▶ SURGERY, DEVICES, AND OTHER INVASIVE PROCEDURES

Scientists are testing a number of surgical approaches in their quest to treat Alzheimer's. Some might belong in a science-fiction novel, but so does a bad day with Alzheimer's.

Brain Chips

We don't think Dr. "Bones" McCoy used this on the *Starship Enterprise*, but he might have. Scientists are developing chip implants that they hope could stimulate the brain's memory centers and serve as backup memory storage sites. Researchers have already placed such chips in the spinal cords of people with spinal cord injuries, giving them limited ability to move certain muscles.

In the case of Alzheimer's and the brain, the memory centers are much more complex than the primitive nerve-muscle junction being tested in spinal cord patients. So it will probably be years before doctors use this technique in people with Alzheimer's.

Deep Brain Stimulation

Here, doctors drill a hole in the skull and implant an electrode that stimulates areas deep inside the brain. It may sound like a scene from *The Manchurian Candidate*, but this is nonfiction: The technique has been used successfully to treat Parkinson's and other conditions, and doctors plan to try it in Alzheimer's patients too.

Transcranial Magnetic Stimulation

You could say this technique used to treat depression has a certain magnetic charm. Doctors deliver a magnetic pulse to the front of the brain via a small handheld magnet to stimulate the cells in specific brain regions. Some studies have indicated that daily exposure over several weeks can lift depression in people without Alzheimer's, but it hasn't yet met the level of proof required by the FDA. Researchers are now testing whether the device might help Alzheimer's patients.

Vagus Nerve Stimulation (VNS)

VNS is a rather unusual procedure, where a surgeon wraps a wire around a nerve in the patient's neck and implants a stimulator under the patient's chest wall. It might help people with Alzheimer's, because VNS stimulates the release of a key memory chemical, acetylcholine. There are problems, though: The procedure can cause serious side effects, including surgical complications such as infections. While VNS is already used to treat depression and epilepsy, most experts in this country are skeptical about its value for Alzheimer's, so it is not likely ever to be used widely here.

► ALZHEIMER'S PREVENTION: FAR AWAY
BUT NOT IN NEVERLAND

No drug at the moment can prevent Alzheimer's. Therefore, your wisest course of action is to focus on maintaining a healthy lifestyle and reducing your risk factors, all discussed in detail in Chapters 16 and 17. So far, researchers have completed only about ten drug-based prevention trials, many of them using the same experimental medications being tested for treating Alzheimer's.

This sneak peek at the future should give you an idea of the wide range of treatments researchers are studying in the hopes of curing this difficult disease. If all goes well, one or more may end up solving the puzzle that is Alzheimer's disease.

PART THREE

► **YES, THERE *IS* LIFE AFTER DIAGNOSIS**

CHAPTER ELEVEN

HEADING TOWARD A NEW NORMAL: LIVING WELL WITH EARLY-STAGE ALZHEIMER'S

Now I am perhaps one of the few men who will ask for directions.
—A MAN WITH A SENSE OF HUMOR *AND* EARLY-STAGE ALZHEIMER'S

To help you learn how to make the most of those days, to help you retain and enjoy the many abilities and passions that define you and your family, this chapter is for you, the person with early Alzheimer's (and we've also snuck in a few sections for family members). A diagnosis of early Alzheimer's explains all the changes in thinking, mood, and performance that you or your family has been noticing and that, perhaps, have been frustrating and frightening you all. But you can be assured that you walked out of the doctor's office as the same person who went in—just with a better understanding of what's going on.

Your diagnosis will require you and your family or friends or colleagues—you're not alone if you ask for help—to adapt to the changes that you undergo. The trick is staying flexible and blame free. In this way, you will find that your life is now about adapting to a chronic condition, creating a new "normal." You will also find that other people with Alzheimer's and their families, as well as support groups and organizations, are available to help.

Your goal is to tailor your response to the changes you notice in your memory, thinking, and ability to do things. If you find yourself a little fuzzy on how to do a task that was once routine or your spouse accuses you of misplacing something, you will feel frustrated. That's normal. But what can also become normal is shrugging off the small stuff, laughing at your mistakes, asking for a little extra room to mess up, and accepting change.

▶ REDEFINING SUCCESS

Success is finding the tasks and hobbies that you can still do and finding new ones to enjoy. One crossword puzzle fiend found that the jumbles puzzle in the newspaper was more his speed now. Fortunately, his housekeeper who was learning English also liked doing them, so they joined forces during a coffee break on the days she came to clean. She had never taken a coffee break at work; he had never sat and chatted with her. But they both laughed when he repeated back Spanish words to her in his terrible accent, and no one expected him to remember the words when she returned the following week.

When it comes to Alzheimer's, success is retaining your values, your purpose in life, your sense of self. If you are lucky, your sense of humor will continue to find expression in your new life. If you are really lucky, you will enjoy camaraderie, coffee breaks, and new pleasures. Remember, there's a good reason we talk about "a person with Alzheimer's" and not an Alzheimer's patient.

As with any new undertaking or change you face in your life, fears and questions will probably come up as you adjust to living with Alzheimer's. You may wonder:

- When, how, and what should I tell others?
- Can I or my family afford this illness?
- What if we have to move?

Bigger questions may pop up as well:

- What next?
- What am I supposed to do now?
- What does memory loss feel like?
- How can I stay "me," make the best decisions for me and for those close to me?

Fortunately, we (and others) will help you answer many of these keep-you-up-at-night questions. As we help you slim down your fears, we'll beef up your appreciation for the many wonderful moments that still lie ahead. Good things and joy can happen to those who have Alzheimer's.

Are we living in fantasyland? Nope. We know that any disease that gets worse over time requires people to face uncertainty, grieve, and adapt to new losses. We know that the embarrassment caused by a "senior moment" differs greatly from the frustration and fear caused by the confusion and memory whiteouts of Alzheimer's. It's just that we have strategies, and you will find others on your own, for navigating these ups and downs. For example, you will discover ways to "outsource" your calendar to someone who can remember to look at it better than you can. You will also outsource jobs that involve complex multitasking like balancing the checkbook, certain household repairs, and complex meals or tasks at work. But what you will retain is your sense of being connected to what you enjoy and love: friends, family, the opera, a warm shower, playing with your dogs. We strongly urge you to

- find ways to increase your time doing what you enjoy
- focus more on what's really important
- learn to let go of the small stuff
- try something you never considered fun, whether it's drawing, dancing, sculpting, gardening, or walking. You may surprise yourself—and your family.

▶ THE EARLIER, THE BETTER

Before we talk more about what to do after the diagnosis, let's back up and talk about the diagnosis for a minute. Until the last decade, mild cognitive impairment or early-stage Alzheimer's was not on professionals' radar and went undistinguished from normal aging. Now advances in early detection and diagnosis have created a demand for programs developed specifically for people in the early stage. Being able to take advantage of those services is a real bonus of an early diagnosis.

An early diagnosis doesn't help if you don't believe it or understand it and don't go looking for help. Alzheimer's makes imagining anything beyond the moment very difficult. Some people just can't accept that they have changed. They may feel that trying harder to remember things or to think clearly will help them "get over" this memory loss. If you have gone to a trustworthy doctor and sought out a second opinion, however, you are better off at least acting as if or assuming the diagnosis is correct. Remember, having Alzheimer's isn't your whole life. You're still a teacher, mother, brother, golfer—however you defined yourself before diagnosis.

Some people worry about embarrassing themselves, making mistakes, losing control, or upsetting their family. Family members fear being embarrassed by their relative, having to think for two, and having to manage both their new and old responsibilities. They may fear getting the disease themselves. Being part of a clinical trial or a support group can help you and your family deal with these concerns and put them behind you. One man with early-stage Alzheimer's was surprised by what he learned from his support group of people with early-stage memory disorders. "We have as many laughs and 'aha' moments as our wives do in their meeting next door."

▶ WHAT'S CHANGING?

Here's a brief introduction to common changes that occur in early-stage Alzheimer's. We briefly mention solutions where they are needed and available; more detailed solutions are described later in the chapter.

Personality Changes

I'm not myself. Some people with Alzheimer's describe losing their spark, their zest for life. Doctors call it apathy, indifference, loss of motivation. It can develop toward one specific activity and vary from person to person. Families notice a reluctance to start new projects or a lack of interest in previous pleasures. Sometimes, Alzheimer's reverses people's personalities. The even-tempered become irritable, the shy become uncharacteristically talkative with strangers, the laid-back worry more, the type A's lose their drive, or the family nurturer stops caring. One father who was always a bit tight with his money started buying his kids gifts.

TREAT THE BLUES

Depression is common in people with memory loss. Alzheimer's can impair the parts of the brain that produce mood-stabilizing chemicals. The apathy of Alzheimer's can mimic symptoms of depression. You will function better, feel better, and have more energy and a longer attention span if you get prompt and thorough treatment for depression and a doctor monitors it over time. Doctors can't cure Alzheimer's, but they can often treat the depression that accompanies it. (For information on medications, see Chapter 8.)

Going with the flow? Your family says you've become inflexible. Change or anything new (other than something on the scale of a new grandchild) is greeted with a sigh at best and, more likely, worry, nervousness, fear, or anxiety.

Solution: Gradually, you and your family will learn that keeping to a schedule and making your day predictable frees you up to relax and enjoy the little surprises as they come along.

On the other hand, some people with Alzheimer's loosen up, relinquish old worries, and trust those around them to navigate the changes with surprising ease.

Mr. Nice Guy? Along with irritability may come a gradual loss of tact, tolerance, and sensitivity to others' feelings. You may not realize how your personality has changed, or welcome comments about it from your family.

Solution: It's usually not a good idea to try to remind a person with Alzheimer's that he or she needs to be more polite. Instead, the goal again is to keep your day as predictable as possible so you are less agitated.

On the other hand, some people with early-stage Alzheimer's begin to appreciate their family and friends more. One man wrote a tribute to his wife and all "caregivers" in advance of the help he was likely to need from her and others.

Memory Blips

Memory storage is full, or at least difficult to access. Your brain seems unable to absorb new information or retrieve what just happened. Some people care, others don't seem to mind. For those who care: Keep reading.

Banana peels. Your family may notice changes in your eating habits or your weight. You may forget to eat or forget that you have just eaten. When one daughter found four fresh banana peels in the kitchen garbage, she accused her dad of being on a banana binge. He denied the charge, banana in hand.

Lesson: Your family needs to keep binge food out of sight.

Double-checking. You are spending a lot of time making sure you haven't made a mistake: checking your list, recipe, math, the lock, the stove.

Solution: Keep reading. This one is tricky.

Old-dog syndrome. You may feel like the old dog in the saying "You can't teach an old dog new tricks." It may seem that the new coffeepot your children gave you for your birthday or the microwave they bought to make your life "easier" doesn't work right or is out to get you, when actually you can't remember how to use it. Not only is it more frustrating to learn new skills, you don't feel up to familiar tasks.

Solution: Consider that you feel well and look the same, and you certainly are not ready for old-dog status. Plan to let the world adapt to you. Dig out the old coffeepot that your spouse so kindly saved. Give the new one to your young neighbor. If your children ask, blame it on the Alzheimer's!

The checkbook tells all. Money matters can become overwhelming, and bills may go unpaid or overpaid. Waiters may benefit from your uncharacteristic, and perhaps unintentional, generosity. At the grocery checkout, it may seem easier to ask the cashier to collect the correct change from your wallet.

Solution: Your adult daughter comes over every week to pay your bills with you, so you take her out to breakfast at your favorite restaurant. She can't believe what great service you get on a busy Sunday morning. But keep reading because getting your finances in order is very important for everyone, including people with early Alzheimer's.

Go slow, brain working. Even routine chores take longer, and any unexpected events become obstacles or distractions. It's easy to lose your place in what you are doing, but you may find something else worth pursuing at the moment. Rushing just discombobulates you even more. Your (nice) spouse asks, "What's the hurry, anyway?"

Thinking Malfunctions

Thingamajigs and whatshisnames. Besides misplacing your keys or cell phone, appointments and facts may go missing. As a result, you may talk less and use the wrong words or rely on favorite, though not always correct, words or phrases. Let people fill in the word for you—they are going to whether you want them to or not.

Attention deficits. You can't stay focused on one activity, conversation, or book like you used to. You get distracted or you easily lose your place. When it comes to the many multistep dances that life demands, from following recipes to shopping to completing a report at work (yes, some people with early Alzheimer's still work), you feel as if you just aren't performing up to your old standards. A wise minister learned to have his wife check to see that he hadn't left anything out of his sermons. He could be as inspirational in his delivery as ever, but a little checking in advance made both of them more comfortable.

"My brain is more like a flashlight than a lightbulb and it can shine on only one thing at a time," explained one man with early-onset Alzheimer's. His solution? He joined an informal support group for people with early-onset Alzheimer's. Together, the group played brain

games and took continuing education classes. "Keeping up with normal people is exhausting and it's easier and more relaxed to go with these folks." [For games, see www.aarpmagazine.org/games.]

"I'll have what she's having." Everyone occasionally decides to go with what a friend or spouse is ordering, but you may have trouble making decisions. Fortunately, one woman was always delighted by her daughter's choices at a restaurant. She enjoyed reminding the waitress "like mother, like daughter," and they would laugh as they routinely split a lunch entrée and a dessert. Making choices from too many selections isn't worth the aggravation. Your relatives may think you have become passive or uncaring, but really you're just worn out from trying to keep things straight all day.

Swiss cheese logic. Everyone has a lapse in reasoning, but now what seems logical to you may make less sense to others. Also, your planning and organizational skills may have taken a hit. It's hard when others question your reasoning. One businessman decided to delegate, telling his colleagues it was "their turn to take responsibility for financial decisions." He chuckled when they struggled to learn procedures he had done with ease.

Abstract ideas such as time may prove difficult to grasp or measure. ("Did she say she would be back in five minutes or five hours? Has it been five hours yet?") Meanwhile, odd notions are impossible to shake. You are sure, for example, that you must go to the bank, yet your wife says it's two A.M. and the bank is closed. Finding ways to control your anxiety is even more important now.

When did they move the grocery store? It's easy to get lost, even in familiar places, yet harder to reorient or find your way back. You may get tired, give up, and go home without ever finding the store. One woman came to the wise realization that the store will be there tomorrow, and it was probably time for her to accept her friend's offer of a ride.

What people with Alzheimer's do about midsentence brain freezes:

- "I don't volunteer for long speeches."
- "I keep quiet, turn the conversation over to someone else, or ask for a prompt."
- "I say, 'Alzheimer's at work,' so people know to fill in for me."

- "I've become good at just letting it go, saying, 'Oh, well.'"
- "Sometimes I swear a bit."
- "I lose whole ideas and just say, 'Well, that's one I missed.'"
- "I ramble on to another topic, sort of like jumping trains."

► HERE'S THE GOLD

Realizing that these changes are taking place, experiencing them, and being told they are Alzheimer's is scary, confusing, and unsettling. The good news is you don't need to just "deal with" all the changes. It may seem hard to believe, but you'll find a new normal. You are still able to enjoy feelings of well-being and belonging, pleasure and joy, just like everyone else. How? By making time for the satisfying, fun, and important activities that you continue to do well. You also need to avoid or spend less time on frustrating activities, which usually are those that involve handling money, planning, and organizing. The surprising rewards of living more in the moment are now open to you.

You may discover that you appreciate what you never appreciated before, like a leisurely lunch, the feeling of warm laundry coming out of the dryer, a political discussion, or a walk down memory lane with your children. Some people with Alzheimer's say they experience life more richly than they did in the past. Some feel less constrained by convention or rules, less bothered by life's "shoulds" or the little hassles that used to upset them.

> *"I don't have time for trivial things like anger—I'm so busy just trying to keep my act together."*
>
> *—A person with Alzheimer's*

► MAKE A LIST, CHECK IT A LOT

A tried-and-true method for keeping up your spirits during early-stage Alzheimer's is surprisingly simple. With help from someone you trust, make a list of events, pastimes, or routine tasks that you enjoy doing or find meaningful, and that you do well with and without a companion. To make this list, think about what you look forward to in a typical day or week. Close friends and family may remind you of other activities they notice you enjoy these days. Now ask yourself and your family, "How can I increase the amount of time I devote to these pleasant events and activities, and decrease the time and energy I devote to frustrating and unpleasant ones?" Be sure to include pleasant activities with your family or close friends on your list, as being social and connected will improve your mood and function. New research has demonstrated links between loneliness and Alzheimer's.

Pleasant activities may involve socializing, reminiscing, volunteer work, listening to music, visiting a museum, going to church, or even housekeeping. You may want to hire someone to mow the lawn, but you'll still do the raking, weeding, or planting, for example. If traveling is on your list of fun activities, plan to go, but adapt your travel plans to fit your new reality.

▶ **Good Advice:** Figure out and follow a predictable daily routine you enjoy. Limit the number of new situations that may confuse or upset you, but stay open to new things you may enjoy for the first time. Some people discover they love concerts in the park, strolls through a museum, or a game of checkers with the right person and at the right time.

You and those around you may be pleasantly surprised to find that you remember a lot from the past and still enjoy intellectual pursuits. After books began to feel too long to follow, one intellectual with Alzheimer's loved listening to taped lectures by university professors and having his children catch him up on the day's news during their phone calls.

▶ **Helpful Hint:** Try to minimize what you have to remember. Label your drawers with what goes where; use a timer to remind yourself when to turn off the stove or go to a meeting; ask your family or friends to call you so you don't have to remember to call them. This will free you up to enjoy the intellectual pursuits you've always enjoyed (or new ones!). People with Alzheimer's are able to learn new skills and information, even when they are in the moderate stages of the illness. If you enjoyed learning before, you probably still do.

TRAVELING WELL WITH ALZHEIMER'S

Being in a different place each night can be disorienting and tiring, so take shorter trips, stay in one place, and take longer breaks between sightseeing excursions or social events. Traveling with a friend or another couple offers many benefits, such as having a companion when you and your spouse would normally go your separate ways (even if that's just to the bathroom).

Pack lightly. Spare yourself the burden of feeling weighed down, mentally and physically, by stuff you may easily misplace. Keep your identification with you at all times. Wear a bracelet or necklace from the Alzheimer's Association's Safe Return program or MedicAlert. You can wear it inside your shirt, and you never have to take it off. Pack medications in pill organizers and take extra pills in case your trip is extended.

If a big trip is impossible, go for drives, explore your surroundings, check out the local sites. Have a picnic. If a disability prevents you from walking, have a tailgate party.

► YOUR RIGHTS

Are others making unrealistic demands on you? Are they excluding you from decision making and no longer treating you as the adult you are but instead as "the Alzheimer's patient"? If you feel this way, you need to let people know. You have the right to

- be informed
- be included in family and community life
- be treated appropriately as an adult
- have your feelings taken seriously
- have medical care that reflects your values
- have the security of a relatively predictable daily routine. (People with Alzheimer's cannot always respond well to sudden

changes or surprises. Buy yourself the T-shirt with the slogan
"Change is good—you do it!")

- be productive and useful
- have meaningful activities
- get outside regularly
- be touched and loved
- be with people who know your life story, values, and traditions
- be cared for by people who understand your condition and its effects on you and your family

► SOME ADVICE WON'T FIT YOU

No two people experience Alzheimer's in exactly the same way. The
disease affects everyone differently. Focus on what works for you
now, even if you need to change your approach later. There is no
"right way" to live with any chronic illness that changes over time.
Most people get Alzheimer's in late middle age or beyond, with a
lifetime of unique experiences under their belt. Those experiences
make you more unlike than like others with Alzheimer's. Find your
own new normal, taking into account your own, your family's, and
your community's strengths and limits.

► **Alzheimer's at Work:** It is not your fault when seemingly simple
tasks become harder.

► REDEFINING NORMAL

Living well with Alzheimer's requires changing expectations and
finding alternatives. If memorizing is a strain, but you have always
enjoyed learning, sit in or audit courses at a local college or community or senior center. Even if you can't remember much of what you
have heard, you will enjoy the intellectual stimulation, discussion,
and camaraderie.

You may have to give up a passion for motorcycles or plans to learn
a new instrument, but look for new delights, such as taking walks,

singing with a group, or participating in a volunteer activity. Maybe you once met your friends for competitive golf games, but now you hit balls at the driving range and enjoy lunch together afterward. One elderly woman gave up her aerobics class and switched to the slower-moving tai chi.

Focus on What's Left, Not What's Lost

Ask yourself what you're grateful for; your list won't come up empty. You may have more items on it than you did before you discovered you had Alzheimer's. You may have many good years before you have significant Alzheimer's-related disabilities. Many skills and abilities remain intact well into the course of the disease. Best of all, the capacity to experience joy and pleasure is particularly stalwart (unless you are suffering from untreated depression or anxiety). The good mood that a pleasant event, visit, or outing creates may outlast the memory of what you did. Fortunately, Alzheimer's disease progresses slowly, giving you time to adjust to it gradually.

FOR MORE GOOD ADVICE

Check out the Alzheimer's Association. Almost all of its chapters have educational and support programs specifically for people with early Alzheimer's or their families. Most of these programs are free.

The association, staffed by professionals knowledgeable about all memory disorders and capable of answering your questions, has an advice center at 1-800-272-3900. You can also go to www.alz.org and look for the section "For Persons with Alzheimer's or Dementia" for great tips and an e-mail forum. Friends who have relatives with Alzheimer's can provide great advice, but their opinions may be specific to their experience.

► **A Word to the Wise:** Trying harder will not necessarily work. Ask for help in the form of reminders, reassurance, or cues.

New Expectations for Your New Normal

During our adult years, we learn a lot about ourselves and don't expect what we learn to change. You may know, for example, that you are a talkative person who works well in chaos and has a temper. Another person sees himself as an introvert who has a great mind for details and loves sports. Alzheimer's will shake up these seemingly stable characteristics and make them less specific or certain.

A good way to ensure good days with Alzheimer's is to anticipate change. The early years are all about modifying, adapting, or at least monitoring expectations of what you can and like to do. The early years are also for planning for your future while tending the present: Tell your family what you need from them now and what you want for the future.

No one can predict what you will be able to do and how you should adjust your expectations. We can, however, provide guidelines for what to expect. Although Alzheimer's progresses slowly, sudden declines can and do occur, triggered sometimes by changes in your family, moves, travel, a hospitalization, or other illness. Brain changes can make you more sensitive, and events and illnesses will make you more confused, scared, or frustrated. You may become quieter and require more downtime.

Finding What Fits

Even though you need more help from others than you did before, you can still help others and live an active life. Make your activities fit you.

- A musician who had Alzheimer's could no longer play his instrument, but he continued to sing with his band.
- A grandfather who formerly preferred his older grandchildren's interests found delight in playing on the floor with a new grandbaby.
- A busy executive found his dog far more entertaining and enjoyable than he ever had before.
- Some gourmet cooks enjoy flipping through cooking magazines, setting a pretty table, polishing the silver, or arranging the flowers when they can no longer cook.

Some families or family members or friends will want to do everything for you, or you may feel they aren't doing enough. With guidance, overly helpful people will eventually learn that they don't have to take over, do everything for you, or take control of everything you do. They just have to be ready to step in, guide, help, or encourage you as your needs change. They also need to anticipate a different type of togetherness. Instead of sharing activities in the same way, you share time together. You will also discover as you and your family outfit your life to fit your new needs that you don't need family members 24/7, nor perhaps as often as you would like. When you have to stop driving or don't want to tackle public transportation on your own, you can wait for rides. (Waiting may be more difficult when you have Alzheimer's, however.)

Remind those around you to

- slow down
- give directions one step at a time
- spell out what comes next
- limit options
- help with decision making
- apply humor liberally

"If I didn't have a sense of humor, I think maybe I'd be dead."
—*A person with Alzheimer's*

Opt for Honesty, Including with Yourself and About Yourself

▶ **Good Advice:** Tell people important to you that you have a memory problem. They won't know by looking at you. It takes a lot of energy to hide your symptoms, and being honest reduces frustration.

To find a new normal, and particularly a new, satisfying normal, you need to be open with others—and honest with yourself—about the disease. You, like many others with Alzheimer's, may have been trying to hide your memory lapses for some time. You don't have to think, talk, or wallow in the problem every second. But do explain your condition to friends or family, who have probably already noticed or been affected by changes in your personality, behavior, and skills. Ask them not to tiptoe around you but to give you credit for doing your best under difficult circumstances.

Before discovering you have Alzheimer's, you may have felt as if you were going crazy. Admitting to yourself that you have a memory disorder gives you the freedom to blame the forgetfulness and confusion on the disease. You may also stop trying to wish away your problems or blame them on a demanding spouse. Now you have time to adapt to or figure out what helps you live with the problems and even thrive in spite of them.

Being open about the disease opens you up to getting help, which is not admitting defeat. It's saying you intend to defy the illness and care for yourself by asking for the right amount of help at the right time. Admitting, for example, that your growing pile of mail now boggles and frustrates you and that you need help paying bills, tells others that you still care about protecting your financial security. If you ask for assistance deciding what to wear and navigating your closet, you are making clear you want to continue to look and dress as you always have (or better!).

Being open about your disease is not always easy. You may find that your friends and family members don't really want to know what you are going through. At the same time, you can feel good knowing that your Alzheimer's isn't bad enough to be so obvious to others. One woman surprised an old friend by asking for help because "I have Alzheimer's." The friend responded, "You don't look like you have Alzheimer's," to which the woman replied, "I wonder what I looked like before!"

> *"I feel tired for no reason, but my friends know Alzheimer's is not my whole life."*
>
> *—A person with Alzheimer's*

Accepting that you have Alzheimer's may change for the better how you view and interact with the world around you. You may decide to stop spending time on people, activities, or jobs that you've actually never really enjoyed or valued. You may stop comparing yourself to others. Some people say Alzheimer's helped them realize they didn't want the stress of being competitive or a perfectionist. They discovered that they wanted to educate people about the disease, by advocating for research, participating in Alzheimer's research studies, or teaching policy makers and health professionals what people with Alzheimer's need from them. You can become part of the solution rather than "the problem." You may decide that this is the time to turn your energies to family, worship, or a favorite cause.

▶ **Be Prepared:** People may offer too much or too little help. Tell them what you need.

▶ YOUR NEW DAY-TO-DAY LIVING

Organizing your day helps your mind make sense of what's going on. Here are tip from people with early-stage Alzheimer's:

- Get out of the house. Go for a walks. Just be sure to pick a safe, well-lit place.
- Choose small groups and quiet places, when possible. Your focus will improve, your stress will defuse.
- If you get lost or confused, ask for help, especially from police.
- Figure out which of your friends are comfortable talking to you about your feelings and what is happening to you.
- Return the favor. Listen to your friends when they need to talk about their problems. You'll have trouble remembering what they tell you, but that doesn't make you less of a friend.
- Don't waste these years while you are still very capable—do what you love, be with the people you love. Tell them you love them.

"I'm unsure, uneasy, perplexed—it may take me longer, but so what?"
—*A person with Alzheimer's*

Alzheimer's makes it difficult to plan or carry out multiple-step projects or even daily routines like making coffee. You may avoid devices that once seemed very familiar, such as the microwave or electric can opener, because they don't seem to work as they used to. You don't like to ask for help or don't know whom to ask. You may feel overwhelmed or frustrated by all the changes to your daily routines.

Getting Organized for Your New Day

Finding your new daily routine is the trick to making sure you have the time and energy to get to the activities and people you enjoy.

Start by getting organized, because even a familiar home can easily become overwhelming. The goal is simple: to make it easy to find things. Ask a friend or family neatnik to help you get rid of old (and new) belongings that you don't need or want.

Throw it out. Dispose of old cleaning agents, garden chemicals, or any other potentially hazardous or just confusing material. Extremely dangerous items like power tools and guns must go, even if you have previously been an experienced hunter or craftsman.

Give it a home. Organize what you keep. Label your drawers and kitchen cabinets, so you know what goes where. It may seem silly, but you'll really appreciate it in the future, as will anyone who comes over to help. (If you're feeling creative, make decorative labels or even go to a ceramics studio and paint knobs with a picture of what's in that cabinet, such as coffee mugs.)

Keep the important things you need throughout your day— wallet, phone numbers (and your phone), pills, keys, toothbrush, glasses, reading material—in the same prominent place. If you will remember to look at it, a notebook or date book with the names of people you know and your schedule comes in handy. Include labeled pictures of friends and family (especially those great friends whose names you keep forgetting).

Clear the pathway, you're coming through. Your house needs to be safe to navigate. Make sure you have good lighting throughout the house, grab bars in the bathroom, and rails on both sides of the staircase. Speaking of stairs, they aren't storage areas. Clear them of all junk.

Move at the speed of you. Alzheimer's can make tending to daily tasks more difficult, because you may forget what you were just doing and what comes next. You tire easily and your thoughts tend to wander. So whether it's getting dressed, making a meal, cleaning the house, or completing your responsibilities at work, you will need—we hope with help from friends or family—to break down your day's chores into bite-size pieces. Focus on one task at a time. Multitasking is overrated (and harder for older persons and people with early-stage memory changes). Limit distractions. You may be more efficient if you turn off the television while getting dressed, for example. Give yourself plenty of breaks and downtime (how bad is that?).

It's great to post reminders for yourself, but also ask others for help. If you worry about being ready for an outing or social event on time, ask a friend, the doorman, or a neighbor to call you when it is time to start getting dressed or to meet your ride. The goal is to reduce the number of worries on your to-do or to-remember list. You want to avoid last-minute rushes that leave you frantic and unprepared to have a good time.

▶ **Good to Know:** Your memory and thinking will vary daily and even hourly. Expect good days when things are easier for you and not-so-good days when it is best to do less.

To make your days as successful as possible, you need:

- Information about the disease and about services available to you and your family
- Acknowledgment from others, including your doctor and other family members, that you are dealing with a memory disorder
- Forgiveness for mistakes you make (including inappropriate or rude remarks)
- Permission to be imperfect
- Support making decisions
- Humor, compassion, and a fresh perspective
- Concrete help, such as a visit, a ride, or help with shopping

Minding Your Body?

Don't look now, but your body may be talking to you. It needs attention. You may be thinking a lot about how to keep your brain functioning, but take time for care of your body too. Your mind works better when your body is healthy and treated well. You can't "fix" your memory, but you will function better when your hearing and vision are all tuned up. Eating healthfully, drinking water with each meal, and getting regular exercise, such as daily walks, will help ward off those everyday annoyances, like constipation, blood sugar fluctuations, dry mouth, and tiredness. A simple infection can increase your confusion and irritability, so getting prompt treatment for ailments is more important than ever—and be sure to get an annual flu shot. You can't prevent all illnesses, but you'll perform better if you take your medications, get exercise, and socialize, whether with friends, family, or colleagues. Lifestyle improvements or changes don't cure Alzheimer's, but they really improve your quality of life.

If you are noticing changes in either your hearing or vision but have passed your annual exams for both, the problem may be with your visual or auditory processing. You can see objects, but judging their distance from you or even identifying them may no longer feel automatic. Or you may hear what people are saying, but it doesn't make sense the way it used to. Alert your friends and family to the changes so they will be patient if you are searching for something in plain sight or asking "What?" a lot. If the changes throw you physically off balance, consider asking your doctor about a walking stick, cane, or walker for added security.

Going to Work—or Not

Are you still working at a paid or volunteer job where you would like to stay for as long as possible? If so, you need to let your supervisor or partners know that eventually you will need to change what you're doing, so you can continue as an effective and productive part of the group. This may involve having someone double-check your work, modifying the kind of projects you work on, taking on fewer tasks, taking more time to complete projects, or working more closely with a colleague.

For example, the director of a community group that delivers meals to homebound people found aspects of her job frustrating when she developed early-stage Alzheimer's. So she teamed up with her husband: He drove and she brought the meals to the recipients' doors and chatted with them. She benefited from having a pleasant routine, while her husband was very glad to share an activity with his wife. (Couples who are dealing with memory issues gain when they find ways to continue being a twosome.) A sales manager with mild cognitive impairment gave up the deadlines and responsibilities of management to become a greeter at a discount store, where he could use his strong social skills and choose his own hours. People with Alzheimer's do best when they are able to complete meaningful tasks each day, and you will feel better if you have chances to give as well as to receive help.

If you are the boss or owner of a small company, you'll need to ask your partners or top employees to handle deadlines, complex decisions, and negotiations. Particularly if you have a family-run business, you may enjoy coming to work for the camaraderie. Your family may feel more secure having you with them at work rather than alone at home.

Truth be told, most people leave their full-time jobs quickly after discovering they have Alzheimer's. They worry that their speed or judgment is declining and they may put others at risk.

"I had to quit as a sales manager because I lost my ability to focus and multitask."

—A person with Alzheimer's

Having Sex—or Not

Sex may no longer belong in the day-to-day or week-to-week category, but nothing about early-stage Alzheimer's precludes sex. In fact, one of the problems facing some couples is that people with Alzheimer's want sex so often that the spouse resorts to sleeping in a different room, relying on "out of sight, out of mind" to solve the problem. This avoids having to reject a well-intentioned partner.

Alzheimer's can also interfere with normal inhibitions and good judgment about where and when to talk about sex or other personal topics. Ask your spouse or friends to help you limit or recover from any comments you may make that are inappropriate.

Alzheimer's or some of the medications used to control its symptoms may decrease the sex drive. Also, some people with Alzheimer's become quite prudish and opposed to references to sex, which can become a problem when you want to see almost any movie not rated G. (The solution: Get the video and fast-forward through sex scenes.)

Safe Sex

Keep in mind that there is nothing about having Alzheimer's or being older that prevents you or your family member from getting sexually transmitted diseases, including HIV.

Giving Up Driving

Driving has probably been a part of your day-to-day life for decades. Particularly outside of urban areas that have dependable public transportation, driving is an adult's ticket to freedom and independence, to say nothing of the grocery store, doctors, and friends. So giving up the keys means more than having to hunt down rides. It means giving up your sense of yourself as an adult in control of your time and activities.

Unfortunately, at a certain point in the disease, Alzheimer's and driving don't mix. Most people with MCI continue to drive. An early Alzheimer's diagnosis, by itself, should not mean immediate loss of all driving privileges. But even early on, the disease impairs judgment, reaction time, visuospatial skills, and problem-solving skills.

Drivers who have Alzheimer's may get lost, scared, and end up missing. By the time the disease has impaired your driving ability, the disease has also undermined your ability to report or judge your on-road safety. Driving is one area that you and your family members can't ignore. Here are some warning signs that driving is becoming dangerously difficult:

- Getting lost more frequently
- Taking a long time to get to nearby places
- Stopping unexpectedly in traffic
- Turning from the wrong lane
- Missing exits
- Driving at the wrong speed

- Confusing the brake and accelerator
- Responding slowly to something unexpected
- Having a lot of fender benders
- Getting tickets or warnings

We aren't holding people with early Alzheimer's to a higher standard for driving than other people. These guidelines apply to everyone.

Note to Families

Driving is one of the earliest freedoms that people with Alzheimer's must give up, and they are generally very reluctant to do so. Here are a variety of approaches to help get someone with Alzheimer's off the roads before he or she has an accident or gets terribly lost:

- Explain the risks and simply suggest that he retire from driving.
- Ask her doctor to recommend no driving, or at least to stop driving for now.
- Tell your family member that if the Department of Motor Vehicles gets reports of poor driving, it may request the driver to come in for testing and eventually take away his license. If need be, issue the report yourself.

The absence of a license may not stop determined adults with Alzheimer's. They have been known to keep driving, including on the wrong side of the street, while muttering, "That doctor doesn't know anything!" Then it's time for Plan B:

- Shave the car keys, substitute another key, remove a distributor cap, or otherwise disable the car.
- Sell or move the car. One family of a taxi driver put the taxi on blocks in the backyard to help him remember that the car was broken.
- Explain that one of the beloved grandchildren needs the car to get to school.

Persistent individuals have been known to fix the car, replace the keys, or even buy a new car. So there's always Plan C, if you have the time: Give the person lots of other options. Look for driving and delivery services, organize rides from neighbors to church or the grocery store, or set up a charge account with a taxi service. See if you can get the same driver each time. Paying for rides may not be as expensive as keeping a car. Some people with early-stage Alzheimer's are eventually willing to give the car to a grandchild, favorite young relative, or neighbor who, in exchange, serves as chauffeur.

One person with Alzheimer's suggested that family members talk to the impaired driver one-on-one over time about the importance of not driving, instead of "ganging up." He asked each of his family members to "take turns once a week learning how to drive *for* me—not just 'drive me.' Remember, it's what you want, not what I want." Also remember that spouses are affected when their partner must turn over the keys. A wife of a person with Alzheimer's said she gets mad when people congratulate her on getting her husband to stop driving. "Not having him in the driver's seat was as much a loss for me as it was for him," she said.

► TAKE A TOUR OF THE HOUSE

As the saying goes, you want to find trouble before it finds you. Walk through your house with a family member to look for the potential risks and danger zones.

The Medicine Cabinet

Are you taking the correct amount of prescribed medicines at the right times? Are you taking over-the-counter products, such as herbal medicines, that may interfere with your prescribed medications or worsen your confusion? Having someone fill your weekly pillboxes, if you have them, may not be enough to ensure that you are taking your pills properly. If you live alone or stay home while your spouse is at work, ask someone to call and remind you. One woman's apartment manager offered to check on her each day at noon and before leaving at five P.M. to help her take the right pills. They both enjoyed the short visits. There are many new devices to help remind people to take medication, but they all need human supervision.

The Kitchen

Are you eating and drinking properly? Your family needs to make sure you have prepared, microwave meals in the freezer and that your kitchen is clean and free of spoiled foods. When you shop, go with a shopping list and, if possible, a helper. People with Alzheimer's often buy too many of one item (two biggies: boxes of facial tissue and pet food) and not enough important supplies.

▶ **Try This:** So that you socialize and eat a good meal every day if you are single or a couple, consider dining regularly at the same restaurant or diner. You will get to know the "regulars" and they will get to know you. (Remember to bring home the leftovers for lunch the next day.)

Some people in the early stage eat all the time because they forget they just ate or don't notice that they're full. Others forget to eat, lose weight, and then end up going through a battery of unnecessary tests for cancer or other illnesses that cause weight loss.

You may be eating more sweets. The drive for sweets in many people overrides the weakening sense of what and when they "should" eat. Have lots of healthful foods around the house and enjoy your occasional cookie or ice cream.

Alcohol is more dangerous. You may forget you already had a drink and have another and another, or that you always have only one shot and not two or more. Some people with Alzheimer's become physically dependent on alcohol without their family realizing it and end up requiring hospitalization to stop drinking. But if you have always been a moderate drinker and someone is making sure you remain moderate, cheers!

You might be forgetting to drink enough water, which may increase confusion. Alzheimer's and aging interfere with the body's thirst-alert mechanism, so make a point of drinking the right amount of water or other healthful drinks. Some medications can cause your thirst to increase, and if this happens tell your doctor. Drinking too much water can also be harmful.

Keep the thermostat on your water heater below 120 degrees to avoid accidentally scalding yourself or others.

If you are forgetting to turn off the stove:

- Consider putting a device on the stove that turns it off automatically.

- Use a microwave, coffeemaker, or toaster oven with an automatic turnoff.

- Take the knobs off the stove to remind you not to use it.

If you have young grandchildren or other little visitors, these safety measures will serve a dual purpose.

Closets

Are you dressing appropriately, including choosing the right clothes for the time of year? Ask a friend to help you organize your closet, to make getting dressed easier. Leave only the clothes in the closet that are appropriate for the season and for the type of events that you normally go to. If you don't need suits and fancy dresses, put those items in a separate closet or storage. If you find yourself preferring the same outfit every day, buy more of them if your budget allows.

The Phone

The phone is your lifeline, but it is also an open door for a scary scenario: Criminals call your home, say they are officials from your bank, credit card company, or elsewhere, ask for personal information, such as your credit card number, and use your credit card or withdraw money from your bank account. It happens.

Here's how to avoid accidentally giving information over the phone or making calls that you later forget and regret:

- Forward your calls to a family member, who will screen incoming calls and pass along messages.

- Let your answering machine take all your calls. Pick up the phone only after you hear a friend or family member leaving a message.

- At a minimum, ask someone to make sure you are on the national do-not-call list to limit telemarketers.

- One caring daughter put a tape recorder on her mother's phone, listened to what the mother had ordered, and then canceled the orders she knew her mother really didn't want.

- If you find yourself getting confused about how to use the phone, including remembering to hang up when you go to check on something, ask for help getting a phone that is easier for you to use. As time goes on, however, not being able to use the phone reliably is one reason that people with Alzheimer's stop living alone. Another reason: calling an adult child or neighbor many times throughout the day and night because you can't remember what time it is or that you just called.

The Front Door

Another route of entry for criminals is, of course, your front door. If you might forget how to respond to strangers who come to the door, such as salesmen, charity or church workers, or people offering to repair your roof or do yard work, put a sign on the inside of the front door reminding you to keep the door locked and not to open it to strangers. Put a sign saying "no solicitors" on the outside.

The Out-of-Doors

Can you leave and return home safely? To answer that question, consider:

- Are you still able to drive safely without getting lost or scared?

- Do you have a Safe Return bracelet or MedicAlert bracelet or necklace? These little pieces of jewelry are very low on the bling scale and very helpful. They provide vital medical and contact information to anyone trying to help you.

- Is your neighborhood safe?

- If you locked yourself out, would you know where to go for help?

Even if you're not driving, you can still get confused on walks and bike rides, while taking public transportation, and when trying to give someone else directions. To make your outings safer, start by changing your expectations. If you expect to remember how to get around the way you used to, you're setting yourself up for trouble. In most towns, you can't rely on old landmarks because of development. Besides, there are probably more cars, exits, and stoplights than ever before to confuse you. Always wear a clear form of identification, wear your house key on a chain under your shirt, and carry important phone numbers.

Danger Zones

As navigating the outside world becomes more difficult, so does getting around inside your house. Have you fallen, lost your balance, or noticed more bruises and cuts on your body? Often, people with memory disorders have problems going up stairs, positioning themselves comfortably in their bath or shower, or even sitting down safely in a dining room chair. To help yourself, try nonslip shoes and two-sided carpet tape. Throw out the throw rugs and remove all clutter in your path.

As the disease progresses, your response to minor disasters, like the toilet overflowing, or true ones, like an injury, may be slow. Ask someone to post in your house clear directions for emergencies. Many people living alone use personal response systems, which enable you to summon help by pushing a button on a necklace. A neighborly neighbor may prove even more helpful, particularly in those situations where you think something is broken but instead it is just confusing to use.

► LIVING ALONE WITH ALZHEIMER'S

Living alone when you have early-stage Alzheimer's is possible if you live near people who can be trusted to look out for you. They don't need to spy on you, but now is the time to ask neighbors, friends, or family to help. You may also need to hire people to assist with odd jobs.

This may be the first time in your adult life that you have had to turn to others for help with day-to-day living, and it will take some getting used to. If you are uncomfortable asking for help, your clergy person, attorney, doctor, family, or friend can do so on your behalf.

You can continue to enjoy the book club, garden club, or golf outing without reading the book, hosting the meeting, or scheduling the tee time. Read what you can of your group's book selection and enjoy hearing about the rest and talking about what you did read. Invite one of your favorite garden club members to take a quiet walk through a special garden. One woman remarked that she noted new growth in a community garden that everyone engaged in conversation seemed to overlook. Another man was surprised that his golf swing actually improved once he stopped worrying about keeping track of the game. He enjoyed demonstrating his new stance and swing.

► IT TAKES A FAMILY AND FRIENDS TO TACKLE ALZHEIMER'S (BUT FIRST YOU HAVE TO AGREE ON WHAT TO DO)

First, get mad at the disease, not at each other.

Dealing with Alzheimer's, as with any problem, can split up families or bring them closer. Family members get angry at one another for not doing their share, for being critical, for being cheap, for . . . the list could go on and on. Instead, try to look at Alzheimer's as a challenge that you and your family will tackle together, recognizing there is safety in numbers, especially when they are all on your side. Particularly later in the disease, when care becomes more demanding, it's all hands on deck.

Alzheimer's gives adult children the opportunity to do full-circle care. That is, their parents took care of them when they were little and now it's their turn to help their parents. Alzheimer's gives couples the opportunity to deepen their appreciation of their shared history, if they call on the strength they have used over the years to tackle tough times.

At first, you may cringe at the thought of your family being burdened by your care, and your family may feel unprepared to provide care. But over time, everyone may define his or her roles, schedules, and abilities. You may relax and trust that your needs will be met and that you still have much to offer other family members.

Isn't It Time We Talk? Family Conversations

The time will come when your family (and you) should talk about tough or complex questions concerning your current or future needs. Have this talk wherever works best—a coffeehouse, your home, a sibling's home. If family members live far away, meet remotely via cell phone conference calling, videoconferencing, or speakerphones. Before the meeting, everyone should together decide on the most pressing topic that needs discussing. For example, it could be how to handle money, medications, finances, or a move. All participants should have a chance to discuss their immediate concerns, their perspective on what is happening now, and what must change to accommodate your memory disorder.

Dos and Don'ts for a Successful Conversation

- Make sure you are included. You are the reason for the discussion and must have a chance to express your preferences, values, goals, worries, or concerns.

- Everyone should come to the conversation with information on options related to the topic.

- This is not a time for opening or resolving long-standing family feuds or grievances, or for catching up with one another.

- Show your appreciation of one another and have a sense of humor. ("Do you know why families are like peanut brittle? It takes a lot of sugar to hold the nuts together.")

- Each person gets equal time to talk about the issue on the table, what he could contribute, and what he hopes will come out of the discussion.

- Develop an action plan that includes what will be done, in what order, and by whom. Get commitments.

- Discuss how you will follow up with one another and whether it will be by phone or e-mail.

- Most families aren't used to getting together for decision making. So keep it simple—this isn't an intervention, therapy, or mediation.

Denial? What Denial?

Family members may surprise one another with the power of their denial.

Denial is a force to be reckoned with in many families struggling with early Alzheimer's. Suppose Dad is showing *very* clear signs of memory impairment and even has a diagnosis of early Alzheimer's from a reliable doctor. But Dad can still work puzzles, beat you at tennis, or even go to work every day. So Dad is really okay to live on his own without help. Right?

Wrong! Denial is a reaction to a difficult situation. It's a way of coping, of holding out hope, of taking time to process what is going on or to get through a particularly stressful time. Denial may be uncertainty about what to do next.

Nevertheless, family members' denial can get in the way of offering needed help to the person with Alzheimer's and keeping him or her safe. It can also make family members suspicious about one another's motives. In these cases, the primary family caregiver may prove helpful by working with or around those in denial as much as possible. Inform the doubters about what's going on and suggest written materials, Web sites, seminars, or Alzheimer's help lines as sources of objective information. Suggest that these family members spend time with their relative, since early-stage Alzheimer's is not always obvious during brief visits or conversations. Suggest that for now they act as if it is Alzheimer's and help with specific tasks that the relative can no longer perform easily. (But make sure they aren't scolding or pushing the relative.)

Advice for Family Members Who Are Far Away

Even though you may feel somewhat helpless and frustrated, family members who live far away from their relative with Alzheimer's can do a lot to fill the gaps.

- Help interview and hire professional care providers or geriatric care managers, or find an assisted-living facility.

- Offer to take over financial matters. Have bills sent to your house, do the taxes.

- Plan to take your relative on short vacations or weekends or have her visit your home.

- To be a valuable contact person, keep a notebook or files with information about his health care, medications, allergies, social services, friends, and financial accounts.

- Before you visit, talk to her about what she would like to do. Arrange for those activities and doctors' appointments in advance.

- When you visit, don't overschedule yourself. Stick to your to-do list.

- Make time for really talking to or at least listening to your relative, who may take a few days to open up to you.

Reality 101: For Family and Friends

People with Alzheimer's generally know that something is changing in their mind and they feel different. However, fear sometimes makes them unwilling to acknowledge their need for help. To help, say, your mother become less defensive and more accepting of herself and of your help, avoid reminding her of her impairments. Think of her as disabled instead of as someone who is deliberately being unreasonable or illogical.

Also, think logically about what you can do:

- The disease is bigger than you, and you can't solve all her problems. You will need to make realistic compromises among competing needs, loyalties, and commitments.

- The disease, not you, makes her unhappy.

- Chronic illnesses often cause people to take their frustration out on family members.

- Alzheimer's symptoms change over time. New problems are inevitable.

- Not all of her symptoms are related to Alzheimer's.

- Define your limits and then call in reinforcements.

- Friends who are unfamiliar with your situation may swoop in on you, trying to help too much, or you may feel your friends have abandoned you and are not helping enough. Don't feel you always have to take other people's advice.

- Find someone with whom you can be honest and discuss your feelings.

- If you regret a decision, remember you did what seemed best at the time, your choices were limited by circumstances beyond your control, and others have had to make the same decisions.

- Avoid making promises that include the words *always, never,* or *forever.*

- People with Alzheimer's have a lot to give, if you let them.

▶ SUPPORT GROUPS: A SOURCE OF INFORMATION, A CHUCKLE, A SHOULDER, FRIENDS

Support groups are for people with a common bond or issue. They usually meet weekly and serve as a place for members to give and receive help, guidance, and information concerning the problem. The groups usually meet in person, over the phone, via e-mail, or in chat rooms. Groups for people with early-stage Alzheimer's are generally led by professionals (nurses or social workers) but are not group therapy. There are groups for caregivers too. Many cybercommunities provide anonymous support for people dealing with Alzheimer's.

Support groups do not seek to change participants but, as the name suggests, to truly support them. Expect to hear "Aha!" or "You, too?!" a lot, if it's a good group.

At meetings, people with early-stage Alzheimer's tend to talk about the loss, anger, misunderstandings, fear, and frustration that clutter their days. They also talk about what is going well for them, such as feeling closer to family and friends or being able to enjoy certain activities. There is often as much humor, storytelling, and problem solving as there is shared grief.

Almost all local chapters of the Alzheimer's Association have support groups for people in the early stage of the disease and their

families. Most last about eight weeks and combine education and
support. Many friendships blossom in these short-term groups, and
couples may continue to meet regularly for mall walking, dinners
out, or other activities. Some early-stage support or education groups
morph into outings or other groups that help everyone have fun and
simply feel normal.

- The Northwestern Alzheimer's Center Culture Bus program
  grew out of their early-stage patients' interest in seeing more
  of Chicago's highlights. Once a month, they load into a van,
  hit one cultural hotspot like the Botanical Gardens, and enjoy
  a day with lunch and tours from docents who understand the
  group's unique needs. See the free downloadable booklet from
  this group, "What Happens Next?" at nia.nih.gov/Alzheimers/
  Publications/WhatHappensNext.htm/.

- The Australian Alzheimer's Society developed Memory Cafés,
  permanent places in a variety of locations for people with
  Alzheimer's to socialize, have coffee, and play checkers.

- The Colorado Alzheimer's Association turned Memory Cafés
  into evening events with dancing, dining, and a little Alzheimer's
  education on the side.

- A California Art Appreciation group visits art museums, taking tours from docents whom a social worker trained in facili-
  tating discussion.

- There's an Out and About group for persons with mild- to
  moderate-stage dementia, similar to the Culture Bus program
  at Northwestern Alzheimer's Disease Research Center.

- A Virginia early-stage support group had a professional leader
  who developed Mind and Body workshops for couples, which
  included mind teaser activities for couples to do as a team and
  funny activities to help them feel more lighthearted, creative,
  and in touch with each other.

Why Join?

Compared with people not in support groups, family caregiver participants report feeling less alone and misunderstood and more
accepting of their relatives' diagnosis. They say the group helps them

find solutions to daily hassles or frustrations. Here's what else family caregivers appreciate about caregiver support groups:

- "Compassion, laughs and camaraderie—that's why I keep coming back to this group."
- "Where else can I say how I feel and have 'fellow travelers' understand how I feel?"
- "I'm an information junkie—these people know every advance and good deal."

The success and quality of an early-stage support group depend in part on the skills of the group leader or facilitators. Here's what you want an early-stage group leader to do:

- make sure the group discusses both the positive and negative aspects of Alzheimer's
- help members feel that their experiences, thoughts, and feelings are supported
- understand but not analyze members' experiences
- help members use humor as a coping strategy
- tie members' comments into themes important to the group
- restate comments made by members as needed, to make sure everyone is understood

Support groups aren't for everyone. If the group doesn't seem right for you, try another group or wait and try later. You may have all the support you need from family, friends, and other community groups, like your men's club or church circle.

► FINANCES AND YOUR FUTURE: DON'T GO IT ALONE

Starting now, you will benefit from additional assistance managing your finances, including paying your regular bills and taxes. Plan for your financial future now, while you are comfortable stating your preferences and participating in decisions. Part of that planning should include asking a trusted person (family or professional) to be your financial and health-care durable power of attorney or your substitute decision maker. See the Resources section for booklets and Web sites on how to do this.

Talk with everyone in your family about your wishes and who should take charge. Put your decision in writing and give everyone who needs to know a copy of your agreement. The person you select may be, but doesn't have to be, the same person who helps you with your immediate banking needs, such as keeping your checkbook in order and your bills paid on time. Have your bills forwarded to that person, if you are having trouble keeping up with the mail. Be sure to tell your family where you keep your financial and personal papers, from your marriage certificate to your tax returns.

One more cautious step: Ask your bank to notify the person helping you with your finances, or another trusted individual, of any unusual withdrawals from your account. You may also want to ask the bank to put a limit on how much money may be withdrawn at any one time. Lowering the limit on your credit card might be a good idea, too, especially if you are having trouble keeping track of it.

If you feel you need a specialized attorney or trust officer to handle your legal and business affairs, you may want to turn to an elder law attorney. These specialists usually charge more than generalist attorneys but can be especially helpful if you have no family, if you do have family but they are likely to fight over what's best for you and your assets, or if you have an unusually large estate (over $3 million). Trust officers generally charge a percentage of your trust to manage your money. For more information, go to the Web site of the National Academy of Elder Law Attorneys (www.naela.com), a nonprofit association of lawyers and others who work with older clients and their families. The American Bar Association Commission on Legal Problems of the Elderly has useful information for people of all income levels (www.abanet.org/elderly/toolkit/home/html).

Before hiring anyone to help you with your finances or around the house, ask a trusted family member or friend to help you screen the applicants. Check with neighbors or close family about whether the person can be trusted. Don't be paranoid, but do be wary of anyone who seems unusually friendly or loyal to you, particularly new people. Also, be very wary of anyone who asks you for a loan or for gifts. A trustworthy professional who comes to your home should have high ethical standards—he or she shouldn't take advantage of someone with a memory disorder by asking for a loan.

Paying for care is one of the early worries that strikes people with Alzheimer's and their family members. Figuring out how to cover your bills and your future needs will become more difficult as the disease progresses. So plan for and anticipate future needs now. Part of this advance planning should include writing your will.

To address future medical issues, you will want to prepare a comprehensive advance directive, a legal document that states what sort of medical treatments you want and do not want. Doctors and your family should refer to it when you are no longer able to communicate your preferences or make informed decisions. In the directive, describe your preferences in general. You don't need to refer to specific medical situations that may or may not come up. To learn more about an advance directive, including what it can—and can't—do, check out the American Bar Association's Web site (www.abanet .org/publiced/practical/directive_writing.html) and the consumer site of the American Hospital Association (www.putitinwriting.org).

These documents won't do any good tucked in a drawer, so make sure you give copies to your family members and doctors. In fact, give copies to more than one family member, friend, and doctor. Many decisions must be made in a hospital emergency room, often before a single family member can be found.

If Alzheimer's appears to be a strong inheritable condition in your family, your children and younger siblings may want to consider private long-term care insurance for themselves, so they can afford costly care if needed.

► FOR FAMILIES AND FRIENDS: WHAT TO DO WHEN YOU FEEL GUILTY, TIRED, AND FRUSTRATED

Guilt: The Universal Force

No chapter on early Alzheimer's would be complete without a section on guilt. We're devoting just a little space to it here, but you may be devoting a lot of space to it in your head. You may feel guilty about something you have done or not done for your relative with Alzheimer's. You may also feel guilty about how you treated or behaved toward him, prior to learning the diagnosis or even afterward. You may feel guilty or ashamed about being embarrassed by your relative. Remember, you're not alone in your guilt, and guilt just means that you want to act responsibly. Your relative probably feels bad about not being able to do everything he once did and for being what he feels is a burden.

▶ **Antidote to Guilt:** Take comfort in knowing that no one is the perfect family caregiver, and only the truly responsible people feel guilty and do something to avoid future problems. Indeed, the family members who are doing the most are the most likely to berate themselves for not doing more. You can even take some comfort knowing that the person with Alzheimer's has a poor memory for what you did wrong (and, unfortunately, for what you did right!).

Fatigue

Exhaustion is a common complaint early on of people with dementia and their families. Both are responding to new demands on top of their normal responsibilities. They are also stressed by their new roles in the family. Fatigue becomes particularly problematic toward the end of the day, when energy and patience are running low.

▶ **Hint:** Don't shortchange your need for nature's fatigue fighters and mood elevators: sleep and exercise.

Frustration and Anger

Even though they aren't the ones with the disease, family members can lay claim to a big share of frustration. They may get annoyed with their relative's new and unusual behavior, and many come to resent the intrusion on their privacy and time.

What to do? Start by putting a reminder sign in your own house that says "Blame the Disease!" or, if you want to be discreet, "B.T.D!"

One man put up a sign on his study door, "Alzheimer's at Work: Prepare to Repeat."

When your once-dignified spouse becomes stubborn, resistant, suspicious, or even racist, follows you around the house, or calls you at work every five minutes, you may start thinking, "I always thought he was a bit ——— [needy, small-minded, you fill in the blank], and now it's really surfacing!" The B.T.D. sign will remind you that this annoying behavior is not a character flaw going public; it's the disease talking. The brain is damaged and isn't working the way it did.

Most family members, some earlier in the course of the disease than others, have an "aha!" moment when they realize that the person with Alzheimer's isn't intentionally being lazy, indifferent, annoying, picky, demanding or ——— (again, your turn). She isn't intentionally ignoring your useful suggestions and requests. (Well, not most of the time, anyway.) It's the disease talking—B.T.D. Moreover, she's not a child—you can't teach her to stop these new "bad" habits.

▶ **Need to Know:** Alzheimer's shrinks people's ability to adapt to new situations.

You need to see how *you* can change, to adapt to his new normal, and how you—or whoever is helping you—can change his environment to fit his new needs. Think about distracting, encouraging, and reassuring him. But then look for ways to take time for yourself, read a magazine, or catch up on a hobby you enjoy or chores that need doing. Couples benefit from separate activities. Ask his friends to take him to lunch or bowling while you do what is important to you, whether it's going to work, having a date with friends, or getting to the hairdresser.

One woman whose husband has Alzheimer's describes living with him as a long, infuriating game of hide-and-seek. "We get a bill, he opens it and misplaces it, or I put letters on the kitchen table to be mailed and they disappear. He can't remember if he mailed them or not. I made a special place for his glasses and keys, but he can't remember to put them there. Then every day he asks me: 'Where did YOU put my glasses, my keys, my wallet?'"

Even though some of his comments, actions, and ideas may seem more than odd to you, they are his Alzheimer's talking.

What to Do When Your Relative Does . . .

Here are nine behaviors that families often complain about and tips on how to handle them:

1. His idea of what he wants is more intense and inflexible than ever, but also he changes his mind a lot.

It's jarring suddenly to be stopped in your tracks when you've been helping him with something and then he changes his mind and announces, perhaps sternly, "I never said I wanted that!" Here's what is going on for him: He forgets what he wants and remembers only the feeling of being sure about . . . something. Be prepared by knowing you may have to stop a project and pick it up later, whether it's an outing, an art project, buying a new outfit, or even making a large purchase.

2. She gets angry easily and at nothing. She doesn't remember your plan to stop after shopping to visit a sick friend. As soon as you arrive, she says, "Haven't you gabbed here long enough?"

Say, "I'm sorry. I know you are ready to go. I will try to wrap this up quickly," or, "Thanks for being patient with us—you know how we carry on." You're not accusing her of anything (like being impatient) or forcing your reality on her (you have been there only five minutes), and you're respecting her feelings. Call your friend privately when your relative is comfortably settled in front of the television at home so your conversation isn't shortchanged and you can get the rest of the story.

3. His appreciation of you ebbs and flows.

It's not worth reminding him of all that you do to help him. It's not that he doesn't appreciate you; it's just that he can't remember what he has asked for or everything you have just done. He will confabulate, meaning he will fill in the holes in his faulty memory with something that makes sense to him. A wise *Peanuts* cartoon once described how Grandpa used to be afraid of forgetting, but now he has a worse problem—he's remembering things that never happened!

4. Her expectations of what others can and should do are unrealistic.

The disease is robbing her of empathy and limiting her appreciation for anything that's not right in front of her. If you're working behind the scenes, you might as well not be working. Her world is getting narrower.

It won't help to tell her how long a request will take to carry out or what else you have to do. Just tell her whether you can or can't do something, or who will take care of it for her.

5. The abstract concept of time, including what times are appropriate to call family and friends, is becoming difficult to grasp.

Alzheimer's causes people to have trouble telling morning from night, because they can't make sense of the usual cues (it's dark outside, it's quiet inside) or they forget what those cues mean. They may also just forget that it's impolite to call at night or that everyone was okay a few hours ago. When you get repetitive off-hours phone calls, tell him you're sleeping, everyone is just fine, and you will talk again in the morning. Otherwise, there's not much you can do, because you want him to have access to a phone.

LIFE WITH A HUSBAND WHO HAS ALZHEIMER'S

"I tell him about an invitation and he refuses to accept. Then a few days later he answers when the friend who sent the invitation calls. 'Of course! I'd love to go,' he tells her. After he hangs up, he is mad at me for not telling him about the party. Responding honestly to him would only infuriate him, so I remind myself what a friend told me after he was diagnosed: 'You will never be right again, let alone win.'"

6. He accuses you or others of betrayal (adultery, robbery, whatever).

Because of his faulty thinking, he's quick to conclude that when something is missing (meaning he can't see it), whoever is around must have taken it. If you go next door for a minute to borrow something, to him it feels as if you've been gone for two days, so he accuses you of having an affair. Don't try to explain that the neighbor is thirty years younger and happily married. He is scared of being abandoned in a world that doesn't make sense to him. If you get angry with him, you are only upsetting him more. Comfort and distract.

7. She has an obsessive need for repetition and reassurance.

She doesn't want to be this way, and she won't always be this way. As the disease progresses, people with Alzheimer's become less demanding. Sadly, they also become less responsive. Keep in mind that dependency does not imply weakness of character or will.

8. He's so slow! It takes us forever to get anything done.

It's frustrating to wait while the person with Alzheimer's completes a minor task, such as drying the dishes or folding the laundry. Distract yourself while you wait and resist doing too much for him. He feels good about helping. Also, he needs the daily practice so he will continue to remember how to do the task. Relearning it would be difficult to impossible. If you must rush off to an appointment, save his job for him to complete when you return.

9. She refuses to help around the house at all, to take care of herself, to bathe or dress properly.

The golden rules for motivating people with Alzheimer's to accomplish a task:

- Ask her politely, as you would anyone else, "Do you have time to help me now?"
- Model or demonstrate what you want done.
- Don't command or demand.
- Compliment, don't criticize.
- Say, "Do what you can do."
- Reinforce, don't force.

We know. Easier said than done. It's also easier to know when to turn the page (when you've come to the end of the chapter) than to know when a person has turned the page from early-stage to middle-stage Alzheimer's. The next chapter, which is written for family members, is about the middle stage. But you will find that people with Alzheimer's can keep one foot in early stage and the other foot (the one with the mismatched shoe) in middle stage.

▶ **Good Advice:** No matter where you and your family member are, stay focused on what's left, not what's lost.

"I advise my friends with Alzheimer's not to be ashamed. We talk to each other, laugh about the good times, and tell lies about how we're doing now."

—*A person with Alzheimer's*

CHAPTER TWELVE

THE MIDDLE YEARS: FINDING PEACE OF MIND

Life is about not knowing, having to change, taking the moment and making the best of it without knowing what's going to happen next.

—GILDA RADNER

As Alzheimer's disease progresses, symptoms change and, eventually, the person has progressed from the early stage to the middle stage. It's a gradual process and not clear-cut. Some changes will be barely noticeable, while others will be unexpected and dramatic. A person in the middle stage may disappear in a minute and get lost in a crowd, or search the house half the night for something familiar, but still read, bike daily, and appear the same to others. (The guise of normality may fall as soon as he tries to do a task that once felt simple and now doesn't.) Another person may continue to play the piano quite well yet be unable to dress herself without a lot of direction and cues.

Most people with Alzheimer's do change in the middle years in four key areas: their behavior, language, sense of time and place, and sleep. Families need to anticipate that Alzheimer's eventually robs people of their:

- Peace of mind. They have a lower tolerance for stress and are more likely to become suspicious, confused, agitated, resistant, angry, or upset.

- Communication skills. Their difficulty in communicating frustrates and exhausts them.

- Sense of time. When their internal timekeeper goes askew, so does their ability to plan, to wait for you to return, and to sleep. As a result, they may go looking for you and, eventually, go missing.

- Ability to maintain a regular sleep schedule. Their sleep may become so erratic that caring for them alone without help is almost impossible.

No matter what specific changes your relative goes through or where your relative is living, in the middle stage families need to get more involved. Consider how you can take the lead in planning her life while maintaining your own life and mental well-being. You want to focus on heading off problems that could affect both you and her, instead of exhausting yourself by putting out fires as they occur.

Your responsibilities change, as you try to catch up or keep pace with the changes he is going through. One wife compared caring for her husband to being the manager of a large and unpredictable project for which she had no expertise. Another older wife explained that waiting for her husband to do anything required the type of patience she has never had and, at her age, isn't sure she will develop.

One husband said that his wife's personality changed as her Alzheimer's progressed, and he felt as if he had to get to know her all over again. She was charming and helpful with casual friends but withdrawn, resistant, sullen, and insensitive with him. Her self-centeredness was foreign to him. He realized that she was unaware of his disappointment, embarrassment, loneliness, frustration, and anger. He had to accept that only he could do the changing now, and remember that she would have done the same for him.

A wife said caring for her husband at home for more than ten years taught her that she was strong enough and kind enough to endure.

She became less afraid and more confident, while learning that always being in control was highly overrated and unattainable. She learned to cut herself some slack and accept that strong enough was not the same as perfect.

Care providers of people in the middle stage of Alzheimer's find themselves having to do more with less energy. They need to feel okay about sharing their responsibilities with others and relaxing their standards enough to retain some quality of life for themselves.

▶ **Consider**: She can't change her behavior or the course of this chronic disease. But you don't have to lose your sense of self as you accommodate her needs.

While you are doubling your efforts to help, it may seem as though your relative is halving hers. She may still look physically able but is doing less and less for herself and others. Remember:

- She didn't choose and doesn't want to be like this, nor does she want to be dependent on you. But because she is becoming less aware of what is going on around her, she may be less grateful for or satisfied with her care.

- She is losing her ability to express or meet her needs to feel loved, secure, and productive. Keep a few extra doses of humor, patience, and compassion in your medicine cabinet. Then you can meet those basic needs without losing your mind.

A man with Alzheimer's chatted with the daughter of a friend. He stood up to leave, hugged her warmly, held both her hands, looked into her eyes, and said, "And tell me something, how do I know you?"

▶ THIS CHAPTER IS FOR YOU IF . . .

If your family member has begun to exhibit some or many of these behaviors and has been diagnosed with middle-stage or moderate Alzheimer's, welcome to your chapter.

- *Who are you?* The stereotypical symptom of Alzheimer's is not recognizing people who were once very familiar. Not everyone develops this symptom, but if it does occur, it's usually in the middle stage. Your relative may fail to recognize or name close friends, family, or care providers. He may also mix up identities, confusing a grown daughter for his wife, for example.

- *And who are you?* You may feel as though you don't recognize him, either. Middle stage can bring changes in hygiene, dressing, and many other aspects of behavior.

- *Where did he go?* You can't leave her alone in a car or any public place, as she may well forget she is waiting for you and take off, thinking she has to go to work or run an errand from long ago. She may also go look for you.

- *Your shadow.* He shadows you or the person he spends the most time with. That person has become his "prosthetic" brain, the person who interprets the world for him, who is his harbor in the choppy waters of his day.

- *You told me already!* Expect to hear the same story, concern, observation, complaint, question, or fear repeatedly. Yet what she can still remember and understand may surprise you. Heading to a doctor's appointment, a mother kept asking her youngest daughter where they were going. The daughter finally said, "Mom, I wish you wouldn't repeat yourself." The mother snapped back, "If I hadn't repeated myself, you wouldn't have been born."

- *Just sit still!* He can't stop moving or touching things.

- *I just don't understand.* She can't organize her thoughts, follow complex conversations or instructions, or complete tasks on her own. She's discombobulated.

- *Filling in the memory blanks.* His imagination picks up where his memory left off.

- *Don't ask.* She may still be able to read and listen to stories or movies, but don't ask what she just read or saw or what it's about. Her comprehension, recent memory, and attention are waning.

- *He gets an idea in his head and he can't let go.* He perseverates and no amount of logic or reason will set his mind free, though a pleasant distraction might.

- *Stand back.* When she feels she isn't being heard or understood, she may resort to yelling, cursing, threatening, or striking out.
- *Help!* He needs prompting, cues, reminders, and a lot of reassurance.

▶ **The Numbers:** Of the estimated 5 million Americans with Alzheimer's, 70 percent are cared for at home, usually by a spouse or daughter. Half of these caregivers live with their relative for the entire course of the illness.

▶ LET'S TALK

To prevent or avoid difficult behavior, rely on the three Rs: routines, rituals, and repetition. People with Alzheimer's thrive on all three.

Here's how to help her communicate when she is having difficulty remembering words, forming thoughts, and keeping her thoughts in mind long enough to express them. Remember, you can't follow all of these suggestions all the time.

Both understanding your family member who has Alzheimer's and being understood by her may be difficult: She is becoming supersensitive to nonverbal cues, your tone of voice, and being rushed. Nevertheless, she still wants to converse, to be understood, and to understand what is going on around her.

▶ **Good Advice:** Tell her, "We're in this together, and I'll help you figure it out." Help her feel that you're on the same team.

A quiet setting may be the most important conversation starter. Minimize distractions and noise, such as television or radio, to help her focus on what you are saying. Don't expect her to follow a group discussion. She might want to be part of the group, as long as she doesn't feel she must contribute. Tell her that you're glad she's there.

Tips for Talking

- Allow her time to process and respond.
- For a little while, be willing to listen to the same question and repeat the same answer.
- Reassure, slow down, smile, and nod.
- Listen and respond to the feelings, not just the facts, he is trying to convey. Say, "You look frustrated," "You look sad," or "You sound mad."
- Speak calmly and clearly.
- Get his attention before you start talking.
- Simplify your message. Instead of "How about lunch now and then afterward we'll . . . ," try "Please join me for lunch now!"
- Try to explain what you mean one step at a time—it's frustrating for you to speak in bite-size or very concrete ways, but it sometimes helps.
- Instead of asking questions, offer suggestions. If she looks as though she needs the bathroom, for example, don't ask if she wants to go. Instead, say, "The bathroom is right here," and show her where.
- Don't help the second he begins to struggle to find a word but offer it before he forgets what he wanted to say.
- If she's having difficulty getting her point across, repeat back to her what you think she's saying. Then ask, "Is this what you mean?" or "Am I on the right track?"
- Use gestures or pictures to better explain yourself.
- If possible, look as if you're listening, even if you feel distracted.
- When you can muster it, use a calm, unrushed tone and pleasant expression.
- Don't talk to him as if he were a child.
- Don't talk about her when she's within earshot. (Remember, Alzheimer's doesn't impair hearing.)

- Avoid idiomatic expressions that could be taken literally or just misunderstood, such as "Hop in," "Jump up," or "Don't go there."
- Use humor and make fun of yourself.
- Don't correct him if he says something inaccurate unless there's a safety issue.
- Try "Let's go" rather than "Do you want to?"
- Don't respond to rude comments or take them personally.
- Use familiar phrases. Try terms or phrases from her work or hobbies. One woman discovered that saying "Everything is squared away" calmed her retired military husband down when nothing else would.
- Don't ask, "Do you remember when . . . ?" Instead, reminisce. A son might say to his mother who has Alzheimer's, "I remember when you let me pull up a chair next to you and help you bake cookies." Or a spouse will admire an outfit that his wife wore at her retirement party.

► DEMYSTIFYING DIFFICULT BEHAVIOR

Unbecoming conduct is usually an expression of unmet needs. Here's how to help your relative be more like the person he or she wants to be.

Although people in the middle stage of Alzheimer's are very different from one another, their challenging behavior generally falls into four categories:

- A loss of control, which includes disinhibition, unusual movements, sleep and appetite changes, and an odd kind of euphoria
- Psychosis, which includes hallucinations and delusions
- Mood disorder, which includes depression, anxiety, and apathy
- Agitation, including aggression and irritability or resistance

Families often talk about how their relatives' anger is more excessive or catastrophic than the problem warrants. Even if your relative was very mild mannered, he may now have a shorter fuse. He may also forget what is appropriate behavior or be unable to control his impulses. He may even threaten to hurt you or strike out. How to prevent or respond to aggression is the number one concern of families and professional care providers.

▶ **Warning:** In the middle stage, Alzheimer's generally limits people's tolerance for stress. Because their reserves are limited, they may get frustrated easily at seemingly trivial annoyances. A woman will jump out of a beauty shop chair in the middle of a comb-out and say, "That's good enough," because something just started to bother her. A normally gracious grandmother will fight with her toddler grandson over where to place the teddy bear.

Try these power tools for defusing anger. Again, don't expect perfection from yourself or your relative. Do what works for you.

- Instead of arguing, agree. It will calm him down, and calm is the prerequisite for cooperation and trust.

- Make eye contact, speak in soothing tones, touch gently.

- Don't try to reason. The disease has impaired her reasoning skills. Instead, divert or distract by taking her for a walk or a ride in the car. Offer her a familiar photo album or security object.

- Preserve dignity. Focus on helping him feel respected and useful.

- Never shame a person. If possible, do your divert-and-distract routine. If, for example, she starts to do something embarrassing such as getting undressed in front of others, simply say, "I bet you're ready for your robe and a snack." Mention two foods she could choose, while covering her with a robe or walking her to the bedroom. She probably is tired, hot, or uncomfortable. If she's prone to grazing at the grocery store, let her push the cart to keep her hands busy.

- Be excessively polite. "I'm sorry to interrupt you. Do you have time to help me now?" It may feel disingenuous, but the situation is already a little unreal, even without you channeling Emily Post.

- Change the environment. Turn off the television, go outdoors, turn on soothing music, get him something to eat or drink, get him something warm to wear or take off a layer.

- Don't blame yourself if you feel rushed, tense, or angry. Just try not to take those feelings out on her, or let her see your tense body language.

- Look for triggers that set off the behavior and work around them. For example, if a bath sets him off, try fewer baths per week. Try giving him a bath in the morning when you don't have exhaustion working against you or try a towel bath with no-rinse soap or shampoo.

- Pick your battles (safety first), and try to ignore what you can't control.

TAKING IT ALL OFF

Alzheimer's causes some people to feel a need to undress or shed clothes in order to get comfortable, and they forget what is public or private behavior. If nakedness happens, quietly cover him or move him to a private place and either distract him or wait it out. People take their clothes off at the wrong times for some pretty good reasons, such as having itchy skin, bothersome labels, clothes that fit poorly, or being too warmly dressed.

Try putting him in lighter clothes with soft seams, such as sweatpants instead of slacks. If all else fails, use clothes that fasten in the back or have lots of buttons, or turn his belt buckle toward the back. But anything that slows down undressing could interfere with getting to the bathroom in time.

When these "solutions" don't work and you're wondering why we even dared call them that, it's time for Plan B:

- Call for help. A fresh set of hands is vital.

- Wait it out. As long as you both are safe and reasonably comfortable, see if this too will pass. He may forget what was bothering him or get tired and fall asleep.

▶ AGITATION

People with Alzheimer's easily get agitated or anxious, and they show it by being restless, pacing, rummaging around, searching, yelling, or refusing to do something. It can be one of the most difficult symptoms for care provider and person alike. Agitation has emotional, physical, and environmental triggers.

Emotional Causes

- She is depressed, anxious, scared, confused, unsure of what's happening.
- He has become highly dependent on someone, and he can't see her and doesn't remember when she will be back.
- She can't communicate or even understand how she's feeling.
- He is having frightening delusions or hallucinations.

Physical Causes

- She's exhausted, hungry, thirsty, in pain, constipated, cold, hot, sick, or suffering side effects from a medication, alcohol, or caffeine.

Environmental Causes

- There are too many people or the wrong amount of stimuli (either too little or too much).
- The surroundings are unfamiliar, so he wants to leave as soon as he arrives. Even a friend's house may feel foreign to him.

When you see agitation developing, there are several things you can do:

- Try to remove whatever is upsetting him or move him to a quieter place.

- If you are in a car, get off at the nearest exit, because he may have a flight-or-fight reaction and bolt from the car.

- Modify the activity. If she is getting agitated doing a task that has become too difficult, change it or switch to something else, saying, "We don't need to do this right now."

- Offer her a security object. Having her beloved *New York Times* in front of her calmed down one older woman, although she no longer read it. Other people might like something soft to hold, such as a favorite shawl, warm tea to sip, or a cat on her lap. Some women enjoy holding dolls or stuffed bears.

- Exercise. If her agitation takes the form of pacing, suggest a better outlet for her energy, such as walking, riding a stationary bike, throwing a ball for the dog, or batting a small beach ball around with a tennis or badminton racket.

- Lock up or get rid of all dangerous objects, especially guns or other potential weapons.

Here are some comforting questions and comments to say when he or she gets agitated. (Keep a copy of this list where others can see it, in case they face the problem when you're not around.)

- May I help you?
- Do you have time to help me?
- You are safe here.
- Everything is taken care of.
- I apologize.
- I'm sorry you're upset.
- I know it's hard.
- I will stay until you feel better.

Try not, if at all possible, to

- raise your voice
- take it personally or take offense
- corner, crowd, or restrain him
- rush, criticize, or ignore her
- confront or argue with him

- teach her what she's not ready for or interested in knowing
- show alarm, make a sudden movement, or surprise him from behind

Agitation and other difficult behaviors sometimes diminish when people move to a high-quality facility for people with dementia. They no longer feel responsible for tasks they don't like or can't handle. ("This is an amazing place—I don't have to do any housework!" was one woman's response when she moved to her new home.) The physical design is suited to their particular needs. You don't want to and can't make your home into a professional facility, but you can

- get rid of clutter or confusing passageways, so he can move around easily
- leave out objects such as letters, photos, souvenirs, books, and small projects that trigger memories or give her something to do with her hands
- turn on his favorite music or a ball game (whatever he's enjoyed in the past)
- enhance natural lighting to remove the threat of darkness or shadows (although some people calm down in a dimly lit room)

Alzheimer's takes people out of the world of words, logic, and reason, and brings them into a landscape of feeling and sensing. Appeal to his senses through art, massage, the pleasant scent of food cooking, warmth, embraces, and, best of all, music. Music is a great tool for calming, motivating, and having fun. Play his favorite upbeat music for getting dressed, and after breakfast, push back the furniture and ask him for the next dance. One wife coaxed her husband to his day program each morning by literally dancing him out of the house and into the car. (She should be nominated for sainthood—most people don't have that sort of energy, which is fine.) Soothing music may help him get ready for bed. Select only music he knows and likes, recognizing that tastes can change, including with Alzheimer's.

► SUSPICIOUSNESS OR FALSE BELIEFS

In middle stage, people lose their hold on reality, and the results can range from sweet to disturbing.

► **All Aboard!** One former naval officer with Alzheimer's treated his floor of a nursing home as his ship and the residents and visitors as his worthy crew.

The two most common false beliefs are that a spouse is committing adultery or someone (usually immediate family) is stealing from him or her. Those ideas come from feeling she no longer has control over what happens to her or her things, fears of abandonment, and general confusion about what is lost or misplaced.

You probably can't talk her out of her beliefs, and trying may anger her more. If she accuses you of adultery, calmly say, "I am a one-woman man. You're stuck with me, hon!" or whatever light response would appeal to her. If she accuses you or someone else of stealing her book, for example, don't pretend you are guilty. Just say, "I understand you need your book. I'll help you get it back." The solution, as usual, is to reassure and distract (even when you feel like walking out the front door!).

He may think that you or other friends and family are imposters, and demand, for example, that they bring back his "real wife." Respond as calmly as possible with, "I'm sorry. Would you mind if I stay here for a while until your wife gets back?" Soon enough he will forget he didn't know you.

If you ever feel physically threatened or in danger (even if she doesn't seem stronger than you), leave the house immediately, call for help or call the police, and explain that she has Alzheimer's. (This is another example of why you must get all guns and other weapons out of the house.)

Realize that on rare occasions the fears and accusations are valid, as people with Alzheimer's are at risk of being taken advantage of. One man in an assisted-living facility for people with Alzheimer's complained that a woman entered his room and woke him up. The staff and family thought maybe it was a case of wishful thinking, but they discovered that one of the female residents was indeed paying him unwanted visits. (More on sex and Alzheimer's below.)

People in the middle stage may hallucinate or see something that's not there, especially if they have Dementia with Lewy Bodies (DLB). Hallucinations are a problem only if they scare or endanger someone. Sometimes people appear to be hallucinating when actually they are just confused, mistaking a mirror image for another person. If the person sees bugs crawling on him and scratches the skin off his arm, he needs medical attention. It might be dry skin, bug bites, anxiety, or hallucinations.

▶ **Note:** When confronting difficult behavior, repeat to yourself: "It's not about me or anything I've done. He's not choosing to be like this." Then give yourself a pat on the back.

Shifting the Focus

When he or she is agitated or angry, discouraged or distrustful, try whichever of these tricks you think might help:

- Rethink. Can you approach the problem in a different way, or even decide it's not a problem?
- Redirect. Distract him or move him to where his behavior won't be a problem.
- Restrict. Keep her away from situations or objects that will threaten her or your safety.
- Reassure. Speak simply and calmly. Touch lightly. Ask few questions.
- Remain realistic. Consider what he really likes and can still do and don't push him past his comfort level. Be real with yourself about your own limits and desires.
- Redefine success. Your goal is to keep everyone safe and comfortable. So if she's wearing her ratty old sweater but she's okay with her appearance, you've succeeded. If she's eating, even if it's ice cream before dinner (again), you've succeeded.
- Register. An ID bracelet or necklace can assist you if he gets lost or if you get hurt when alone with him.

FINDING HIS COOPERATIVE SIDE

When a person with Alzheimer's doesn't cooperate, it's usually because he feels frustrated, confused, scared, or physically uncomfortable. Spell out, step by step, where you are, what you are doing, and what will happen next. For example, say, "After this appointment we will go home and have your favorite soup." Limit his choices but acknowledge his preferences. "I know you want to go home, so we will skip the rest of our errands for today." Keep noise or confusing stimulation to a minimum.

If he's suffering from Alzheimer's-induced apathy, meaning that he lacks enough motivation, energy, or interest to engage or start any new activity, you or a friend can gently coax or encourage him to try something small. Too much stimuli will cause him to withdraw. For any activity you choose, assume he will need you to begin the activity with him. Also schedule lots of breaks to accommodate his short attention span and your needs as well. If he gets tired, the apathy may return and he may need to rest or stare out the window for a while.

What seems like apathy—he's gazing out the window and unwilling to budge—may not be. We don't know what's going on in his mind, and he might be remembering some wonderful times from long ago. Or his mind may be blank.

▶ WATCH OUT FOR WANDERING

▶ **Caution:** Don't leave a person with moderate Alzheimer's alone for even a minute in public.

People with Alzheimer's are at high risk of wandering off, of leaving and not telling anyone, and of becoming lost. Why does it keep happening, even to extremely vigilant care providers? Because it's impossible never to take your eyes off a person. Because it's hard to believe that your relative is at the point where she would walk away. But someone who is still able to dress herself and make polite conversation could very easily disappear while you are chatting with the salesclerk. (If she does, alert the staff immediately so they can watch the doors.) She's going someplace she thinks she should be. She might even be looking for you.

She could be watching you one minute, get distracted, and then forget where you are. So she goes to find you. She may go looking for you if you leave her alone for "just a minute," because to her a minute seems like an hour. She may get up in the middle of the night, think it's morning, think she has a job, and go to work, even if she hasn't held a job in years.

Predicting if your relative will wander or when is almost impossible, but there are clues. She is more likely to wander if her recent memory is very bad, if she has a poor sense of how much time has passed, or if she is impulsive.

Ways to Protect Your Relative

In Public

- NEVER let him out of your sight, when you're walking or biking on busy streets or in a park. People literally vanish in a crowd. Urban dwellers are so used to homeless people that they may not think to help your relative, even if he ends up on their doorstep.

- In public, hold hands or latch arms. One woman who holds on to her husband's arm in public was pleased when someone commented that they looked like newlyweds.

On Vacation

- If you are in a hotel, put a knob cover on the door and, if possible, disguise the door. One woman slipped out of the bed she was sharing with her daughter, unlocked the door, left the hotel, crossed a major highway, and walked into a gas station. Thankfully, the attendants thought to call the hotel, even though the woman didn't know where she was staying.

At Home

- At home, use knob covers as well, move the door latch out of sight, or disguise favorite exits with a Japanese screen.
- Ask the neighbors to tell you immediately if they observe her looking lost or confused, and teach them how to gently guide her home.
- Get a room monitor, so you can listen for him at night or if you go into another room during the day.
- If necessary, install alarms on your doors that ring when the door is opened.

Always

- Make sure your relative is wearing an identification bracelet or necklace. It's suitable (and critical!) for men or women.

If She Does Disappear

This can happen no matter how careful and conscientious you are. Don't blame yourself—or her. Take action quickly.

- Notify the police, neighbors, family, and friends. If she's wearing a Safe Return bracelet, which she should be, dial the toll-free number service immediately. Never wait, assuming she will return.
- Check places she talks about needing to go, like her old job site or her church.
- She can get farther than you think. Stories abound about excursions that people with Alzheimer's have taken on their own. One man bought a plane ticket with a credit card and flew across country—in his pajamas. He was noticed only when he refused to disembark. (This was before 9/11 and such strict airport security.)
- Have current pictures ready so others can identify her.

- In the unlikely event that she isn't found quickly, have an un-washed item of clothing available for use by search dogs and a print of her favorite shoe (on aluminum foil, kept in the freezer).
- Immediately put up posters of her, as someone may recognize her and call you.

When you find her, don't scare her by explaining the danger of what she did. She will probably beat you to it. "Where were you?! I looked for you everywhere!" Just be happy to see her again.

GOING "HOME"

People with Alzheimer's often say, "I want to go home," even if they still live in their home of many decades. This yearning probably comes from being unable to recognize current surroundings or people. They want the comfort and familiarity that make them feel at home.

How to respond? What usually helps if you have a minute is to say, "Okay, let's go," then drive him or walk around the block. When you come back in the house, say, "We're home!" Another option is to acknowledge his feelings. In a reassuring voice say, "You really miss home. Where is home? Tell me more about your home." Let him reminisce. One woman with Alzheimer's told her husband, "Home is where I remember things." Physically bringing him back to his childhood home doesn't usually help, because he may not recognize it. Having photographs of friends, family, and pets from over the years may make it feel like home.

► WHEN NO ONE'S GETTING ANY SLEEP

Normal aging often disrupts people's sleep patterns, and Alzheimer's disrupts them even more. Your relative may sleep either more or less than normal, and his sleep cycle will change. He may be unable to stay asleep at night for very long and doze off frequently during the day. He may have trouble moving from a dream to waking. This is a time when he is at risk of wandering, because he is disoriented, afraid, or needs something, such as help getting to the bathroom. Certain medications and Lewy Body Dementia may make dreams more vivid so he wakes up confused, mistaking dreams for reality.

The cause of his sleeping problems may be nothing more than headlights shining through the window or itchy skin. But you will probably have to do some sleuthing to solve his sleep disturbances. Start by looking at his sleep habits.

- Does he have a set time for going to bed and waking up? Don't be rigid, but try to establish times that are as close as possible to when he would go to sleep or get up on his own.

- What does he do when he wakes up in the middle of the night? Discourage television and suggest reading or listening to quiet music instead. A small glass of warm milk may help.

- Is he getting enough exercise during the day? Exposure to a little sun during the day, say on a midday walk, helps promote nighttime sleep.

- How much and when is he napping? He may be getting worn out trying to make sense of everything during the day and need a nap. Short naps in the mid- to late afternoon are helpful.

Next, investigate his sleeping environment.

- Are his nightclothes and bed comfortable? Some people feel constrained under blankets and need them untucked. A mattress that was once just right may now feel too hard or too soft.

- Does he like his bedroom? Make it inviting, cozy, and special. One man who always liked bright colors regularly showed off his yellow bedroom and bright orange bedspread to visitors.

- Does he feel lost in the dark? A night-light will help.

- Is he afraid or lonely going to sleep by himself? Sit with him until he falls asleep, or try a security object like a favorite pillow or throw.

- Is he hungry? Offer him a snack at bedtime, but avoid foods that may upset his stomach, such as fried foods, alcohol, spicy foods, and peppermint.

Finally, avoid stimulants.

- Is one of his medicines keeping him awake? Ask your pharmacist or doctor if any might be a stimulant. If so, don't give it before bed.
- Is he losing his tolerance for caffeine? Caffeinated soda, tea, or coffee, and even dark chocolate eaten later in the day have enough caffeine to disturb sleep.
- Are noises bothering him that he once ignored, such as traffic?

SLEEPING PILL ALERT

Don't give him a sleeping pill or any over-the-counter product that will make him drowsy without his doctor's permission. In fact, don't give him *any* medicine without his doctor's okay. People with Alzheimer's are very sensitive to medications. He could be taking a medication that doesn't mix with the one you're handing out.

► MEDICATIONS: WHEN BEHAVIORAL TECHNIQUES DON'T WORK

She eats well and gets exercise, her home provides a soothing environment, the doctor has ruled out any medical problems, you've tried communications skills, reassurance, and diversion tactics, and she still is agitated, sleepless, or showing other signs of being unhappy and unsettled. Don't wait until things get worse. Talk to a doctor about what medications might help. A nonsedative medication, such as an antidepressant, may make a big difference to her and your quality of life. (For more on medications to treat behavioral problems that arise in the middle stage, see Chapters 14 and 15.)

If you suspect that your relative needs medication, go to a doctor who knows your relative well and can do a thorough review of her pills and general health. The doctor must be experienced with treating the kind of problems you are facing and be available for follow-up appointments to see how your relative is doing on the medications. Over time, dosages need adjusting, and medications may need to be dropped or new ones added.

▶ **Counting on Kindness.** When someone with Alzheimer's is being difficult, try not to remind him that something is "good for him" or tell him how great he used to be.

▶ TAKING CARE OF PERSONAL CARE

I base my fashion taste on what doesn't itch.

—GILDA RADNER

Here's how to (and here's to) making baths and dressing pleasant parts of the day.

Bathing and grooming are an important part of your family member's day and use a lot of her limited energy. Stay true to the way she cared for herself before getting sick and use the products she preferred, but also make changes that will make your job easier.

Although some people with Alzheimer's (and some without it) would rather skip the daily rituals that keep us looking, smelling, and feeling presentable, it's up to you to see that your relative's basic hygiene needs are met. You may find that she can do a lot for herself but still needs assistance. Even if she is physically able to care for these matters on her own, no amount of physical strength can replace the mental muscle it takes to organize and remember the multiple steps involved in these seemingly simple tasks.

▶ **Try This:** She may just need help getting started, so guide her hand with your hand as she brushes her teeth or combs her hair. Once she gets going, step back and admire her efforts.

If she tries to handle grooming tasks without help, she may become frustrated, upset, or distracted and quickly wander off to do something more satisfying, such as stare out the window. So try giving step-by-step directions, such as, "Put the toothpaste on the tooth-brush," followed by gentle cues.

You will need to find a balance between helping and letting her do for herself. When you do a task for her, say, pulling a shirt over her head, she will soon forget how and, in most cases, not relearn it. You are also limiting her opportunities to help herself.

On the other hand, you don't want her to waste her energy or your patience doing something that is difficult and uninteresting, such as brushing teeth. You also don't want her to lose her teeth (which can happen when she is not brushing the back molars, where food lodges).

▶ **Dental Dos:** If she's resisting brushing her teeth or doesn't seem to like it, try a different toothbrush or toothpaste. Regular dental care, particularly to make sure dentures fit well, is important.

Steps to Bathing

One of the most common times people with Alzheimer's get mad or hurt their caregivers is when they feel their privacy and control over what's going on are being threatened, such as during bath or toilet-ing time.

To Help Make Bathing Pleasant

- Collect everything you'll need, such as soap, towels, powder, and comb. Keep hair dryers and razors out of his reach. Make sure the tub or shower stall has secure grab bars and a no-slip tub mat.
- Have both the bathroom and water temperature the way he has always liked it, but don't depend on him to judge tem-perature.
- If needed, use a shower chair and a handheld showerhead.
- If he is concerned about privacy, put a towel over his lap or shoulders and wash underneath or let him wash himself. Expose only one part of his body at a time.

- If he seems anxious, tell him what you are doing as you go along, encourage him by saying how well he is doing, and distract him with stories from the past. He may prefer to have music on or the opportunity to hold a soft cloth in his hands.

- He may enjoy putting lotion on his skin or, if you feel comfortable, having you apply it. (He may also really need lotion to prevent dry skin.)

- A bath or shower two or three times a week is plenty, unless he is incontinent. Buttocks and genital areas need daily cleaning. You can use disposable wipes.

If you've made sure the bath feels private and comfortable and she still resists bathing, here are some tips:

Tactics for Overcoming Resistance

- Don't ask if she'd like to take a bath or remind her that she needs one. Just say her bath is ready and it's just the way she likes it, then lead her to the tub or shower.

- Figure out what time of day works best for her. If she is resistant, drop it and try later.

- Try to understand her concerns. After days of refusing to step into the shower, one woman with Alzheimer's finally said to her care provider, "Why are you pushing me in there—it's raining!"

- Ask someone else to try helping her bathe.

- Go into the bath or shower with her. You can both wear bathing suits if being nude together isn't appropriate.

- It's okay for her to get in the tub dressed or in a robe. She may be willing to take off her wet clothing while in the tub or shower.

- Try alternatives to a regular bath or shower, such as a sponge bath or just washing and rinsing off with a wet washcloth and a no-rinse shampoo.

▶ **Good Advice:** While helping with dressing or bathing, check for any skin problems, such as dry skin, rashes, sores, or bug bites.

BEAUTY PARLORS FOR ALL

A regular outing to the beauty parlor or barber can be pleasant for men and women and a good way to get hair clean and nails clipped. If your relative resists going, tell him or her that you or a favorite grandchild needs a haircut. Be sure to follow through on what you promise. A regular appointment at an old-fashioned beauty parlor is lot less expensive than a home care aide to wash his or her hair for $18 an hour.

The Finishing Touches: Shaving or Makeup

Shaving, makeup, and other beauty rituals are where you can have fun. Men have personal preferences regarding shaving protocol, as women do regarding makeup, so indulge them. If a man has always used after-shave, keep it part of his routine. In the middle stage of Alzheimer's your relative can probably still wield his razor successfully and safely, but you will need to guide his hand back to missed places. You need to find a balance between helping him look good so people won't judge him, letting him do it himself so he won't forget how, and *not* driving yourself crazy every morning trying to get the man shaved!

A woman may feel as if she's forgetting something if she doesn't have her mascara on or feel undressed if she's not wearing jewelry. If you don't help her with both, her final look may be clownish. But as with shaving, you need to find the happy middle ground between letting her do for herself, keeping her presentable, and maintaining your sanity. If your relative is no longer interested in makeup, skip it unless it's important to you or other family members. If she still wants to shave her legs and under her arms, it's time to employ an electric razor for both. But as some women age, their body hair naturally thins and may not be noticeable.

All Dressed—Finally!

Here are some tips for how to help him get dressed without wearing yourself out.

Some people with Alzheimer's really like to be well dressed and ask frequently if they are wearing the right clothes. Others, for a variety of reasons, resist dressing and you're lucky just to keep them in sweatpants and their favorite shirt or T-shirt. If your relative is willing to wear only one outfit, buy duplicates of it. If he enjoys picking out his own outfits, keep only clothes in the closet that are appropriate for the season and his activities.

To avoid getting into a struggle over clothes, redefine your idea of success: He does not look silly, he is clean enough, and he is physically comfortable—not too warm or too cold and his clothes aren't chafing him. Compliment him when he's done dressing, even if you wouldn't have made the same choices. When you are having guests over or going out, help him dress nicely to ensure an easier reception by others.

Dressing Tips

- Lay out the clothes in the order they are put on, with underwear on top.
- If the only thing standing in the way of a woman dressing herself is a bra hook, offer her a camisole or undershirt instead. A bra that hooks in the front is easier than one that hooks in the back.
- Stockings and panty hose are difficult to get on. Offer knee-highs or tube socks.
- If a zipper and buttons are making pants difficult, try elastic-waist slacks and pullover jerseys.
- Avoid clothes with tight elastic, such as some socks or pants.

If you are helping him dress, limit his choices. Don't ask him what shirt he wants but instead give him two to pick between. Present him with one article of clothing at a time. Give him plenty of time to dress, particularly for finding those annoying armholes. Respect his privacy as much as possible.

MIRROR, MIRROR ON THE WALL . . .

People with Alzheimer's see their image, but the "What's wrong with this picture?" doesn't register. So they may look at themselves in their bedroom mirror, then proceed downstairs with zippers undone, three shirts on, and no pants.

A mirror can also be frightening. Some people see themselves and think the image in the mirror is a stranger or someone following them. Others enjoy the "companionship." When one woman saw herself in the mirror, she very politely said, "I remember your face, but my dear, I'm so sorry I can't place your name. It's good to see you again."

Toileting

Many people with middle-stage Alzheimer's continue to use the bathroom just fine, with only minor faux pas like forgetting to flush or wash their hands. But some people do have accidents because they do not or cannot ask for the help they need, and they can't find the toilet or use it properly. Incontinence usually comes later in the course of the disease. What your relative needs now are simply regular reminders or cues about how to use the toilet.

How to Help

- Look for signs that she has to use the bathroom, such as fidgeting with clothing, pacing, sudden mood change, pausing while she is speaking and looking around (for the bathroom). Then gently suggest she use the bathroom and, if need be, take her.
- Help her undress and sit comfortably on the toilet if needed.
- Leave the bathroom as soon as possible so she retains her sense of dignity and privacy.

▶ **Try This:** Asking to serve as his or her escort service (to the bathroom) may save both of you later embarrassment.

➤ BEING ACTIVE

"What am I supposed to do today?" The surprising but correct right answer to this question is, "Not much!" The family, not the person with middle-stage Alzheimer's, tends to be bothered by boredom. Asking "What am I supposed to do now?" more likely indicates fear rather than boredom and a need for reassurance that he or she isn't forgetting or missing something important.

Families often try to keep their relatives too busy or leave them directionless. Think broadly about your definition of an activity. Perhaps for your relative at this point getting bathed, dressed, and having breakfast are all mentally and physically stimulating and challenging activities.

People with Alzheimer's get very upset if they think they are supposed to be doing something that they are not doing. Adapt a task to fit their needs, but make sure the task is one that any adult would do. For example, say, "Do you have time to help me set the table—here are the plates." (You may still end up having to set the table for her.) You can also give them tasks that relate to their old job. A former teacher may appreciate being given spelling tests to check or some other assignment. Always assure them that they are right on target.

Move It

Staying mobile is one of the keys to staying healthy and happy. How to keep your relative moving will depend on his or her and your abilities. Whatever approach you choose, try to make it dependable and as much fun and pleasant as possible for both of you, so it will feel comfortable and reassuring instead of new and challenging. Here are some options:

- Go for walks, including in the mall if the weather or your streets aren't good for senior striders. Walking the same route gives you a chance to see other regulars. Use a pedometer and record increases in distance or speed to reward yourselves. Just remember that his balance will worsen over time, so offer him an elbow before a fall tells you he needed it.

- If he does fall, instead of trying to hold him up, ease him gently to the ground. If he is injured, make him comfortable and wait for help.
- Go to the gym together. At a gym, she can look and feel normal when she does the exercises that don't require too much thinking, such as the stationary bike. You'll get a chance to exercise as well.
- Exercise earlier in the day to avoid disrupting sleep.
- Dancing at home does count as exercise.
- If she'll be more comfortable exercising at home, buy a stationary bike. You can buy used ones. Just make sure she has the balance to stay on and you set the speed. Watching television or listening to music while exercising may help her exercise longer.

▶ **Take Note:** Television can be very disturbing for people with Alzheimer's, because they may feel as though whatever is happening on the television show is happening to them. Select cheerful, fun shows without complex plots, such as nature shows, musicals, or sports.

Chores as Distracting Activities

Suggest that he or she try doing these chores, even if you don't need them done or you have to redo them afterward. Doing them with you or another relative or friend makes them even more enjoyable.

- Kitchen duty: everything from rolling out cookie dough to peeling carrots
- Clipping coupons
- Sorting anything—poker chips, buttons, socks, laundry, coins
- Planting seeds, raking, watering flowers
- Arranging flower bouquets
- Sweeping and dusting
- Polishing silverware or shoes

- Folding clothes
- Washing dishes
- Grooming the pets
- Rolling yarn in a ball
- Sanding woodwork
- Emptying the garbage

▶ **Good Idea:** Leave small projects, such as scrapbooks in process, laundry to fold, coins to wrap, or a favorite jigsaw puzzle, out on the table for him or her to do alone or with you.

Your relative may also enjoy looking out the window; listening to music; looking at magazines or picture books on travel, art, fashion, sports, or nature; or playing with a pet.

You may wonder how much you should encourage or help your relative to keep up her former hobbies, work, or interests. The answer is as much or as little as you both have energy for, but you will have to modify the activities so she can do them without feeling embarrassed or frustrated. If she's very apathetic, however, you may not be able to help her muster the interest.

> The family of a lawyer who had Alzheimer's worked it out with his office so he could go to work every day, sit at his desk, and look through his mail and journals while his secretary, who now worked for others in the office, kept an eye on him. He felt dignified and content.

Try an Outing

Alzheimer's doesn't mean you forget how to play.
— *THE ALZHEIMER'S ASSOCIATION*

It's a good idea to get out of the house, as cabin fever can afflict everyone. Plus, errands are unavoidable, so making them as pleasant as possible is key.

- Plan, to go out when he is well rested, and stop for snacks or drinks.
- Limit your errands to one or two a day.

- Never leave her alone anywhere or even let her out of your sight, as she may wander off, even if she hasn't in the past.
- Visit the bathroom regularly.
- Keep a change of clothes, snacks, and extra water in your car or a purse or backpack.
- Make sure he wears warm clothes. Alzheimer's lowers people's tolerance for discomforts, such as feeling cold or hungry.
- Make plans that you can adjust easily, in case her mood doesn't match the moment.
- If you are dining out, choose a quiet or familiar restaurant, pick times that are less crowded, and invite only a couple of friends.

When looking for activities outside the home that he or she may enjoy, consider the following:

- Try events where it won't matter if he, and any guests or grandchildren you bring along, talk or move around, such as outdoor concerts or sporting events.
- Join volunteer activities, such as helping in a food kitchen. Plan on modifying the activity so she can do it, or you or a friend may want to work with her.
- Go to museums or historic points of interest, which often trigger old memories and interesting conversation.
- Some people who stopped attending or never attended religious services take pleasure in going.
- An old-fashioned drive in the country or just around the neighborhood can be soothing too.

Don't let your fear that he may make a mistake in public stop you from trying a potentially enjoyable activity. If something goes wrong, try to stay calm. He's more sensitive to your response than to the mistake. Try to ignore any rude comments or stares that may come your way and revel in the kindness you will encounter.

When a woman's father and two young children became a bit unruly all at once in a restaurant, an older man offered to help, saying, "I hope my daughter is as nice as you when I'm old!"

An elderly man found that when he took his wife, who had Alzheimer's, to church, everyone complimented him on how nice she looked and took no notice of her strange commentary.

► MAKE NEW FRIENDS AND TRY TO KEEP THE OLD

Staying connected to people who are important to you and your relative is not easy but is worth it.

Many family members of people with Alzheimer's find that friends stop calling or visiting. They feel uncomfortable and unsure how to interact with her, or they may feel scared and sad. They decide it's okay to stop calling, since she wouldn't remember the phone call anyway. You may need to look for additional or new friends, such as from a support group.

A VISIT TO REMEMBER

You visit me, your friend who has Alzheimer's. You bring something for us to enjoy together. Maybe a photograph album of a trip we took together or of a trip you just took. Maybe dominoes. Maybe some songs to play on the piano or music to listen to together. Maybe something good to eat. I'll ask for some tea to go with it. We go for a drive to see a nearby sight. You ask me questions and smile when I respond, and all my answers feel right. You tell me about people I knew, things we did together, about politics and golf. I feel smarter than I have in a long time. I'm tired when you leave. When my daughter calls and asks how my day was I say, "Great. A friend visited!" "Who?" she asks. "A friend," I say, smiling.

What her friends and acquaintances need to know is that she would be cheered by a visit or fun activity long after she can remember the event, plus you would certainly remember the kindness. People with Alzheimer's sometimes "rise to the occasion" and put on amazing performances for favorite friends, seeming almost like their old selves for an hour or so.

To encourage her friends, tell them when she's free for visits or outings and how much she enjoys seeing them. Make a brief tip list for visitors on how to communicate with her, what she likes to eat, how often she needs escorting to the bathroom, and any other details to make the visit or outing a success—including safety tips about wandering. That list will need to be updated as the disease progresses.

► SEXUAL INTIMACY IN THE MIDDLE STAGE?

The easy answer is yes, and then it gets complicated. People with Alzheimer's have romantic attachments and sexual feelings, even as the disease progresses. The part of the brain that hollers at us to at least get cozy with another human remains functional for quite a while. But problems with diminished drive or what spouses describe as forgetting how, where, and with whom to have sex may begin early in the course of the disease.

As with people of all ages and conditions, men with Alzheimer's may lose the capacity to attain an erection, women may have problems with lubrication, and both parties may have difficulty with loss of libido. But these problems play out differently under the influence of Alzheimer's. For example, the man may forget he just tried unsuccessfully to maintain an erection and try again. The couple may think they have a new relationship problem that is actually an Alzheimer's-related problem.

How long the sex drive survives may depend on both a person's condition and the importance he or she placed on physical intimacy before the onset of dementia. Not everyone will pursue sex, as changes in their brain from Alzheimer's or antipsychotic or antidepressant medications may dampen their interest or abilities.

People with Alzheimer's sometimes behave in ways that others misread as sexual. They may, for example, suddenly undress if they are warm or itchy or fiddle with a zipper when they have to go to the bathroom. Alzheimer's also causes people to misread cues, so when a care provider says, "It's time for bed," the person with

Alzheimer's may read that as a welcome invitation for companionship. Even touching in the context of helping someone dress may be perceived and acted on as a sexual advance. This is especially painful for teenage children, as their once very appropriate parent may make sexual advances after Alzheimer's begins to destroy their judgment.

▶ **Consider:** As the disease progresses, the person's world is becoming increasingly confusing. He or she may feel lonely and misunderstood.

About 10 percent of people with dementia have frontotemporal lobar dementia, which is characterized by a loss of impulse control, including sexual impulses. Instead of the typical first memory symptoms of Alzheimer's, patients have improper judgment about sexual behavior, such as making lewd comments to strangers or family in public.

Loss of impulse control creates some of the biggest problems for any care provider, particularly unsuspecting spouses. Alzheimer's can cause disinhibition, which means your spouse may be making the moves on you (or others) all the time, at the wrong times, or in public places. People with Alzheimer's may forget that they just had sex and want it again. And again.

Despite their mental impairment, people with Alzheimer's may feel ashamed or angry if they can't perform sexually, and their partners may feel guilty or disappointed. Then again, a well partner may not want to have sex or be intimate after having helped change her sweetie's clothes or wiped his mouth for the hundredth time that day. For couples that are relatively young when dementia upends their lives, the issue of intimacy is even more poignant, especially with children or other family members in the house.

If you or any children are uncomfortable about inappropriate advances, be clear and firm about it. Intimacy between adult couples can be maintained in new ways (touching, massage, kissing, or hugging), but the well partner must take the lead in setting the agenda, frequency, type, and place of sexual intimacy. Above all, try to ensure privacy for self-stimulating behavior or alternative sexual practices to save *everyone* from feeling embarrassed, fearful, or intimidated. You may need to seek professional help, and the family member with

Alzheimer's may need medication or alternate ways of meeting his or her needs for sensory stimulation. Sex is a tough issue for spouses and children, especially because you cannot talk about your sexual relationship in the ways you talked previously, now that Alzheimer's is in the picture.

► YOU DESERVE CARE TOO

Repeat often:

- Other good people feel the same way I do.
- New problems will occur even if I do everything perfectly.
- There is no obvious right decision.
- My choices are limited.
- My family, like all families, will disagree with one another sometimes.

Try as often as you can to make number one (that's you) number one on your to-do list. If you are exhausted, angry, frustrated, or in poor health, you won't be the person you want to be. Besides, you owe it to yourself and your family members to enjoy good times and good health. We'll introduce you to common signs of compassion fatigue and offer a refresher course on self-care.

Taking care of someone with Alzheimer's is stressful. Caring for your relative may make you proud or give you a sense of purpose. You may feel glad you are able to set an example for younger generations or keep him in his beloved home. But you also have a lot on your mind:

- Your relative's personality changes and unpredictable behavior
- The day-to-day chores
- The responsibility of thinking and acting for two people
- The nagging fear of what might happen next

All this can be very difficult, even with lots of help and support. You may find yourself asking, "What about me?" and "Can I survive this as long as he does?"

How You May Be Feeling

Anger and resentment are common feelings to most family members—and don't forget the guilt for feeling angry and resentful, because, as you keep telling yourself, she can't help the way she is. All anger is important to pay attention to. Everyone who has provided care for a long time is very familiar with it. Be sure to check out the Resources chapter for books on anger.

Feel Familiar?

- Embarrassed by your relative, even though you love her and want to protect her
- Ashamed of yourself for (see above)
- Angry at the doctors and other people for letting you down
- Guilty for neglecting your relative, your children, your spouse, your employer . . .
- Did we miss anything?

Well, this is what you may be missing: a sense of pleasure, motivation, privacy, intimacy, friends, hobbies, your identity, "the old you,"—— (fill in the blank)

So True. Get through today, fix things tomorrow.

If you ignore your negative feelings and losses for too long, your "Get-help-now!" indicator light is going to start flashing. Signs that it's about to go on:

- Instead of feeling tired occasionally, you feel depressed often.
- Instead of feeling busy, you feel overwhelmed, as if you are on a treadmill and can't get off, or as if you are losing your grip.
- Instead of her being on your mind, she has taken over your thoughts.
- Instead of having some downtime, you have no time to think.
- The problems you are facing have grown from minor to major.
- Instead of help, all you are getting from your family is criticism.
- You are abusing alcohol or food, sleeping too much, or using drugs to get through your day.

- Instead of just getting frustrated, you are losing it.
- The health and appearance of you or your relative are deteriorating from lack of attention or interest.
- You wish you could run away or that your relative would disappear.
- You feel like a failure.

▶ **Be Careful.** Self-destructive behavior is taking your frustration out on yourself.

Don't ignore your blues. If you or your family members think you are suffering from depression or anxiety, talk to your doctor and seek treatment. Time is not a cure for depression or anxiety; neither will it just "go away." Nothing will seem doable or pleasurable until your mental health is restored. Also, don't hide. Your relative's behavior may be unpredictable and erratic, so you avoid going out with him or her in public. But staying home usually makes matters worse. Everyone gets cabin fever, which increases the risk of anger and neglect. Remember, your relative feels alone, too. Take some of our suggestions below to end the isolation.

Add Meaning to Your Days

You may know not to sweat the small stuff, but too often we ignore the big stuff, like friends, forgiveness, and faith. Get the big stuff in order and the details (with some planning, nudging, and help) will fall into place.

Find someone to confide in. One source is an Alzheimer's support group (for more on support groups, see the previous chapter and contact your local chapter of the Alzheimer's Association).

Learn to forgive. Everyone, including you, your relative, other family members, friends, and doctors, will make mistakes. Work on forgiving people for disappointing you. Start by forgiving yourself when you make mistakes.

Set limits. If you feel exhausted, lower your expectations and examine your priorities. Say, "Sorry, I can't," more often.

Have a sense of humor. When you find yourself laughing at some of the, well, very funny mistakes that people with Alzheimer's make, don't think, "How could I?" Laughter provides relief and hurts no one, as long as you are discreet.

Take comfort in your spiritual beliefs and moral values. You may discover that they deepen as you continue caring for your relative.

Create a sanctuary. Turn a room, or just a corner of a room, into your cozy spot that reminds you to relax and enjoy. Decorate it with photos or art; keep a little supply of your favorite chocolates, nuts, or low-fat snacks nearby, along with a book, music, a journal, or sketch pad. You decide. It's your place.

Don't miss out on a minute to relax. Getting the mail? Read it outside in the sun. Making dinner? Put on some music. Waiting for him or her to finish? Close your eyes and remember a special time. Getting your hair cut? Ask for a new do, maybe highlights. Letting the cat out? Peek outside—see the stars? Learn the constellations.

Use a computer. It's your connection to friends and the outside world. If you don't have a computer at home, use the one at the library.

Caring for Everything Below the Neck

Taking care of your body improves your outlook.

- Exercise. If you haven't done so already, start an exercise program (get your doctor's okay first). Walk, either outside or in a mall; work out at a gym; use a stationary bike or exercise video at home. Your relative can join you in all of these, though you may want some time to yourself. Don't give up hitting golf balls or tennis balls if it's your passion. Favorite sports activities, even fishing, are as important as achieving a "target" heart rate.

- Eat a healthful diet.

- Learn ways to relax, such as meditation.

- Get a massage. People with Alzheimer's have been known to give great back rubs or massages. Trading places as "caregivers" is good for you both.

- Take a yoga or tai chi class or get a yoga video.

Take the time to do whatever makes you feel put together, and more like "the you" you like.

CELEBRATE YOUR RELATIONSHIP

If you are caring for a spouse, family member, or special friend, celebrate being a couple any way you can: hold hands, use loving words, have candlelight dinners. No matter what your relationship with the person you are caring for, visit places that hold meaning to you both, celebrate birthdays and anniversaries of special events, continue (with modifications) your family traditions.

If your relative no longer talks at dinner and you miss the conversation, it's okay to put on music or watch a movie during dinner or invite a friend or young neighbor who doesn't cook to join you. Some partners resort to talking to the dog or cat or the evening television weatherman during meals. At least they are never rude!

Caring for Your Financial Health

Part of taking care of yourself is taking care of your finances. Becoming a care provider can change your financial picture. If you were working full-time when you took on the responsibility of a relative with Alzheimer's, you may have cut back on your work hours, decline a promotion, or quit working entirely. If you haven't officially cut back on your hours, you may find yourself "absent on the job." You are there physically, but you are worrying about what is going on at home and not what's going on at work. You may be losing the positive self-image that comes with successful work.

Think hard before giving up that full- or part-time job or business to provide more direct care or supervision for your relative. You may lose your health insurance, retirement benefits, or tenure. Your job skills may decline and you may miss essential social and intellectual stimulation. Getting private health insurance can be difficult and expensive, particularly if you have or are at risk of having a medical condition.

If you are taking over the finances for the first time or merging your money with your relative's, start by making a budget. Don't forget those small expenses that add up. You may be surprised at how many household items or gadgets are "broken or lost" when

Alzheimer's is at work. Ask family members to help offset the costs of care or to take over the paperwork, endless phone calls, or more frustrating aspects of your day. Our Resources section lists groups and Web sites that provide information on how to determine eligibility for a variety of public and private benefits. You and your relative may qualify for help, even if you never needed it before.

PAYING FOR IT

Some states are experimenting with "cash and counseling" programs where they give families cash, in the form of vouchers, and counseling on hiring friends or even other relatives who want to help but can't afford to quit their day jobs.

► CHILDREN AND OTHER FAMILY MEMBERS

Alzheimer's is hard on everyone in the family, not just the person who has it or the primary care provider. Young children in particular are often confused by the changes in their grandparent. They may say Grandfather is funny but also resent that he absorbs so much of their parents' time. Children need simple explanations about why their grandfather interrupts conversations, reads the same thing on the ketchup bottle over and over throughout dinner, and isn't interested in them "like before."

- Explain that Grandfather has a disease, he has not always been like this, and he does not want to be this way. The disease is not catching, but it doesn't go away.
- Talk about what he was like as a younger man and share the stories you grew up with.
- Display pictures of the children with their grandfather when he was healthier.
- Tell them that Grandfather still loves them more than anyone in the world.

- Show them how they can make him smile or laugh. If Grandfather can still get a joke, give them jokes to tell him. One little girl learned to say that she and her sister were her grandmother's best medicine.

- Give the children small jobs to help Grandfather, such as turning the television on for him, bringing him his newspaper, playing a song they learned on the piano, or showing him their homework. He may have long-dormant drawing skills or enjoy a game of checkers.

- Praise and reward the children for helping with Grandfather.

- Be understanding if they don't want to be around him. Reassure them that their feelings are normal. Books and videotapes for children about Alzheimer's may help (see the Resources section).

- Try to make enough time for your children so they don't feel too resentful of their grandfather's needs.

- Never leave children in the care of a person who has middle-stage Alzheimer's, or vice versa.

► GETTING HELP FOR YOURSELF

Accept help when it's offered and look for it when it's not. Request assistance caring for your relative before you are desperate for it. If you wait, you may not have the time or mental stamina to find good quality help when another crisis strikes. What if someone else in your family became ill? What if you become seriously ill? When under stress, you are at greater risk than normal of getting sick.

One advantage of building your support system early is that other people, including professional care providers, can give you a fresh perspective on your relative's problems and capabilities. Someone else may find that he has abilities that he isn't using. Also, if you get help before his Alzheimer's advances, his new care providers will have a chance to know the "real" him.

► **Take Note:** It's almost impossible to convince some family members to let go and others to help.

Roadblocks to Getting Help (Detour Directions Provided)

The biggest obstacle to finding good care is the lack of high-quality, available, and affordable options. However, families can be their own worst enemies when it comes to getting help. They tend to get less help than they need or seek the wrong level of care. For example, they may think their relative could live in an apartment of an assisted-living facility, when he or she actually needs to be in a special facility for people with Alzheimer's. Here are some other "reasons" for not getting help:

"He doesn't want to go to adult day care."

Most people don't, until it becomes familiar and predictable. Also, if he's not happy there, he may not be happy at home either. To get him to go, explain that the staff would appreciate him helping or that it's "just for a few weeks."

"She says she's not ready."

Don't expect her to make the right decision in a timely fashion. Accept that she has changed and needs you to make important decisions for her.

"They won't appreciate or understand him."

Neither will you if you don't take a break.

"Those people are unreliable, they never show up on time."

Some services are more reliable than others. You may not luck out on the first try. One family used four agencies before finding one that provided great caregivers for many years.

"I don't really trust nursing homes or home care agencies."

A little mistrust is good, but only if it means you find the best aide or home, not if it means you do without. Many families are amazed to discover that their relative improves in the hands of a professional. Do a lot of research before you choose help, then monitor your relative regularly.

"No one cares for her the way I do."

That's true, but it's not necessarily a bad thing. Being around others, she will discover new interests. One wife was a little dismayed to see her husband happily dancing in the living room of his new group home with a (male) singer who came regularly to entertain the residents.

"We can't afford help."
This is the rainy day for which you or your relative has saved.

"We're saving our pennies for a rainy day."
It's pouring.

"I promised to care for him until 'death do us part.'"
Ensuring that he receives the help he needs now *is* caring for him.

"We take care of our own."
Your relatives developed their cultural traditions of caring for their own under different conditions, when family members lived together or nearby, didn't work outside the home, and had fewer older relatives with disabilities at one time. Also, using help does not mean you will be less involved; you are just expanding her care options.

"That's what we have daughters for."
Do your daughters agree? Unless they truly want to give up their existing responsibilities and pastimes, they won't provide quality help. If they aren't the primary care providers but instead regular visitors, your relative will enjoy their attention and show them off to his friends.

"I should be able to do this on my own."
Erase that from your rule book, and replace it with, "No shouldas, oughtas, or couldas."

One obstacle to getting help is not knowing where or how to start. The will is there, but not the how-to. Ask yourself:

- What would help me be the best advocate for him now?
- What does she need that I find hard to provide?
- Whom would we both trust?

Then think about what option would work the best for you both. Do you want to hire a companion to come to your home, or would she prefer the activity of an adult day program to someone she might view as an unnecessary bodyguard? Many people with Alzheimer's feel stressed by the need to entertain or keep a helper busy. Would a housekeeper to help you with chores be most useful? Communities differ greatly in the type and quality of available programs. Call your local Alzheimer's Association or county department on aging to learn about your options.

Sometimes people need help but don't go looking for it (even when their well-meaning children have given them a list of people to call), because they don't know what to expect of or ask from the service or provider. Will a "companion" feed my husband or just sit with him? Will a housekeeper keep an eye on my wife or just do laundry? Service providers should be happy to explain their expertise, limits, and skills and answer all of your many questions. You should request references, a written contract, or information on the service before you interview anyone.

▶ **Note:** No single program or service will be the right one for the entire course of the disease.

Family Help

Usually in families, one member is it when it comes to care, even if the person with Alzheimer's lives in a residential care facility. In fact, rarely do all family members take an equal or even a "fair share." Try to divide responsibilities equitably, rather than equally. For example, a daughter can take over money matters, while a son or older nephew can be in charge of doctors' appointments and other medical needs.

As an alternative to moving a relative to a residential facility, some families pass the impaired family member from one relative to the next. It's usually an effort to share responsibility, or a response to the primary care provider dying or getting sick. It's also usually a bad idea. A person with Alzheimer's needs a stable, familiar care provider and home environment.

▶ **Our Take:** Having one person as the primary care provider is easier on the person with Alzheimer's, but the care provider still needs lots of support, recognition, and backup from family and friends.

When you ask for assistance, don't just say, "I could use some help." Instead, be specific. Ask someone to take your relative to a doctor's appointment or for a haircut, and for lunch afterward if he has the stamina (mental and physical) to enjoy a two-part outing. Some families are fortunate to have a "support team" of neighbors, club members, or church members who agree to "adopt" the family, with each volunteer choosing one activity he or she prefers to do.

Consider setting up a weekly or monthly schedule and asking for volunteers to fill regular spots. You can post your schedule on a free Web site, and friends and family can choose, using their computer, the times they want. Your helpers are much more likely to stick with a commitment if they choose something they enjoy and can do easily.

Ask your friends or family helpers to come to your house, since most people with Alzheimer's don't adjust well to a new environment, even if it's just someone else's living room. Some people do like a change of scenery, but don't count on it.

When you leave her in the care of others, give detailed instructions on her daily routine, preferences, habits, recurrent worries, favorite expressions, and people she refers to often. Be honest about difficult behaviors, including eating inappropriate foods, wandering, undressing, or missing the toilet. Don't leave out anything for fear of scaring off the person or not respecting your relative's privacy. The helpers will discover the problems eventually anyway. Also, put away anything such as bills or personal materials that you don't want others to see.

Ask for the help you need. If you need a load of laundry done while you're away, say so. If someone handy is coming over, point out the leaky faucet or other little odd job that needs fixing. If you'd like them to pick up a prescription at the drugstore when they take your relative out for lunch, leave them some money and a note. If they can't or don't want to, they'll say no.

If helpers do what you ask but not the way or as well as you would, relax your standards. They can't be you. If a helper fails to show up, or shows up late, you may feel like you no longer want to use outsiders. But try not to fall into that way of thinking. Be patient and look for reliable support. It is critical to your mental and physical health.

► FRIENDS AND FAMILY AREN'T THE ONLY SOURCE OF HELP

You can hire trained, certified aides or companions through licensed agencies to come to your home. Home care aides from certified agencies start at eighteen dollars per hour and usually insist on a four-hour minimum visit. Before agreeing to hire anyone, volunteer or professional, check his or her references. Also, expect to kiss a lot of frogs before you find the perfect candidate. It's not easy to find someone you and your relative trust and like. Nor is it always easy to pay for professional care. If your finances don't allow for paid help, check the Alzheimer's Association and state family caregiver support programs for information on subsidized or voucher programs for in-home and day services.

A federally subsidized program for families whose relative is going to a day service and coming home at night is Program of All-Inclusive Care for the Elderly (PACE). Some programs offer in-home care at night and on weekends for people who go to day services. Other programs actually provide overnight and weekend care at the daytime site. In the future, you may have to pay assisted-living or nursing home expenses ranging from $4,000 to $6,800 a month, so now is the time to save if possible.

Adult Day Service and Respite Care

Adult day services offer recreational activities, outings, meals, and social contact and sometimes nursing services for isolated and frail people, including people with Alzheimer's. They can be very beneficial but are often underused, because families assume their relatives won't like the program and won't go. But many people with Alzheimer's actually benefit from and come to enjoy the scope and range of activities, especially the opportunity to be part of a group of new friends. It just takes time.

Recent evidence suggests that if a person living with a family caregiver at home attends a quality day program more than twice a week, there are measurable health benefits both for the person with Alzheimer's and for the family caregiver. A quality private program may be sixty-five to seventy-five dollars a day without transportation, but that's cheaper than having an aide come to your home. Many day programs have multiple private and public sources of funding for those who can't afford to pay full fare.

When deciding on a program, look way beyond price and hours of operation—check out the level of care, safety, and services. Ask about financial assistance and transportation options. Visit the program and stay long enough to listen in on conversations, talk to the staff and participants, and watch how the staff treats and converses with everyone. Make sure that the program staff is experienced with people with Alzheimer's, as well as trained, caring, and creative. The program needs to be certified, licensed, or surveyed by some governmental agency.

If you are just looking for a break from caring for your relative, or if you are going away for a few days, check out nursing homes or assisted-living facilities that take temporary residents on a space-available (but preregistered) basis. Such facilities can also address specific problems, such as helping your relative adjust to new medications, heal after an illness, or withdraw from alcohol or medications.

Getting Cooperation

To encourage your relative to try a day program, you may need to tell him that he's going to a class or a club, or ask him if he'd volunteer at the center. But first convince yourself that it's the right thing to do.

Then stay true to your decision. If he complains, don't argue. Just say, "They are expecting you" or "I hope you will try it while I am at work" (or wherever he thinks you are going). Once you get him there, the staff will need you to tell them how to help him get comfortable. When it's time for you to leave, they should reassure him that you will return for him. If all goes well, by the time he's forgotten that you are coming back, he'll have forgotten that you are gone!

Start with two or three days a week and add more days slowly. Once a week is too infrequent for him to become comfortable at the center.

As with everything that a person with Alzheimer's tries, if it doesn't go over well the first time, try again a week or two later.

How to Leave

Whether you are leaving him at a day facility or at home with an aide, there's no one right way to leave. Try different approaches, from a proper good-bye to casual comments about "going to throw in another load of wash" and then leaving quietly. Some people with middle-stage Alzheimer's separate easily, but most don't.

Try to use the time away to really recharge your batteries. Paying bills or cleaning the house rarely recharges batteries!

NOT THE PERSON HE WAS

When hiring people through a local agency to come to your home, you may discover that your relative has become homophobic or developed prejudices against different racial or cultural groups or people who are overweight. Even seniors who once prided themselves on opposing racism, for example, may become overtly racist. Alzheimer's-driven prejudices are common and hurtful. You can't change the person, so simply apologize to anyone he has insulted and alert future service providers to the problem.

Care Managers

If you are having trouble finding someone to help you care for your relative with Alzheimer's, if you need help overseeing and managing your relative's care because you are far away, or if you have a particularly complicated situation, a professional geriatric care manager can help you assess the level of care you need and help find, evaluate, and monitor the people to meet those needs. Many care managers are nurses and social workers who can see you through all stages of the disease.

But—and this is a big but—they are expensive. They charge $350 to $500 for an initial assessment and recommendations, and $75 or more an hour thereafter. You will want someone who is trustworthy and experienced enough to be worth the money. To find a care manager, check out www.caremanager.com. When you interview candidates, ask to see their credentials. Also find out exactly what tasks they do themselves and what they "outsource" to others. For example, they may have assistants who take your relative to a doctor.

Some care managers are also financial planners who can suggest ways to improve your cash flow, identify tax savings, review investments, or make suggestions to keep a larger portion of your investments in lower-risk, easily accessible money market or short-term bonds. Often, care managers have a network of trusted referral sources such as elder care attorneys and home care agencies.

► HOSPITALIZATION HAPPENS

People with Alzheimer's usually end up in the hospital because of an emergency, such as an injury from a fall, or from an illness or medication reaction that went undetected. Doctors try to keep people with Alzheimer's out of hospitals because it's so disorienting for them and fraught with potential risks. Hospitalization increases the risk that a person with Alzheimer's will fall, get an infection, or become delirious. But sometimes hospitalization is unavoidable.

To make her visit to the hospital emergency room easier, have a bag packed with everything she will need for an overnight stay, even when she is home and well, including:

- A copy of her medical history
- Extra medications
- A list of her medications, including over-the-counter medicines, and food allergies
- Medical insurance information
- Health-care proxy
- An advance directive

Include a change of clothes and toiletries for yourself, your medications, a cell phone, important phone numbers, snacks, and a note explaining the person's dementia and particular preferences or needs in case you can't talk to the staff in private.

Call a friend or family member to meet you at the hospital, to keep an eye on and comfort her while you are filling out the medical forms and talking to medical staff. Write down her symptoms so you won't forget one.

Once You Are at the Hospital

- Preferably where she can't hear you, tell the staff right away that she has a memory problem.

- If needed, give the staff some communication tips so they can question her more successfully. For example, you might say, "She responds best to Dr. Smith or Cynthia" or "She can hear fine—please don't yell."

- If the medical staff is talking about her as if she weren't in the room, ask that they speak to both of you.

- You or another family member, friend, or private duty nurse should stay with her all night. The regular nurses cannot watch her closely enough and she may get confused or hurt trying to get out of bed, even if she hasn't done so before. When one older man with Alzheimer's fell while getting out of his hospital bed unsupervised, he—accidentally and quite painfully—yanked out his catheter tubes.

- Try to be at the hospital in the morning, when medications are given, procedures take place, or doctors make rounds.

- Leave a note if your relative can read: "Honey, you fell and broke your hip. Please rest until I can get back."

▶ **Take Note!** Any sudden change in her confusion levels or awareness may signal a medical problem, such as a urinary tract infection, pneumonia, or other infection. Get care *immediately*.

▶ WHEN A MOVE IS A MUST

It's often after a hospitalization that family members realize that their relative has to move to a home or facility that offers greater care.

Making Room in Your Home

When someone you love, feel protective of, or simply feel indebted to can no longer care for himself, it's instinctive and generous to invite him to live with you. But it's not always a good idea. Ask yourself these questions before issuing an invitation:

- How well do you get along? Living together can exacerbate differences.
- What do others say about your plan? Will relatives be helpful or resentful?
- Is your home large enough for everyone to still have privacy and to adapt to your relative's changing needs?
- Do you have a Plan B, if *you* get sick, hurt, or, God forbid, die?

If your relative does move in, make sure you

- set limits—you can't do everything for him
- have a routine, but be flexible
- help him take on some household chores (even if you have to redo them)
- be ready to compromise
- give everyone time to settle in
- have a backup plan if the arrangement doesn't work

Residential Facility

Families of people with Alzheimer's consider many factors when deciding where their impaired relative should live (see alz.org/SNAP for Seniors, a national dementia-specific senior housing database). When the well-being and safety of all involved are put first, the family often decides to move the relative to a residential facility. The primary care provider may not feel ready to let go, however.

Like many of her peers, eighty-year-old Jill felt bad about moving her husband until her kids explained they feared losing two parents to one illness. The children helped her accept that the stress of providing care was taking a visible toll on her health.

But Jill also needed them to listen as well. She was sad to lose her husband. She wanted to be a couple, as they had been for fifty-plus years. She was lonely, tired, and scared. His move to a nursing home felt like a death to her, yet in no way protected her from grief when he did die.

Reasons to Move Your Relative

- Your health is failing.
- She needs more care than you can provide.
- He won't leave you alone.
- Neither of you is sleeping at night.
- She is becoming aggressive, and medication and behavioral interventions aren't helping.
- He is becoming less mobile.
- She is falling often and you must call for help to get her up.
- He is aggressively resisting all attempts at care.
- You are exhausted.
- You have no other sources of help.
- You want your life back.

Deciding that she needs to move from her home or yours is one of the most difficult decisions you will make. Families are under stress no matter where their relative lives, but the stress is worse right before a move. The decision brings up conflicting feelings. You may feel guilty but also, perhaps, relieved. You worry about the quality of the facility yet also dread the expense of a top-notch one. You worry about missing her or being lost without her. You feel as though you failed to live up to commitments or to make her well or happy, yet you know you've tried to do your best.

Unfortunately, this is when friends and even family members say the most insensitive things, like, "Well, she won't know the difference" or "Now you can take care of yourself" or "I could never do that to my mom." (We're not exaggerating.)

Paying for It

If or when the time comes to move, you will need a plan for how to pay for a residential facility. Many families can't afford private nursing home care and are just over the income and asset limit to qualify for Medicaid. Medicare does not cover nursing home or assisted-living costs. There is a big "no care" zone for many people with moderate- to late-stage Alzheimer's.

Some families have been advised to give away their assets to their children, so they qualify for a nursing home that takes Medicaid. This isn't a good idea. For one, there aren't a lot of facilities that accept Medicaid, and even fewer high-quality ones. Second, for up to five years after the parent dies, Medicaid can ask for the money back from the children to pay the nursing home bills. (Medicaid will not, however, expect the surviving spouse to give up his or her home, nor does Medicaid expect children who have not received their parent's money to pay for a parent's bills.) A better option is to move your relative into a good facility, pay the fees as long as you can, and when you run out of money, turn to Medicaid. The facility may well accept Medicaid then, since your relative is already a resident.

Ready to Move

To make the move easier, learn about possible residential facilities for your relative before the need arises. If there is an emergency, you may have little time to prepare. Also, the move will be easier if you are somewhat familiar with the facility or staff. You may need to get on a waiting list for a quality facility, particularly if you are in an area where few facilities exist. You may want to take him with you when you visit a place; it depends on whether the visit would interest or upset him. If you know someone living in the facility, make it a social visit. At some point prior to being admitted, however, your relative will have to meet the admissions staff.

Moving your relative to a residential facility is difficult, because in the back of your mind you are thinking, "This is the last stop before the final stop." But that's not how your relative is seeing it. The disease can sometimes free people from an awareness of their own mortality. If you've found a good place and you advocate regularly for your relative, it will be a home where he is safe, encouraged, stimulated, and respected.

► IN SUMMARY

As your relative's Alzheimer's worsens, your role as care provider or family member gets harder. It also becomes even more important and worthwhile. Family members who care are forever changed by the experience, and sometimes in good ways. Family members tell us they

- feel more passionately about life and their families
- commit more fully, with greater patience and compassion, having made many tough and complex decisions
- learn to live with the "gray" uncertainties of life, giving up the simple black-and-white sense of control that never fits experience
- are less concerned with trivial, insignificant, or surface fluff
- find it gratifying to share what they have learned with others
- are strong enough to "seize the day"

PART FOUR

► **WHEN IT'S MORE THAN MEMORY LOSS**

CHAPTER THIRTEEN

CHANGES IN BEHAVIOR AND EMOTIONAL WELL-BEING

*For an actor there is no greater loss than the loss of his audience.
I can part the Red Sea, but I cannot part with you . . . If you see a
little less spring to my step . . . you will know why. And if I tell you
a funny story for the second time, please laugh anyway.*
— ACTOR CHARLTON HESTON ON ANNOUNCING HIS DIAGNOSIS OF
ALZHEIMER'S IN 2002

If your relative is suffering from depression, anxiety, insomnia, apathy, agitation, hallucinations, delusions, or other emotional or behavioral symptoms, this chapter—and a great deal of sympathy—is for you.

"A little more irritable" is how Angelina described her husband to his doctor, when they went for a checkup. Lyle, a sixty-seven-year-old retired science teacher, had been in good spirits prior to his recent diagnosis with early Alzheimer's. "He gets really anxious two or three times a day for about ten to fifteen minutes, usually when he forgets something, and he can't sit still—he's sort of agitated and nervous."

Just three months later, Lyle had lost interest in his hobbies and was preoccupied with worries about his health and finances. Despite having previously been a sound sleeper, he was waking regularly at three A.M. in a panic, his heart racing. His anxiety was also making his memory worse and, for the first time in his life, led him to consider suicide as a way out.

Angelina was scared of leaving him alone. When he was napping, she finally called his doctor, who convinced her to bring him in under the pretext of having a routine physical. At the visit the doctor diagnosed him with an anxiety disorder and panic attacks. He recommended breathing exercises and some medication. The doctor convinced him it would "help him relax." Lyle went along with the treatment, to everybody's relief.

Stories of subtle or dramatic personality changes are common in the world of MCI and Alzheimer's. Sadder yet, the behavioral and emotional problems can grow worse as the brain's health declines over time. Fortunately, the drug treatments for these symptoms have improved, though the drugs that are available are still imperfect and most have not been as widely studied in people with Alzheimer's as have memory drugs. As Chapters 11 and 12 explain, some of these problems can be alleviated through nondrug means, and you should definitely explore these before or at least while trying medications.

Left unrecognized and unchecked, emotional and behavioral problems can get to the point where the person no longer enjoys life, alienates family and friends, is a risk to himself or herself and others, and can no longer live at home. To reduce the behavioral and emotional symptoms of Alzheimer's, you need:

- Early recognition and treatment
- Flexibility and patience on the part of the family
- A pinch of good luck

With these, you will find a new and more peaceful normal.

► **Take Note:** Studies show that untreated behavior problems in people with Alzheimer's—especially wandering, aggression, and agitation—are more likely to lead to institutionalization than poor memory and confused thinking.

► HOW COMMON ARE THE BEHAVIORAL AND EMOTIONAL WOES?

The answer is *very*. A recent large study of people with dementia, including Alzheimer's, found that three-fourths of the group had experienced depression, apathy, irritability, or some other psychiatric problem within the last month. Meanwhile, half of the group had two or more of these symptoms over the last month and slightly fewer had experienced three or more.

Even though so many people suffer from these ills, medical experts haven't described and categorized them as thoroughly as we would like. While one doctor may see a patient as being depressed enough to require medication, another might view the same patient's symptoms as normal, everyday blues.

Sometimes the person with Alzheimer's fools a doctor, particularly a doctor who isn't so experienced with Alzheimer's. Your relative may act like Prince Charming in the doctor's office and a grumpy old man at home. (People with Alzheimer's may be on their best behavior for brief periods, but the disease prevents them from keeping it up.) Also, guilt or shame may keep people in the early stages from reporting their symptoms.

► RECOGNIZING DEPRESSION

Depression is one of the most common symptoms of Alzheimer's, affecting about 20 percent of those with Alzheimer's, compared with only 8 percent of nondemented older people. In addition to making life more difficult for the depressed person and his or her loved ones, depression can worsen memory in the following ways:

- It impairs concentration and, therefore, learning.
- Stress and depression may damage nerve cells, adding to the damage already caused by Alzheimer's.
- Depression may worsen some medical problems, such as heart disease.

- Autopsies of people with Alzheimer's reveal that those who were depressed had more plaque in their brains than the non-depressed individuals.

Depression usually starts out more gradually in people with Alzheimer's than in other older people—and may also look more like anxiety, agitation, or extreme apathy than what you think of as depression. A good test for depression is to get the attention of a person with Alzheimer's, then ask a question and start counting. If it takes a long time for her to respond, she may be depressed. Nondepressed people with Alzheimer's are usually very eager to answer, even if it's not an accurate response. Alzheimer's can also cause people to become obsessively guilty (or delusional) about something that happened long ago.

▶ **Note:** Appearing sad is not a requirement for being depressed when you're older or when you have Alzheimer's. Many people with Alzheimer's deny feeling sad or depressed.

Having several of the following symptoms for a few weeks or more could be a sign of serious depression and warrants a call to the doctor who is treating your relative's Alzheimer's:

- Being unable to feel pleasure or enjoy much of anything. If you ask your relative whether a special outing or a visit from a beloved out-of-town relative would please her, she might say, "Not really."
- Being sad, tearful, terribly discouraged, worrying excessively.
- Withdrawing from normal activities and people.
- Having unexplained physical symptoms, including aches and pains, low energy, lost libido, trouble sleeping, an increase or decrease in appetite.
- Being unusually agitated and irritable, and having trouble concentrating.
- Having suicidal thoughts or feeling like a burden and that life is not worth living.

▶ **Note:** Don't be afraid to ask your relative if she is having these thoughts and feelings. You won't make her feel suicidal or worthless just by asking about it.

When you talk to the doctor, you want to find out if your relative needs to be seen right away. You also need to ask if that doctor is the right person to assess and treat your relative's emotional well-being. The following may indicate that your relative should be assessed and treated by a geriatric psychiatrist or behavioral neurologist, *and* that he or she may need emergency care or hospitalization:

- Talking about suicide, "going to sleep and not waking up," or "just ending it all"; saying "life is not worth living" or voicing specific plans to end one's life
- Drinking a lot
- Being very uninhibited, such as spending too much money or being too sexual
- Hallucinating or having delusions
- Getting very confused
- Acting manic—being very down or very up
- Violence or any behaviors that put the person or others in danger

▶ **Take Note:** Depression will worsen memory, concentration, and thinking speed. In extreme cases, depression can masquerade as Alzheimer's, a condition called pseudodementia.

Irena, a former art teacher who had mild cognitive impairment, developed depression in her sixties. Her depression worsened her memory. When she went for a checkup and took a memory test, the depression lowered her score so much that her family doctor thought she might be suffering from early-stage Alzheimer's.

Irena says, "I was feeling terribly sad and down after losing my husband of thirty-five years. He made such a difference in my life and really helped me with my memory. I wasn't even enjoying spending time with my four-year-old grandson, whom I adore. I was also getting very absentminded. My internist gave me a memory test, which I did poorly on. He thought I might have progressed to early Alzheimer's and sent me to a geriatric psychiatrist, who asked me a lot of questions and gave me more tests. Although my memory was still poor, he said my problems looked more like depression, and he started me on an antidepressant. It took a while to work, which really disappointed me, but I think that now it has helped. Best of all, I'm doing better on my memory tests, and the psychiatrist said I haven't progressed to Alzheimer's."

Grief after a major loss is a normal part of bereavement, and people with Alzheimer's or MCI are no different in this regard. When the grief persists and interferes with the person's daily functioning, it's time to consult with a doctor about possible treatments. For people in the early stage of Alzheimer's, a combination of psychotherapy and medication may be most helpful. The big problem for many families, however, is when people with Alzheimer's refuse both.

Studies of people's brains indicate that depression may actually shrink memory centers in the brain and weaken the connections between nerve cells. Therefore, early treatment of depression is key to preserving memory as well as quality of life.

► APATHY

Apathy often goes along with depression. Although very different from procrastination, apathy steals people's motivation to join in or begin daily activities and eventually causes them to become quite withdrawn. It can arise from chemical imbalances in the brain, as a side effect of some medications, or from small strokes that damage the brain's motivation centers. When you ask a person with serious apathy how he is feeling, he may say blah and indifferent, or that he has no feelings good or bad.

Apathy is difficult to differentiate from depression and many primary-care doctors don't make the distinction. Yet a doctor will need to hunt down the cause of the apathy, such as strokes, thyroid problems, or vitamin deficiencies.

► SUICIDE RISK

In the weeks following a diagnosis of Alzheimer's, family members need to watch their relative closely for signs of depression, anxiety, alcohol abuse, or suicidal thoughts or behaviors. If your relative is saying something, even in a joking tone, such as, "I want a consult with Dr. Kevorkian," take his words seriously. Suicide is not rare in people with Alzheimer's, and there have been cases of high-functioning people with early-onset Alzheimer's or MCI who committed suicide. A prior history of depression, manic depression, drinking problems, and serious medical conditions or pain increases the risk for suicide. So if your relative is giving you reason to worry, tell the doctor right away.

If your relative spends a lot of time alone, such as in his basement shop, make sure you check the area and dispose of or lock up any firearms or potentially dangerous items. Ask your family member directly if he has had suicidal thoughts after his diagnosis, whether he has considered any specific suicide plans, and what he thinks makes life worth living. His answer to the last question could help you and your doctor get some joy back in his life as the depression is treated.

► RECOGNIZING ANXIETY

Alzheimer's makes people prone to anxiety, which often goes hand in hand with depression. Common symptoms of Alzheimer's-related anxiety are:

- Excessive or unwarranted fearfulness, worry, or panic
- Specific worry about the future, such as about health, finances, or a move
- Fear of being by oneself or of being with a group

The anxiety often manifests itself as repetitive questions about the person's own health, future care of children or spouse, or an upcoming appointment or visit. (Anxiety medications are discussed in Chapter 14. Lifestyle and daily management tips for helping your anxious relative are in Chapters 16 and 17.)

► SLEEPLESSNESS AND ALZHEIMER'S: AN EXHAUSTING MIX

Here's a statistic that will keep you up at night: In a group of 205 people with Alzheimer's, 24 percent woke up family members regularly and 9 percent had nightmares or nighttime fears. The sleep disturbances seen in Alzheimer's include:

- Sleeping too much or too little. People with Alzheimer's can go on wakefulness and sleeping binges, such as staying awake nonstop for two or three days and then sleeping twenty-four hours.
- Too many daytime naps
- Waking up early and not being able to get back to sleep
- Having difficulty breathing while sleeping, usually because of sleep apnea
- Sleepwalking and wandering

Causes of and Cures for Sleeplessness

Many factors contribute to sleep disorders in people with Alzheimer's, including damage to the brain's sleep chemicals and sleep centers, depression, and other medical problems. But just like anyone else, they will have trouble sleeping if the conditions aren't right—if their rooms are too bright, too noisy, or the wrong temperature, if they had too much tea before bed, or if they took too many naps that day. However, they can't describe or solve the problem as well as a person without Alzheimer's.

Sleeplessness is worth solving, because sleep is so important for proper brain functioning, including for consolidating memories and repairing nerve cells. Also, sleep disturbances are one of the major predictors of nursing home placement. Family caregivers' patience and stamina can't survive indefinitely with interrupted sleep. If you've not succeeded on your own in improving your family member's sleep, ask his or her doctor for a referral to a sleep specialist, who will assess all aspects of his or her sleep patterns, including:

- The quality of sleep—is it deep and restorative?
- Length of sleep

- Time it takes to fall asleep
- Wakeup time
- Leg movements
- Nighttime breathing problems
- Snoring
- Use of sleep aids
- Daytime alertness

The specialist may recommend a polysomnogram, a test that diagnoses sleep disorders. It can detect sleep apnea, a potentially fatal blockage in the airway that affects about 30 percent of people with Alzheimer's. People without dementia get it, too, but slightly less often. Apnea poses a particular problem for people with Alzheimer's, because their brains may fail to signal the respiratory system to do its job. In addition, apnea may worsen the effects of Alzheimer's by starving the already struggling brain of oxygen.

The good news is that a lot can be done to treat this condition, including wearing a device over the face, called a CPAP, that flows oxygen into the nose and into the airway. It works, but it's very annoying for some people to use. Surgery may also help. Apnea is more common in people who are obese or who have high blood pressure, so treating these conditions can help reduce or eliminate the problem.

Other conditions that can affect anyone, restless leg syndrome (RLS) and periodic leg movements (PLMs), are what their names suggest: uncontrollable movements of the legs during sleep. Researchers don't know what causes these conditions; they may be hereditary or linked to nutritional or chemical deficiencies or both. They are treated with medications that increase a brain chemical called dopamine.

► DELUSIONS, HALLUCINATIONS, AND RAGE

Alzheimer's can cause the behaviors we fear most in ourselves and others: anger, rage, and aggression. People with Alzheimer's may shout, curse, shove, push, and more. The disease can also cause a relentless agitation; people become literally unable to sit still, much less lean back in a chair and relax.

Psychosis is a mental disorder or state where the person's mind is out of touch with reality. At least 40 percent of people with Alzheimer's have psychosis over the course of their illness. With Alzheimer's, it's marked by:

- Hallucinations—hearing, seeing, smelling, or feeling things that aren't there or having a distorted version of what is there. The most common psychotic hallucination is seeing people, usually intruders, in the room.

- Delusions—unshakable and irrational beliefs, such as thinking a parent or spouse is coming for them, the police are after them, or their children are stealing from them.

- Paranoia and unwarranted suspiciousness—such as thinking frequently that the care provider is poisoning them with medications, or believing, despite a complete lack of evidence, that a spouse is having an affair.

These complex and disturbing behaviors and conditions can prove very dangerous. A person may act in response to a hallucination, strike out in a rage, or to try to protect herself physically. It's not usually what people around her say or do that causes these behaviors; it's the illness brewing in her brain. Changing the social or physical environment or how you speak to the person (see Chapter 12) can reduce symptoms, but it won't cure them.

WHAT IF HE'S NOT IMAGINING IT?

Particularly if you don't live with your relative, make sure that his "delusions" are really distortions and not something that actually happened. One elderly man with mild Alzheimer's complained that someone was stealing from the shed after he and his wife went to bed. His wife was worried that he was hallucinating and called the doctor about what to do. The doctor asked whether he was exhibiting other odd behaviors or having delusions. If he seemed okay otherwise, it was probably nothing to worry about. But tired of her husband's complaints, the wife stayed up late one night to see what was going on. A bear was coming from the woods and raiding the garbage! Thanks to his curious wife and reasonable doctor, the husband avoided being put on unnecessary antipsychotic medications. Others aren't so lucky.

If nondrug approaches to control your relative's emotional or behavioral symptoms have failed, you may be ready to call her doctor about medications. But the first thing the doctor should do is to rule out the many possible medical or drug-related causes of psychosis. For example, if someone is hearing odd sounds or ringing in the ears, it may just be from taking a large dose of aspirin or antibiotics or from an ear infection. Even deafness in one ear can cause a person to "hear" music, a type of musical hallucination. A small stroke can cause someone to sound as if he is speaking in a foreign language. Toxicity from high doses of steroids, which have been prescribed for other medical conditions, can sometimes cause irritability or aggressive behaviors. So do not automatically assume odd behavior is a natural progression of Alzheimer's. It could be something that needs medical treatment.

▶ TAKE NOTES

If you can find the time for a week or so, keep a diary of your relative's symptoms to show the doctor. You are probably an expert now on her symptoms, yet they are new to the doctor, who should look over your notes to get a picture of what is going on.

In the diary, describe your relative's worrisome, odd, or otherwise disturbing behaviors, moods, or patterns that weren't present pre-Alzheimer's (don't bother with the weird stuff she did when she was "normal"). Note if she's glum, sad, anxious, withdrawn, irritable, or all of the above. Write in the diary whenever you have a chance, so you can draw a complete picture of what is happening. The more accurate and detailed you are in your description, the more helpful it will be to the doctor.

► **A Bonus:** Keeping a journal can help you feel more sane and in control, too. You will know you aren't imagining the extent of your relative's problems.

Be sure to include the following information in your diary:

- Start date
- The frequency, timing, and predictability (or not) of the troublesome behaviors
- The severity
- The duration of the symptoms and whether they wax and wane or are continuous
- Possible triggers
- What makes them subside
- Whether they are getting worse over time
- If and how they pose a safety threat
- How they interfere with your relative's day-to-day functioning
- Any medication changes or changes in health
- Strategies you've tried

INSIDE THE BRAIN

When someone you know well is behaving in a way that is foreign, you can't help but wonder what is going on in his brain. Well, a lot is going on. Just as plaques and tangles damage a person's thinking and memory centers, those hallmarks of Alzheimer's cloud the brain's limbic system, a collection of structures deep in the brain that help to regulate emotion. Plaques also tend to build up in the brain's frontal lobes, the area generally considered in charge of attention and impulse control. Blockages in vessels may be depriving the brain's emotion centers of adequate blood, causing strokes. All of these can lead to the depression, apathy, and other emotional and behavioral changes that accompany Alzheimer's.

► DON'T FORGET YOURSELF

As a care provider or just an observant family member, you may suffer emotionally from having a relative with the behavioral and emotional problems of Alzheimer's, particularly if your relative is one of the unlucky ones who do not respond well to or refuse medication or lifestyle interventions. Don't ignore your own needs. When you feel yourself becoming depressed, angry, or anxious, or find yourself engaging in destructive behaviors (such as excessive eating, heavy drinking, and so on), take yourself to your doctor. Also check out the previous chapter for information on caring for the care provider.

CHAPTER FOURTEEN

MEDICATIONS FOR DEPRESSION, ANXIETY, AND SLEEPLESSNESS

If you ask what is the single most important key to longevity, I would have to say it is avoiding worry, stress, and tension. And if you didn't ask me, I would still have to say it.

—GEORGE BURNS

Maybe you're seeing your mom become more anxious or fearful, or your husband being depressed, withdrawn, or irritable—not at all the cheerful guy you married. Men who never hit anything other than a tennis ball are slamming their fist against the table, and women who never yelled are cursing their grandchildren! Alzheimer's makes them do it, and it makes the person and everyone around him or her suffer.

In this chapter we get down to details of which drugs appear most effective at tackling the unenviable conditions that often tag along with Alzheimer's—the depression, anxiety, or odd behaviors. But we do so with a big warning label: Our top choices for treating these ills don't come from a pharmaceutical company. They are the nondrug approaches (described in Chapters 11 and 12)—the sooth-ing, the comforting, the distracting, the managing, the hands-on care providing—that family and friends do for people with Alzheimer's.

Always try nondrug approaches first, but once you have ex-hausted those options—and before you, as the care provider, become exhausted—it's wise to consider psychotropic medications, which treat problems like anxiety and depression. When used properly, such medications can be very important in the fight against emo-tional and behavioral problems. In addition, the nondrug and drug approaches are compatible and often successful teammates.

Studies show that getting successful treatment, which includes social support for families, can delay or prevent moves to nursing homes and improve caregivers' emotional well-being and their con-fidence as caregivers.

► WHEN IS IT TIME TO SEEK TREATMENT?

Consider medications when your relative

- has not responded well to behavioral strategies
- wants to try medication, and your doctor agrees it's a good idea
- is having difficulty just getting through the day
- has become a physical or emotional threat to himself or her-self or others
- is diagnosed with delirium, major depression, psychosis, or bipolar disorder, which all respond well to medications
- has taken medications successfully in the past for the problem

If you are reluctant to see your relative taking yet another pill, keep in mind that some conditions, such as delirium, psychosis, and severe depression, don't go away without medication, and delaying treat-ment can be dangerous.

If the medications work, they can make everyone's life easier. Think about how helpful it would be for everyone if your relative's sleep schedule settled down, so he's not getting up—and waking you up—in the middle of the night. Consider what you could get done (or simply enjoy) in a day if your relative was even a little calmer or happier. For example, when one grandfather started taking an antipsychotic, his daughter was able to bring the grandchildren over for visits again. At their best, behavioral drugs foster a climate of well-being for the entire household. Medications don't always work, nor do they eliminate the need for the nondrug interventions, but medications may help nondrug interventions work better.

> Anne, a former physician's assistant, had been diagnosed with Alzheimer's for four years when two common and really distressing symptoms took hold of her: suspiciousness and delusions. She accused her husband of stealing her things, demanded that he leave their house, and even tried to hit him when he helped her bathe. She also began conversing with characters on her favorite television shows as if they were real. In fact, her husband joked, she had some good advice for a couple of the characters on *Days of Our Lives.*
>
> David took Anne to a psychiatrist, who prescribed the antipsychotic medication Abilify. Within two weeks, Anne calmed down, slept better, and became much more trusting. The doctor and her husband decided to keep her on the medication for three months and reevaluate her need for it monthly.

► AT THE DOCTOR'S OFFICE

When you're talking with the doctor, ask if a medical condition besides Alzheimer's or another medication could be triggering your relative's behavioral or emotional problems. Doctors might just blame everything on the most likely or obvious cause, the Alzheimer's. Write your questions down before you go, and take notes or record the conversation if you're worried about missing something during the appointment.

Thyroid disease, bladder infections, vitamin B deficiency, constipation, and other conditions can cause anxiety, confusion, and agitation, particularly in someone with Alzheimer's. Have your doctor screen for these and any other medical issues he or she thinks are relevant. Medications could be part of the problem. Certain drugs, or combinations of drugs, can spark reactions such as confusion, agitation, and delirium.

Ask if these emotional or behavioral problems are a sign that your relative has something other than Alzheimer's. Some kinds of dementia resemble Alzheimer's but have different causes and treatments. For example, Lewy Body Dementia causes extreme sensitivity to certain older antipsychotic medications.

SUICIDE RISK

In rare cases, antidepressants increase suicidal thoughts or agitation. This response, in some cases, indicates that the person suffers from bipolar disorder, which may require adjusting the treatments. If you are concerned that your family member is at risk for suicide, stop reading and call your doctor or 911 right away.

Even when they've ruled out other possible medical issues, many doctors won't start a psychotropic medication unless a family member or the person with Alzheimer's requests it. So make sure you and your relative state your wishes clearly. If you are already under the care of an Alzheimer's specialist, go to him or her. However, if your primary-care doctor isn't experienced in treating psychiatric illnesses or you're not statisfied with the care you're getting after a few weeks, consider a geriatrician, a geriatric psychiatrist, or a physician with experience treating older people for psychiatric illnesses.

Compared with specialists, general practitioners may not be as up-to-date on the available treatments, especially since dosage guidelines for psychotropic medications don't describe when or how to use these drugs to treat people with Alzheimer's. Specialists who are doing their job well rely on the latest scientific publications and their own experience to determine the correct drug and dosage, and to adjust them as needed.

Before starting a medication, it's crucial for the patient to undergo a psychiatric and mental status evaluation. The exam helps ensure an accurate diagnosis and treatment plan, plus provides a baseline for monitoring behavioral changes over time. The exam takes from ten to thirty minutes and involves answering questions about the type and severity of the problems. (Here's when you would turn to the diary, if you've been able to keep one, on your relative's behavior and moods.)

Many doctors don't make as much effort to get people off of psychotropic drugs as they might. The longer a person stays on a medication, the greater the risk of developing side effects. New side effects can emerge after months or years of use. But it's also important not to quit before you get the benefits.

Never stop the medication without advice from your doctor. Unlike most medications, psychotropic medications need to be assessed, ideally, every two weeks. If you can't make a follow-up appointment in that time, put a note on your calendar to call the doctor and update him or her on your relative's progress.

At the end of every visit, ask the doctor what diagnosis he or she is giving your relative, the reason for recommending a psychotropic medication, or the reasons for continuing it after your relative improves.

► LEARNING ABOUT MEDICATIONS

It may take a little digging to get the full story on a drug's effectiveness and side effects. Researchers are more likely to publish positive findings, and until recently, pharmaceutical companies were not required to report the number of studies a behavioral drug had undergone, or the results of those studies, to the general public. Doctors who consult for companies have an advantage over other doctors, in that they learn about the results of companies' investigations and use this information when treating their patients.

Today, scientists and drug companies are more up-front about research results. Since 2006, all of the major pharmaceutical companies have been posting summaries of key positive and negative drug studies. The results are not always easy for a layperson to understand, however. Most are posted at clinicalstudyresults.org, a common site used by major pharmaceutical companies. Others appear on the companies' own Web sites (for example, www.lillytrials.com/results).

The FDA now requires that drug package inserts include any negative findings relating to the drug's FDA-approved use. For example, the FDA has approved the use of antidepressants for treating depression, although not in people with Alzheimer's. Therefore, the insert doesn't need to include information from negative or positive studies on Alzheimer's patients. For added protection, ask your doctor if he or she is aware of any negative studies on the drug your relative has been given.

▶ **Keep in Mind:** People have different body types, metabolisms, genders, size, and medical histories. Because of this, a drug that works well for one person may be ineffective for another.

▶ THE FDA AND THE MEDS

Thanks to twenty-five-plus years of research, doctors now have a choice of about twenty medications, including antidepressants, sleeping pills, antianxiety drugs, and sedatives (also called benzodiazepines), mood stabilizers, and antipsychotics. None comes with guarantees; all come with side effects.

They also come with a couple of caveats: Not all are approved by the FDA for use by people with Alzheimer's. Does that mean the FDA expects doctors to forgo prescribing them to people with Alzheimer's? No. The FDA doesn't tell doctors what drugs to prescribe to patients. If the FDA has not approved Drug X for use by people with Alzheimer's, it just means that not enough conclusive research has been published to meet FDA approval.

But doctors often have to treat conditions for which there are no FDA-approved drugs. In these cases, doctors resort to off-label use. For example, doctors have assumed that because antidepressants work for many people without Alzheimer's, they should work for people with the disease. Fortunately, they often do.

► EFFECTIVENESS

Some people with Alzheimer's respond amazingly well to the first medications they try. Others derive little benefit from any of the drugs, forcing doctors and caregivers to patch together a combination of drugs and lifestyle techniques just to get everyone through the day.

Once again, the key is finding a specialist who knows enough about the disease and the possible drug choices to create and monitor a wise and informed treatment plan for your family member. Check with your local Alzheimer's Association, friends, and family doctor for names of people to call. (Also, check Chapters 4 and 5 on getting a diagnosis—the same suggestions apply to finding good treatment.)

The art of treating Alzheimer's symptoms requires careful monitoring of medications and a willingness to change medications and dosages as needed. You want a specialist who will work with your family over the years, not just diagnose, write a prescription, and hand your relative back to a primary-care doctor.

Most studies on the effectiveness of antidepressants don't look specifically at people with Alzheimer's. However, one small study compared Zoloft to a placebo. Thirty-three percent of patients on Zoloft reported full relief, and 46 percent reported partial improvement, compared to 20 percent and 15 percent, respectively, for patients taking the placebo.

People often need to try more than one antidepressant to find the one that does give them complete (or sufficient) improvement. Because the brain changes of Alzheimer's are so serious and these drugs haven't been studied enough in this population, it may take extra effort to find the right medication.

How Long Does It Take to See Results?

Antidepressants take two to four weeks to work, though they may kick in sooner; antipsychotics take about one week; and sleeping pills or sedatives may take effect within thirty minutes. If the problem is so severe that you or your relative can't wait for an antidepressant or antipsychotic to start working, ask the doctor for a medication, such as a fast-acting sedative or injectable form of the drug, that can help in the meanwhile.

▶ SIDE EFFECTS

Every medication has them, so keep an eye on how your relative responds when he or she begins a new drug. Talk to your pharmacist and read about the prescribed medications, to make sure you're up-to-date on possible side effects and drug (and food) interactions, as well as correct dosages. Still, even if you are fully informed, you won't know the full effects of a particular drug until the person takes it. The risks and uncertainties associated with psychotropic drugs are higher for older than for younger individuals, because it's harder for the aging body to metabolize many drugs.

One woman was startled when her dad's physician prescribed an antidepressant that was known to cause sleeplessness, even though her father had had a long history of insomnia. Even the best doctors can make mistakes. It's particularly important to do your homework on medications that are intended for people with Alzheimer's, because they may be unable to tell you how the drug is affecting them.

Some drugs cause temporary side effects while the body adjusts to this new ingredient in its system. For example, antipsychotics may cause restlessness, and Wellbutrin may cause some anxiety. Adding a second drug to block these side effects for the few adjustment weeks may make the difference between a person staying on the medication and quitting.

When to Call the Doctor

If your relative is experiencing side effects, let the doctor know right away. The doctor may ask you to ride it out a little longer or to stop immediately; you won't know until you call.

Alcohol

People who are taking antidepressants should generally avoid alcohol, since the combination may diminish alertness, coordination, and the mood-boosting effects of the medication. Alcohol impairs memory and reduces brain activity—people with Alzheimer's certainly don't need that. However, if your relative drank moderately before starting antidepressants and would like to continue to enjoy its relaxing effects, his or her doctor may say it's okay.

Dosage

One way to avoid or limit side effects is to start with the correct dosage. An experienced doctor will take a cautious approach to prescribing psychotropic drugs. He or she will start at a low dose and then increase it gradually, assuming that side effects are not a problem. If you think the doctor has prescribed too high a dose too quickly, speak up.

Because Alzheimer's affects many brain chemicals, people with Alzheimer's may react differently to the medications than people without Alzheimer's. Plus, most drugs are tested on younger, healthy individuals. For older people and people with Alzheimer's, a wise doctor will follow the golden rule: Start low, go slow.

► THE COSTS

Prescription benefit plans generally reimburse for most costs of psychotropic medications, if the doctor has adequately documented the reasons for prescribing it. Doctors do, however, need to provide stronger evidence than if the drug was being used for an FDA-approved use.

Prices for most medications range from pennies to five dollars per day. The price varies depending on the type of drug and dosage, as well as the pharmacy and state where you purchase the drug. Some newer medications such as the Emsam (selegiline) patch, an antidepressant skin patch, are much more expensive. Generics and less expensive drugs are available, but few studies have compared generic and newer drugs. If cost is a concern, ask the doctor or pharmacist about generic options or free samples. Although they don't publicize it, companies have programs to provide free medications to people whose income falls below a certain level.

BEATING THE BLUES ON FOUR DOLLARS A MONTH?

Wal-Mart, Sam's Club, and Target offer several generic antidepressants and antipyschotics at a flat price of about four dollars for a month's supply in most states. This is good news, but some of the drugs that these discounters make available are not recommended for Alzheimer's patients, including the older antidepressants. So if you are taking a new medication or are paying too much for an existing medication, check with your doctor to see if any of the discounted medications would be right for you. Of the four-dollar-per-month drugs that these stores offer for treating behavioral problems, the one we recommend most is citalopram (a generic equivalent to brand-name Celexa).

▶ MEDICATIONS

The era of modern psychopharmacology began about half a century ago with the serendipitous observation that tuberculosis drugs induced euphoria and allergy drugs caused sedation. Researchers also discovered neurotransmitters (serotonin, dopamine, and norepinephrine), chemicals in the brain that affect mood. These discoveries led scientists to develop the first generation of drugs, including Elavil, Pamelor, and Mellaril, specifically for treating depression and psychosis. In the last fifteen years, scientists have developed newer psychotropic drugs, including Zoloft, Lexapro, Cymbalta, and Abilify, to overcome some of the limitations of the older drugs.

Today's Drugs	Uses
Antidepressants	Depression, apathy, anxiety, sleep, agitation, pain
Benzodiazepines	Anxiety, agitation, insomnia
Sedatives/hypnotics	Insomnia, agitation
Antipsychotics	Hallucinations, paranoia, agitation, bipolar disorder
Mood stabilizers	Agitation, mood disorders, pain
Stimulants	Apathy, depression, low energy, daytime sleepiness

Fifty experts recently agreed on the best approaches to treat depression in people with dementia, including Alzheimer's. Their top five choices:

1. Antidepressant medication alone

2. Antidepressant plus a cholinesterase inhibitor, such as Aricept, if the patient is not already on one

3. Antidepressant plus psychotherapy

4. Antidepressant plus the memory drug memantine (Namenda), if the patient is not already on it

5. Electroconvulsive therapy (ECT) for intractable depression (rare)

(Modern ECT differs significantly from what you saw in *One Flew Over the Cuckoo's Nest*. It involves inducing a controlled seizure under anesthesia, and can be highly effective for people who do not respond to medication, although it can temporarily worsen memory problems for some.)

Despite this consensus statement on the best approaches to treat depression in people with Alzheimer's, treatment for behavioral and emotional problems is far from uniform across the medical profession. To treat anxiety, doctors may use an antidepressant, an antipsychotic, a benzodiazepine, a mood stabilizer, or even some combination of medications. Why? We still do not have enough evidence to support one approach over another.

Stopping or Changing Medication

As Alzheimer's progresses, symptoms change and, therefore, so does the need for medications. Symptoms may resolve gradually or even spontaneously, or get worse. If your relative is mildly agitated or aggressive, she may become more so as the disease diminishes her ability to talk, or she may develop hallucinations or paranoia. These symptoms may require a combination of an antipsychotic drug with an antidepressant. If her agitation resolves spontaneously, which does happen, then she may be able to completely stop whatever anxiety drug she was taking.

Your relative may need to continue taking an antidepressant for six to nine months after her depression resolves to make sure it doesn't come back.

▶ **Warning:** *Always* consult your doctor before changing any drug regimen, especially when psychotropic medications are involved. Stopping medications can cause withdrawal reactions, including dizziness, diarrhea, or painful tingling sensations in the body. It can also cause symptoms to flare up dangerously.

▶ OUR TOP CHOICES FOR ANTIDEPRESSANTS: SSRIS—CELEXA, ZOLOFT, LEXAPRO (AND THEIR GENERICS)

Our first-pick medications are called selective serotonin reuptake inhibitors (SSRIs). They target the brain's serotonin system, which modulates mood, emotion, sleep, and appetite. In people with depression, the nerve cells in the brain are not exposed to enough serotonin, so SSRIs are designed to make better use of the serotonin that the brain produces.

SSRIs are our first picks because studies of people without Alzheimer's show that this class of drugs is generally safe and effective in treating depression in older people. They have also been better studied in people with Alzheimer's than other antidepressants. For most older people, the side effects of these drugs are manageable. Finally, they are much safer than older antidepressants if your relative accidentally or intentionally overdoses on them.

As with all drugs, side effects are usually milder if the patient starts with a small dose and increases slowly. However, side effects are unavoidable for many people. The common side effects, many of which may be mild or go away as people get used to the drug, are nausea, diarrhea, loose stools, anxiety, dizziness, sleep disturbances, dry mouth, weight loss, sweating, vivid dreams, tremors, headaches, sexual problems, agitation, and apathy.

One less common but notable side effect is a drop in sodium levels, which causes nausea, vomiting, headaches, and confusion. If your relative is on an SSRI, consider getting his or her sodium levels checked regularly.

In rare cases, people have a very strong reaction to SSRIs, where normal side effects are magnified significantly. This rare reaction usually happens only if a person is getting too high a dose or is also taking other drugs that enhance the antidepressant's effect. Drugs to watch out for are some migraine medications, including Imitrex, and the antidepressant Emsam (selegiline).

Celexa (citalopram) and Zoloft (sertraline)

Celexa helps reduce behavioral problems and depression in people with Alzheimer's—not enough to meet FDA standards, but enough that many doctors prescribe it for their Alzheimer's patients. Studies show that Zoloft also reduces behavioral symptoms and improves daily living. Both come in generic forms.

Lexapro (escitalopram)

Lexapro is the left half of the citalopram (Celexa) molecule, the half that drug company researchers felt had the most effect on the serotonin system. While it hasn't been as well studied as Celexa in people with Alzheimer's, it's a good choice because it's similar to citalopram. However, it is much more expensive than generic citalopram.

Prozac (fluoxetine)

Most people are familiar with Prozac, one of the most widely dispensed antidepressants in the world. Although the FDA has approved Prozac for use in older adults with depression (although again, not for those with Alzheimer's and depression), it is farther down on our list because it lingers in the body for weeks after the person stops taking it. Also, it can interact negatively with other medications during that time. On the positive side, a generic form of Prozac is widely available. A drug called Symbyax (which combines fluoxetine and olanzapine) is also available for treating complicated depression but is not as well studied in older people.

Paxil (paroxetine)

Until a few years ago, Paxil was one of the most widely used drugs to treat depression and anxiety. Its main drawback was that it was somewhat more likely than some other SSRIs to interact with some common medications such as beta-blockers or codeine. Stopping this drug abruptly can lead to side effects such as dizziness or tingling. It is now generic.

▶ **Note:** As of this writing, a thirty-day supply of fluoxetine, paroxetine, and citalopram can be purchased at Wal-Mart, Sam's Club, or Target for four dollars. Of these, most specialists prefer citalopram for use in older adults.

Wellbutrin XL

Some antidepressants take a multifaceted approach to lifting depression or easing anxiety. One example is Wellbutrin XL (bupropion), which targets norepinephrine and dopamine, both neurotransmitters that, like serotonin, affect mood, attention, and more. Called a selective catecholamine (norepinephrine and dopamine) reuptake inhibitor, Wellbutrin can be mildly stimulating. It helps people feel more alert, focused, and motivated—a boon for Alzheimer's patients who suffer from apathy or daytime drowsiness. It doesn't dampen sexual performance or libido as much as other SSRIs. Doctors may prescribe Wellbutrin along with an SSRI (such as Celexa) if the SSRI isn't working on its own. Generic bupropion is also available.

The downside of Wellbutrin XL is that it is one of the least studied antidepressants in patients with memory problems. Its side effects include dry mouth, constipation, weight loss, and increased blood pressure. It may also spur on anxiety, panic, or jitteriness. It is not recommended for people who have had seizures, head injuries, anorexia, or bulimia.

Cymbalta and Effexor

These drugs, called serotonin and norepinephrine reuptake inhibitors (SNRIs), work on two brain chemicals, so doctors hoped they would work better than other antidepressants. The jury is still out, but so far it looks as though SNRIs are at least as useful as SSRIs.

Cymbalta (duloxetine) helped lift depression in older adults (not with Alzheimer's) *and* improved their cognitive test scores. It also effectively treats general anxiety problems and painful nerve problems associated with diabetes. Effexor XR (venlafaxine) is widely used to treat depression. The more common side effects of SNRIs include nausea, constipation or diarrhea, high blood pressure, and dry mouth. People with certain blood pressure or urinary conditions or glaucoma should avoid these drugs. People with liver problems and those who drink alcohol regularly should avoid these drugs. A generic venlafaxine will be available soon.

Remeron (mirtazapine)

A unique class of antidepressant, Remeron boosts the release in the brain of the antidepression chemicals neuroepinephrine and serotonin. In addition, it helps prevent the nausea, diarrhea, and appetite loss caused by memory drugs such as Exelon. It works as both a sedative and an appetite stimulant.

In very rare cases, Remeron causes people's white blood cells to drop dramatically. It should not be taken by people with low white cell counts such as those with certain cancers. Also, if your relative is taking this drug and develops fevers or infections, his or her blood should be tested.

Emsam (selegiline)

Emsam works by increasing the levels of serotonin and dopamine in the brain. It is the only antidepressant that comes in a patch form. Patients who require the higher doses of Emsam must avoid certain foods (aged meats, cheese, beans, and beer) to keep their blood pressure under control. Also, they can't take other antidepressants until they have been off Emsam for two to four weeks. It is also the most expensive of the lot. Therefore, Emsam is not as widely used as other antidepressants.

► STIMULANTS

Most people can get by with a cup or two of coffee to start their day, but people with Alzheimer's who suffer from debilitating depression and apathy may benefit from prescription-strength stimulants. However, the evidence is still very preliminary. Best known for treating attention deficit disorders in children, the drugs include **Ritalin** (methylphenidate), **Concerta** (methylphenidate HCl), and **Adderall** (amphetamine salts). These drugs can be addictive, so people with a history of alcohol or drug addiction should avoid them. Among other side effects, they can reduce appetite and increase blood pressure and agitation. Recently, concerns have also been raised over the cardiac safety of some stimulants.

Doctors use the stimulant **Provigil** (modafinil) to treat the daytime sleepiness that results from nighttime insomnia. Increasingly, they are also using it to improve older people's mood, energy, alertness, and concentration. On the downside, Provigil can cause nervousness, headaches, nausea, chest pains, rash, or confusion.

MAKING SIDE EFFECTS WORK

All drugs have side effects, but one person's negative side effect is another person's positive one. Someone with insomnia needs a slightly sedating antidepressant, whereas a chronic napper needs the slightly stimulating option.

► TRICYCLIC ANTIDEPRESSANTS

This group of antidepressants is less widely used today. Tricyclic antidepressants (TCAs) were developed before SSRIs and were once the only choice of psychiatrists. TCAs target three or more chemical systems in the brain. Two TCAs, **nortriptyline** and **desipramine,** are as effective as newer drugs at easing depression and insomnia. However, TCAs can have serious side effects, including impaired memory (as if an Alzheimer's patient needs that!), irregular heartbeat, urine retention, dry mouth, and uneven blood pressure. The level of these medications in a person's blood needs to be monitored every three months or so. The main advantage of these older antidepressants is their low cost, since they are generic.

Another older antidepressant, **Desyrel** (trazodone), is often used to treat insomnia, and doctors combine it with other antidepressants to increase their effectiveness. However, this practice doesn't do as much good as was previously believed. Desyrel has its share of side effects as well.

► **Note:** A thirty-day supply of nortriptyline and trazodone can be purchased at Wal-Mart, Sam's Club, or Target for four dollars.

Not-So-Golden Oldies

We recommend that you stay away from the following older antidepressants:

- Elavil, Endep, Tryptanol (amitriptyline)
- Anafranil (clomipramine)
- Prothiaden (dothiepin hydrochloride)
- Adapin, Sinequan (doxepin)
- Tofranil (imipramine)
- Gamanil, Lomont (lofepramine)
- Vivactil (protriptyline)
- Surmontil (trimipramine)

▶ EASING ANXIETY

Anxiety comes in many forms, as do antianxiety medications. Anxiety may be causing your relative to feel generally nervous, agitated, or uneasy; to perseverate (keep repeating the same thought or behavior); or to suffer panic attacks or be fearful. He may need daily medications for his anxiety symptoms, or get by with taking something just when his anxiety gets really bad, say, when he feels (or you see) an anxiety or panic attack coming on.

Again, anxiety medications have not undergone full-scale tests on people with Alzheimer's. But hands-on experience tells us they are often very helpful and, in some cases, essential to keep people with Alzheimer's safe, comfortable, and at home.

SSRI or SNRI antidepressants (discussed above) are also our first-choice medications for treating long-term, chronic anxiety, including:

- panic disorders, generalized anxiety, and phobias
- anxiety that is accompanied by depression

The doctor should prescribe a short-acting sedative to provide immediate relief until the antidepressant is doing its job.

Buspar (buspirone) treats symptoms of mild anxiety by increasing the activity of serotonin. Buspar's main advantage is that it is well tolerated. (Although it boosts serotonin activity, it's not an effective antidepressant.) It is one of the drugs that can be purchased at Wal-Mart, Sam's Club, or Target for four dollars a month.

Benzodiazepines are effective sedatives. They help reduce occasional panic attacks, agitation, or situational anxiety, such as the panic that people with Alzheimer's can experience when in a crowded store or on a plane. Benzodiazepines also help with insomnia. But sedatives are addictive, so use judiciously, only when really needed and for as short a time as possible.

Ativan (lorazepam), a benzodiazepine, is our first choice sedative for older people, because it has a short half-life, meaning it doesn't linger in the body after the person stops taking it. It also is less likely than other benzodiazepines to be addictive, because it doesn't cause euphoria. Other similar drugs that may work well are **Serax** (oxazepam), **Dalmane** (flurazepam), and **Klonopin** (clonazepam).

It is also a common practice for doctors to prescribe anxiety drugs, such as Ativan, and sedating antipsychotics, such as **Haldol** or **Seroquel** to people with Alzheimer's who suffer from acute anxiety or agitation that does not respond to other measures. In an emergency situation when someone with Alzheimer's needs to be sedated quickly, doctors can safely use injectable forms of some of these drugs. People usually stop taking the medicines after the acute agitation or anxiety is resolved.

One medication used rarely for people with Alzheimer's is the sedative **Valium** (diazepam), the sedative that made an appearance in the 1969 movie classic *The Valley of the Dolls* and at the same period in many people's lives. Doctors still prescribe it to treat anxiety, panic symptoms, and nervousness, but it may be more addictive than shorter-acting sedatives.

Errors Doctors Make When Prescribing Sedatives

- Ignoring memory status or sensitivities when selecting a sedative
- Prescribing more than one at a time
- Prescribing too large a dose
- Prescribing a sedative to treat depression
- Not monitoring the drug's effects
- Not knowing when or how to stop the medication

If you think your relative is taking too much of or the wrong sedative, consult with her doctor or pharmacist. Under a doctor's supervision, tapering off these habit-forming medications may help her feel better and even improve her memory slightly by clearing the fog that the long-term use of these drugs can roll in. Once again, however, never stop a medication without the doctor's approval. The side effects of going cold turkey can vary from mild insomnia to seizures and delirium.

► LOOKING FOR A GOOD NIGHT'S SLEEP

Sleep is critical to our health, including our ability to think and remember. Fortunately, there are new and truly improved sleeping medications for long-term sleep problems such as insomnia or nighttime wandering. But before turning to medications, try the home-based strategies described in Chapter 11 on early-stage Alzheimer's.

If home-based methods don't work, prescription medication, including antidepressants, sedatives, and sleeping pills (called hypnotics), are worth trying. Sleeping pills work by suppressing the REM, or dream, stage of the sleep cycle and shifting the person into a deeper one. Depending on how long a particular hypnotic medication stays in the body, it will help a person either get to sleep or sleep through the night.

► **Note:** In most situations, antipsychotic medications are inappropriate if used just to treat sleeping problems.

Though we recommend getting a prescription for a sedative or hypnotic if your relative is having serious sleeping problems, we'll warn you right up front that they are far from perfect.

- They essentially slow down the brain, including memory, attention, motor coordination, and the ability to process information quickly.
- They may make sleep problems worse or cause vivid dreams when people stop taking them.
- The body develops a tolerance to them, so people regularly need to increase their dose to get the same effects.
- They impair balance and driving abilities.
- People who have breathing problems can't take them.
- They can be dangerous if taken in combination with alcohol.

It is extremely important to go to bed within fifteen minutes of taking a hypnotic medication. In some cases, the brain may not be able to form any new memories until the drug wears off. If your relative is sleeping, she won't notice that effect. But if she doesn't fall asleep right away, she may quickly become confused and forget who and where she is.

Hypnotics may have other side effects too. If she stops taking one of these drugs, her body may "rebound" by trying to catch up on missed sleep cycles. Plus, you have to be alert for possible nocturnal rambles, as people on sleeping pills have been known to walk, go on eating binges, and even drive while they're sleeping.

▶ **Heads-Up:** Some medications to treat Alzheimer's or depression may occasionally cause insomnia, nocturnal delusions, or vivid dreams. A doctor unfamiliar with these effects may mistake them for a worsening of the Alzheimer's and prescribe a higher dose of the offending drug.

Sleep Medications

Lunesta (eszopiclone) is one of the most widely used hypnotics. Its advantages are that it doesn't wear off as much as some others during the night and it appears to remain effective for long-term use.

Sonata (zaleplon), another popular sleeping pill, wears off after about four hours, so it is more appropriate when the trouble is falling asleep rather than getting up in the middle of the night. It works quickly.

Ambien and **Ambien CR** (zolpidem) are two forms of another widely used hypnotic that works quite well. They are longer acting than Sonata, so they can help people to get a full night's sleep. The CR stands for controlled release, meaning it helps people get to sleep and stay asleep. Generic zolpidem is available.

Alternative Sleeping Aides

Over-the-counter medications such as **Tylenol PM** and **Benadryl** make people sleepy, are less addicting than prescription drugs, and can be used easily and on an as-needed basis. Benadryl may impair memory, however, if taken daily for long periods. Taking high doses of Tylenol may damage the liver, especially if you drink alcohol.

These over-the-counter sleep aids can help treat mild insomnia short term but they are not meant for long-term use. And even for nonprescription medicines, you must get the okay from your relative's doctor before giving them and never combine them with other sleeping drugs.

Antidepressants with a sedative quality, such as **Trazodone** and **Remeron,** as well as antipsychotics such as **Seroquel** (discussed in the next chapter), also can help people with Alzheimer's slumber more peacefully. In fact, Trazodone is a top choice for long-term treatment of insomnia, as is Lunesta or Rozarem.

Natural Sleep Aids

In the quest to find safer and more effective sleep agents for people with Alzheimer's, scientists have been working on products and methods that mimic **melatonin,** the brain chemical involved in bringing on sleep.

As we age, the amount of melatonin in the brain decreases. In fact, some studies suggest that taking melatonin, which you can buy as a supplement, may help restore the body's natural sleep rhythms. It's worth a try. However, a clinical trial of 157 Alzheimer's patients with insomnia found no benefit to using melatonin.

One of our first picks of all sleeping medications (not just the natural ones) is **Rozarem** (ramelteon), which works with the body's melatonin system. Compared with hypnotic drugs and benzodiazepines, Rozarem is much less likely to be addictive or to cause a hungover feeling, dependence, or rebound problems. It can be more easily taken or stopped as needed. However, it too has side effects. For example, it interacts poorly with antifungal medications and, if used for weeks, may slightly change the body's natural levels of the hormones cortisol and prolactin.

Another potential "natural" treatment for sleep disorders is not a pill at all. **Bright-light therapy,** also used to treat depression, involves sitting in front of a special light, usually in the morning. The effectiveness of bright-light therapy for treating insomnia in Alzheimer's patients is inconclusive. To increase your odds of success, work with a sleep specialist who knows the specific times and amount of light therapy to administer.

For the more serious emotional and behavioral difficulties that sometimes accompany Alzheimer's, turn to the next chapter.

CHAPTER FIFTEEN

FINDING A CALM IN THE STORM: MEDICATIONS TO TREAT THE WORST BEHAVIORAL SYMPTOMS

Without memory, you are unmoored, a wind-tossed boat with no anchor.

—PATTI DAVIS, WRITING ABOUT HER FATHER, RONALD REAGAN

In 1901, Dr. Alois Alzheimer began seeing a fifty-one-year-old patient who couldn't remember her entire name, her husband's name, and other seemingly obvious information. Within a few years, the patient developed delusions that someone wanted to kill her. After the patient's death, Dr. Alzheimer did an autopsy on her brain and saw the plaques and tangles that would eventually define the disease we now call Alzheimer's.

As Dr. Alzheimer discovered, memory loss is eventually joined by confusion and possibly anger, rage, aggression, relentless agitation, a distorted sense of reality, hallucinations, and more. Dr. Alzheimer didn't have much in his black bag to treat these horrible symptoms. He recommended getting rid of stimulants in the environment that trigger agitation, which is still apropriate. Other techniques in that era included warm baths or moist wrappings to soothe agitation, enhancing the patient's physical comfort, hypnosis, sedatives, or, as a last resort, mild electric current applied to the head.

But by the 1960s, antipsychotic medications, developed to treat schizophrenia, were being used to treat people with Alzheimer's as well.

Since then, researchers have developed newer antipsychotics, and many doctors now have a lot of experience using the medications. However, the Food and Drug Administration has not approved the use of antipsychotics for the emotional and behavioral symptoms of Alzheimer's, because there have not been enough conclusive studies to meet the FDA's criteria for efficacy. But as we explained in the previous chapter, that doesn't mean the drugs are ineffective or shouldn't be used. The drugs are frequently used successfully for just this purpose.

Antipsychotics are often the only recourse family members and doctors have for treating behavioral problems. But they can have side effects, especially when used for months or years, such as stiffness, weight gain, dizziness, blood pressure changes, and the less common ones, including increased cholesterol and triglycerides, hormonal changes, high blood sugars, and tardive dyskinesia (TD), which is a serious nervous system disorder that causes involuntary jerks, grimaces, and tics. Moreover, the drugs are too often ineffective.

These drugs should be used, therefore, only after

- ruling out other alternatives, such as nondrug therapies
- determining that there is more to gain than lose concerning a person's well-being and safety

ALICE: BEFORE AND AFTER ANTIPSYCHOTIC MEDICATION

Four years after being diagnosed with Alzheimer's, Alice, sixty-six, began accusing her beloved husband of forty-two years of stealing her things, demanding that he leave their house, and even hitting him. She also began talking to television characters

(continued)

as if they were old friends. Using a variety of strategies he learned from a social worker, her husband tried to reassure Alice and keep her calm, but his efforts weren't very successful. After ruling out any sort of infection, which in a person with Alzheimer's can cause irritability and odd behavior, her doctor prescribed a small (0.25 milligram) dose of the antipsychotic medicine Risperdal, gradually increasing her dose to 1 milligram over four weeks. Her husband continued to use the strategies he learned from the social worker, but now they actually seemed to work. Alice and he both slept better at night, and she wasn't as suspicious. Her side effects were few, but the doctor went ahead and lowered her dose after a few months and continued to monitor her for side effects.

► OPTIMIZING EFFECTIVENESS, MINIMIZING RISKS

A major government-funded study tested three popular newer antipsychotic drugs (**Zyprexa**, **Risperdal**, and **Seroquel**) to see how well they reduced the often persistent and disruptive problems of psychosis, agitation, and aggression in people with Alzheimer's. Surprisingly, the drugs did not prove to be much more effective than a placebo. Between 26 and 32 percent of people on one of the medications improved, compared to 21 percent of the study participants who received the placebo. Further, the side effects of Zyprexa and Risperdal offset the drugs' slight edge in terms of benefits.

So why do doctors still use them? Several previous studies had suggested that the drugs may work, so some doctors are still relying on those findings despite the negative studies. There are no other treatments. And sometimes the drugs do help. So we do—very cautiously—recommend trying them, but *only* when other approaches or medications fail.

You and your physician can increase the odds of a sucessful trial of an antipsychotic medication in a variety of ways. Sometimes it takes tweaking the dosage, changing the timing of the medicine, trying different medications or combinations, and of course continuing to use nondrug interventions. Again, get help from a specialist or a general practitioner who has experience using such agents.

An experienced physician will err on the side of caution by prescribing drugs for as short a time as possible and at as low a dose as possible. To minimize side effects during waking hours, doctors usually (though not always) prescribe antipsychotics to be taken at bedtime. It may seem strange to take them at night, but the effect will still be there during the day. Because of the drugs' potency, doctors sometimes prescribe them on an "as-needed" basis. That means you would give them to your relative only when he or she really needs it, rather than every day.

► ASK THE DOCTOR QUESTIONS

If the doctor prescribes an antipsychotic drug, ask:

- What is it for?
- Why did you choose it?
- Have you considered an alternative?
- How long will my relative need to be on it?

Also ask how often your relative will be checked for:

- movement disorders, restlessness, and stiffness
- worsening of cholesterol levels and triglycerides
- hormonal imbalances
- diabetes
- heart-rhythm changes
- blood pressure changes
- swallowing difficulties
- weight gain
- blood clots
- side effects specific to the individual drugs

If the antipsychotic drug works for your relative, then over the next few days or weeks he may be less paranoid and have fewer hallucinations. As a result, he will be calmer and less agitated and have a better quality of life. He may sleep better also (but there are far safer drugs for sleeping problems).

If your family member doesn't begin to improve after a few weeks—or if he experiences bad side effects right away—don't hesitate to call the doctor, who should change the dosage or try another medication quickly.

Two Are Rarely Better than One

Some doctors may prescribe two antipsychotics at once, thinking that two drugs will target different brain areas or cancel out each other's side effects. However, no evidence supports that approach, and you should question your doctor or get a second opinion if your doctor recommends it.

► WHICH DRUGS WORK BEST

For your reference, here is a primer on antipsychotics, warnings included. (The worst side effects of antipsychotics we list at the end of this section.) All have been linked to an increased risk for diabetes, changes in cholesterol levels, movement problems, stiffness, blood pressure changes, and drowsiness. If your relative has trouble swallowing pills, you'll appreciate that some of the medications can be given as injection or liquid.

Risperdal (risperidone)

One of the most widely used and studied antipsychotics for people with Alzheimer's, Risperdal treats hallucinations, paranoid thinking, agitation, pacing, and aggression. Nevertheless, not all clinical trials have shown that it helps Alzheimer's patients. Two studies showed it was partially helpful and one found it was no better than a placebo. As is true for many medications, it's unclear why some people benefit from this drug and others don't.

If your relative does benefit from the drug, the doctor will probably keep him or her on it for another week or two to ensure that symptoms don't return, then start to withdraw it *gradually* (to avoid withdrawal symptoms). Generic versions will likely be available in 2008.

Side effects: Although it is among the most widely used antipsychotics, Risperdal has the worst reputation among the newer antipsychotics for causing stiffness, restlessness, blood pressure changes, dizziness, and hormonal imbalances that can cause breast enlargement or tenderness, breast milk secretion (including in men), and loss of libido.

Zyprexa (olanzapine)

Zyprexa has a very different chemical makeup from Risperdal, making it less likely to cause stiffness. It has been studied in six trials of people with dementia (mainly Alzheimer's), with mixed results. It treats the same symptoms as Risperdal and is as effective for people with Alzheimer's.

Side effects: Zyprexa can cause significant weight gain and may increase the risk of diabetes (signs of diabetes are increased thirst, frequent urination, and increased appetite). The drug can also raise LDL cholestrol and triglyceride levels. Some people can gain thirty pounds or more on Zyprexa, so if your relative is overweight or has diabetes or cholestrol problems, keep a close eye on his or her numbers. Other common side effects include drowsiness, dizziness, dry mouth, and runny nose.

Abilify (aripiprazole)

Abilify has become more popular, as it appears to be as effective as Risperdal and Zyprexa yet has fewer metabolic side effects. Abilify has been studied in five trials for treating behavioral problems of dementia, but the results were mixed. Preliminary evidence suggests that it may also help lift some kinds of depression. An injectable form is available to treat acute agitation.

Side effects: It is similar to the other antipsychotic drugs but causes far less weight gain and fewer cholestrol and blood sugar problems than Zyprexa. It is also less likely to cause hormonal (prolactin) elevations than Risperdal. Common side effects include restlessness, nausea, anxiety, insomnia, and constipation.

Seroquel (quetiapine)

Seroquel is believed to have fewer neurological side effects (such as stiffness and tics) than other antipsychotics, but it requires higher doses to produce the same benefits. Because it is sedating, Seroquel often is prescribed when a person also has anxiety or insomnia, and doctors tend to give it on an as-needed basis.

Side effects: Seroquel may increase the risk of cataracts, according to animal studies, but so far this does not appear to be a problem in humans. It can cause weight gain and makes some people drowsy.

Invega (paliperidone)

The newest antipsychotic on the market, Invega is an active ingredient of Risperdal and, therefore, is likely to have similar efficacy and safety.

Haldol (haloperidol)

Unlike most of the antipsychotics developed many years ago, this old-timer still warrants consideration. It's well studied, inexpensive (currently four dollars a month at Wal-Mart, Sam's Club, or Target), and when used at the proper dose Haldol is just as effective as newer agents. In the past, doctors tended to prescribe it in overly high doses, leading to a higher risk of stiffness, tremors, and TD (for more on TD see below). It is primarily used to treat acute agitation in emergency settings or to treat people who cannot afford one of the newer drugs.

Side effects: Haldol has side effects similar to other medications, but it may need closer monitoring for tics, muscle stiffness, cardiac side effects, and hormonal imbalances. It can cause drowsiness and light-headedness.

Rarely Recommended Antipsychotics

Clozaril (clozapine)

Clozaril can cause dangerous side effects, including low white blood cell counts, fainting, and heart problems. For these reasons it is the only antipsychotic drug that requires mandatory blood testing on a strict schedule. However, it may be less likely to cause neurological side effects, so doctors sometimes use it as a last resort for people with Parkinson's disease or Lewy Body Dementia, for whom certain drugs such as Haldol can cause dangerous reactions.

Geodon (ziprasidone)

Geodon is not recommended for Alzheimer's because it is not as well studied in the elderly as the other drugs. It may cause a rare heart complication and it can't be taken with a long list of medications. On the plus side, it appears less likely than Zyprexa to cause weight gain or to increase blood cholestrol or sugar.

In particular, elderly people should avoid three older agents: **Thorazine** (chlorpromazine), **Mellaril** (thioridazine), and **Serentil** (mesoridazine). They can cause serious heart and memory problems.

TREATING THE SIDE EFFECTS

If stiffness or tremors cannot be eased by reducing the dose of the antipsychotic drug or changing to another drug, then doctors may have no choice but to add an "anticholinergic" drug, such as Cogentin (benztropine mesylate), to your relative's regimen. In general, people with memory problems should *avoid* anticholinergic drugs, as they can harm memory and interfere with the effects of Aricept, the common Alzheimer's medication. Cogentin can also cause dry mouth, constipation, and urinary obstruction.

▶ THE MOST SERIOUS (AND LESS COMMON) SIDE EFFECTS

In addition to the problems described above, antipsychotics can cause even more serious side effects, especially if someone has been on a drug for months or years.

One of the most serious is tardive dyskinesia (TD), which can lead to stiff muscles, involuntary twitching, grimacing, neck contortions, and other disabling symptoms. To make matters worse, doctors easily miss its early signs, including tremors, twitching, and restlessness. If your relative develops any of these symptoms, tell your doctor *right away*. The disease won't get worse after the person stops the medication, but it won't go away, either. Unfortunately, TD can develop without warning and is difficult to predict. All antipsychotics can cause TD. Neuroleptic malignant syndrome, a rare but potentially fatal drug reaction, is another concern. It causes a fever, muscle stiffness, confusion, and other symptoms.

If you are concerned that your relative is developing signs of TD, a ten-minute exam, Abnormal Involuntary Movement Scale (AIMS), can detect it in the early stages. Doctors sometimes overlook the importance of this test. If your relative is on an antipsychotic, ask that he or she be given this test at every doctor's visit.

RISK OF DEATH

A review of seventeen studies of elderly people with dementia showed that 4.5 percent of study participants taking an antipsychotic died during the course of the study, compared to 2.5 percent of participants taking a placebo. Heart failure and respiratory problems caused most of the deaths.

The review also revealed that, compared with people taking a placebo, participants taking Zyprexa, Abilify, and Risperdal were two times more likely to have a brain stroke (ranging from mild transient weakness to serious fatal strokes). In 2005 the

FDA added a warning label to these medications concerning cardiac and stroke risks.

The sober truth is that the best antipsychotics for treating the painfully severe behavioral and emotional symptoms of Alzheimer's carry serious risks. Yet psychosis can be dangerous or even life-threatening for the person and others. Therefore, as a measure of last resort in serious cases, we don't hesitate to prescribe an antipsychotic for a short time for our own patients.

► MOOD STABILIZERS

Manic depression, now commonly known as bipolar disorder, can also cause agitation, aggression, mood swings, or irritability in people with Alzheimer's, including in the early stages. The condition must be treated with drugs called mood stabilizers instead of or in addition to antipsychotics. Mood stabilizers on the market include **Lithobid** and **Eskalith** (lithium), **Carbitrol** (carbamazepine), and **Neurontin** (gabapentin).

Depakote (valproic acid) and **Tegretol** (carbamazepine) are anti-seizure medications that doctors once used widely to treat agitation in people with Alzheimer's, but recent studies have shown that they are not especially safe or effective for that purpose. Moreover, they require regular monitoring via blood tests to make sure they are not reaching toxic levels. Therefore, these drugs should be used only in special situations:

- Your relative has a history of seizures.
- Antidepressants or antipsychotics are not working.
- Your relative has dramatic and unstable mood swings.

Ingrid and her brothers used to joke with their German father, Oscar, that he always operated like the trains in his homeland (on time). Not even four kids made him late for work, the theater, or a plane. His attention to time was an endearing and amusing quality—until Alzheimer's took over the controls. When his daughter arrived at one P.M., as promised, to take him to a doctor's appointment, she was met with anger and frustration. "You're late!" he scolded. Sure enough, when she got home, a message was on her answering machine: "Where are you?!"

The family got him an easy-to-read watch, a wall clock, and a big calendar and put up signs telling him to *reeeeelax*. But those props proved useless. He didn't understand them, began to mistrust his exhausted wife, lost all ability to keep track of time, and thought the family was plotting against him. He became agitated and literally could not sit still. The family consulted a psychiatrist, who met with Oscar and listened to the family's experiences.

The doctor diagnosed Oscar as suffering from psychosis. He prescribed Risperdal for daily use, along with the antianxiety medication Ativan (lorazepam) for when the going got really bad. Oscar (and his family) were lucky. He responded remarkably well to the treatment within a few days. The medication had side effects, including dizziness, but they didn't outweigh the relief he got.

▶ WARNINGS

Because antipsychotic drugs can be both life-saving and life-threatening, the federal government has developed prescribing guidelines that doctors must follow. *The guidelines cover the following mistakes that doctors make:*

- prescribe antipsychotic drugs to treat minor behavior problems such as occasional insomnia, mild anxiety, or wandering
- prescribe an antipsychotic over the telephone without seeing the person
- start someone on an antipsychotic drug without going over the risks of the drug with a family member
- recommend a combination of antipsychotic drugs
- continue antipsychotic drugs for months after the behavior has improved
- put someone on an antipsychotic medication but fail to monitor him or her for neurological problems such as stiffness or tics, weight changes, or hormonal or cholesterol problems

- promise the drugs can keep Alzheimer's from getting worse as quickly
- say the newer antipsychotic medications are far superior to the older (less expensive) versions

When using antipsychotic medications, it's more important than ever to find a doctor you can trust to answer all of your questions and monitor side effects carefully.

PART FIVE

► **A BRAIN-HEALTHY LIFESTYLE**

CHAPTER SIXTEEN

WHAT'S GOOD FOR YOUR HEART IS GOOD FOR YOUR BRAIN: DIET, EXERCISE, AND SUPPLEMENTS

Be careful about reading health books. You could die of a misprint.

—MARK TWAIN

We've been hearing for years about a "heart-healthy lifestyle." But is there such a thing as a "brain-healthy lifestyle," and can it make a real difference?

Whether you have Alzheimer's disease yourself or are a family member wondering, "Am I next?" there are choices you can make about your lifestyle that may reduce your risk of getting Alzheimer's disease, delay its onset, slow its forward march, or ease its symptoms.

If you are taking care of someone with Alzheimer's, you have the most to gain from living a brain-healthy lifestyle and the least amount of time to do so. We recommend that you read the prevention strategies described here and work with your physician to launch as many of them as necessary (and as you have time for). Exercise is particularly important: It has one of the best track records of the strategies we discuss and will probably give you the biggest return on your investment of time and energy.

▶ AVOIDABLE RISK FACTORS FOR MEMORY LOSS

Seeing how many risk factors apply to you may jump-start your lifestyle changes. We've put them into categories to make them easier to read, but many fall into more than one category. For example, obesity is an illness, but it's also part of a sedentary lifestyle.

Your Diet

- High-fat diet
- Diet lacking a healthy mix of proteins, fats, carbohydrates, minerals, and vitamins

Your Lifestyle

- Being sedentary
- Having hobbies or jobs with high risk of head injury
- Not wearing seat belts
- Not sleeping enough
- Being under chronic stress
- Being lonely
- Not having mentally stimulating or engaging leisure activities

Your Habits and Addictions

- Heavy drinking, alcoholism
- Smoking

Your Physical Well-Being

- High blood pressure
- High blood sugar
- High cholesterol or poor lipid profile
- Clogged arteries
- Obesity
- Poor lung function
- Sluggish thyroid
- Vitamin deficiencies
- Taking medications that slow thinking as a side effect

Your Mental Health

- Worrying excessively
- Being depressed

▶ **Take Note:** Swedish researchers are developing a new scale to help doctors assess middle-age patients' risk of developing dementia in the future. Check it out at www.medpagetoday.com/Neurology/ICAD/tb/3737.

Instead of adopting a brain-healthy lifestyle, many people who are at risk for Alzheimer's disease or who have been diagnosed with mild cognitive impairment or Alzheimer's do one of the following—all of which are mistakes:

- Spend a lot of time and money on false leads that promise protection
- Wonder about natural ways to keep their brains healthy without doing anything about them
- Assert "It's all in the genes" and there's no preventing Alzheimer's disease, so don't try

We'll tell you what you can do to help protect your brain. But unlike the less-than-scientific memory "experts" who populate the

Internet and elsewhere, we make no guarantees, no false promises. We wish we could give you a magic bullet to delay or prevent Alzheimer's disease. But until rigorous and repeated research studies yield that long-held secret, we will have to stick with strategies that are safe and merely promising. However, thanks to research on the early effects of Alzheimer's on the brain, we are better able than ever to determine whether treatments are working. We also know that what's good for your brain is good for the rest of you as well.

Top Lifestyle Strategies for Protecting Your Brain

1. Avoid or treat strokes, heart disease, diabetes.
2. Treat depression and anxiety.
3. Exercise.
4. Follow a heart-healthy diet.
5. Stimulate your mind.
6. Engage socially with others.
7. Reduce stress.

The media regularly reports on the results of large observational studies, in which researchers try to determine the differences between groups of people who develop Alzheimer's and those who don't. But the most reliable evidence about how to at least delay Alzheimer's comes from clinical trials that provide direct comparisons of lifestyle changes in similar people. We have tried as much as possible here to stick to the hard evidence.

Legitimate anti-Alzheimer's strategies attempt to do one or more of these things:

- Reduce amyloid plaques or tangles in the brain
- Reduce cholesterol plaque in your arteries to prevent strokes
- Improve the reserve capacity of your brain so you can lose some nerve connections and still operate well
- Reduce your risk of developing vascular disease or inflammation
- Protect the brain from cell-damaging "oxidative stress"

- Improve signaling between nerve cells
- Correct chemical imbalances in the brain
- Improve blood supply and growth factor levels in the brain

Because of the emerging links between Alzheimer's and heart disease, our prescription for protecting your brain encompasses well-tested guidelines for avoiding heart disease, stroke, and diabetes so you can protect your heart as you protect your brain. That's a two-for-one bargain you don't want to pass up.

▶ **Before You Start:** Don't change your habits based on just one study or headline. Talk to your doctor first and do a little research on your own, on the Internet or at the library.

▶ DON'T ENDORSE HELPLESSNESS: TAKE ACTION

Until recently, when it came to Alzheimer's—unlike other common illnesses—the medical community practically endorsed helplessness. In contrast, doctors have strongly encouraged women to do monthly breast exams and get regular mammograms. If a woman develops any suspicious lumps, she sees a specialist—her regular doctor doesn't try to treat her. If she has a family history of breast cancer, her doctor may encourage her to participate in clinical trials or genetic studies of breast cancer. Doctors are expected to take the same approach to heart disease and diabetes, regularly testing patients' cholesterol, blood pressure, and blood sugar, and sending patients to a cardiologist or an endocrinologist if the numbers look suspicious.

What do we do for Alzheimer's? Even if both your parents have Alzheimer's, you've probably never been told to see an Alzheimer's specialist such as a neuropsychologist. Yet Alzheimer's moves along the same slow trajectory as heart disease and benefits from some commonsense early interventions. If you are at high risk of getting Alzheimer's disease or are just worried about your memory, you may want to see a specialist to learn how to address your personal risk factors and discuss possible research studies to join. Don't waste your money on a battery of memory tests until you get close to the age when your family member developed Alzheimer's or you show signs of memory loss. But it's never too early to build up your defenses.

Which Came First?

When you hear or read about the latest finding on how to prevent Alzheimer's, think of the chicken and the egg. For example, studies show that people who stay socially active have a lower rate of Alzheimer's. But the question that should pop into your head is: "Do people develop Alzheimer's because they aren't socially active—or do they actually lose their friends and drop out of activities because they have undetected Alzheimer's?" The disease can creep quietly through the brain, damaging brain cells before memory changes occur.

Sometimes it's hard to believe what you read about eating right or exercising, when your uncle Joe smoked, ate poorly, and never exercised, yet had a long life free of dementia. Uncle Joe doesn't disprove the risks of his lifestyle or the findings from prevention studies. He simply demonstrates that the large group studies can't always predict the outcome for a particular individual.

► AVOIDABLE AND UNAVOIDABLE RISKS

Some causes of Alzheimer's are inescapable, while others, research is suggesting, are subject to change. Consider the following research findings from studies of twins. Twins can tell us a lot about the cause of various diseases because twins share almost the exact same genes and, often, have similar home lives.

The study showed that the identical twin of someone with Alzheimer's is almost twice as likely to develop Alzheimer's as the fraternal twin of someone who has the disease.

However, the twin who developed Alzheimer's first was more likely to have one or more of the following risk factors. Notice that these risk factors are somewhat in our control.

- Anxiety
- A previous stroke

- Vascular disease
- A lower level of education
- Less exercise
- Less socially and intellectually engaging work
- The loss of a tooth to infection prior to age thirty-five. (Losing teeth doesn't cause Alzheimer's, but the infection may cause inflammation, which increases the risk of Alzheimer's.)

It's true you cannot avoid the biggest known risk for developing Alzheimer's: old age. Ten percent of people over age sixty-five have Alzheimer's, and the figure doubles every five years after that.

But even if you can't prevent Alzheimer's, try to delay it.

A Family Disease

If two or more of your family members have Alzheimer's, or if the disease struck when they were in their fifties or earlier, you may have one of two hundred rare genetic mutations that greatly increase a person's risk of developing Alzheimer's. Called either APP or presenilin mutations, they show up in a simple genetic test and almost guarantee that the carriers will develop Alzheimer's by their sixties.

Clearly these individuals need to be very proactive about delaying Alzheimer's. If you are in one of these families, you can ask your family physician to refer you to a specialist (neurologist, psychiatrist, or geneticist) or an Alzheimer's Disease Research Center to participate in a study that can help you or your family members. (See www.nia.nih.gov/clinicaltrials for listings.)

A few childhood experiences increase a person's risk of getting Alzheimer's as an adult, including having a head injury that knocked you out. Repetitive mild head injuries, such as from sports, also increase your risk of developing Alzheimer's, particularly if you are genetically susceptible. Having very little formal education appears to set people up for Alzheimer's later in life as well.

► CUSTOM-DESIGN YOUR BRAIN INSURANCE PLAN

When reading about what delays or lowers your risk of developing Alzheimer's, you may wonder: What *doesn't* help? Frequent participation in activities as routine as playing cards, walking, going out with friends, doing crossword puzzles, or eating healthy is supposed to guard your brain. Even eating curry or dark chocolate or drinking moderate amounts of red wine might help protect the brain against Alzheimer's.

The list of possible Alzheimer's preventatives is lengthy because researchers aren't yet sure what helps. Your job is to tackle your individual risk factors. For example, if you have a lot of cardiovascular risk factors, you will want to focus on a heart-healthy diet. Try to follow as many of the recommendations as you can. If you try too much at once, you'll just stress out. Consult professionals (for example, a doctor, trainer, dietician) before you start an exercise or dietary program to make sure that you set realistic goals and develop a safe and effective program.

Some people may find themselves thinking, "It's not worth it—I'd just as soon die a few years earlier or get Alzheimer's a year or two earlier than have to exercise all the time or try some crazy approach to reducing my risk." That's one way of approaching the problem, but one we (surprise!) don't endorse. We're not prescribing a hair shirt or hot coals. Just think:

- Do you walk your dog? Take an extra lap around the park, pick up your pace and, voilà, you've exercised. Bring along a friend; being engaged with others appears to reduce the risk of Alzheimer's.

- Do you consider blueberries on your cereal a punishment? Or what about a trip to the farm stand to pick up homegrown tomatoes, which you'll marinate in a little olive oil and vinegar? No one is forcing cod liver oil down your throat; we prefer to get our omega-3 fatty acids from fish, such as salmon, herring, or sardines.

Sam noticed a bocce game in progress just outside the new retirement condo when he and his wife, Mary, moved in. Sam hadn't played bocce since visiting his dad in his old neighborhood. The guys in the condo welcomed him to join in their game. He was surprised that they didn't seem to notice that he had early Alzheimer's. The more he played, the more bocce buddies he made, and they called him to make sure he didn't miss a game. Sometimes they also went to lunch together. His life had some of the structure, purpose, and even fun that he thought he had lost at the time of his diagnosis. His wife noticed that he seemed more attentive and energetic. He did tell his new buddies about his diagnosis, who took it in stride. Even his doctor commented that he seemed cheerier.

Exercise, diet, and mental routines can all be personalized so they are not only healthy but also satisfying and enjoyable. We'll concentrate on getting your body in shape in this chapter, and move on to mental exercises in the next.

▶ WHAT'S BAD FOR THE HEART IS BAD FOR THE BRAIN (USUALLY)

We used to think there was no stopping heart disease. Now we know you can reduce your risk of having a heart attack or stroke through lifestyle changes and medication. The same may be true for Alzheimer's disease. Your heart and your brain benefit from similar care and nurturing, and they both suffer from a Big Mac attack or a couch potato existence. But protecting your brain is a little more complicated than just following heart-healthy guidelines.

- You can have a healthy heart and still have blockages in the brain vessels.
- Compared with the heart, tiny regions in the brain control much more vital functions and so may be more sensitive to plaque in blood vessels and to blood clots.
- We take for granted that LDL cholesterol (the bad kind) raises one's risk for heart attacks and strokes, but the brain's memory centers need a certain amount of cholesterol to maintain healthy nerve connections.

THE FLIP SIDE OF CHOLESTEROL

Can very low cholesterol levels be dangerous as well? We don't know. The brain needs cholesterol to function, particularly to make hormones and for cells to communicate. Studies suggest that lowering cholesterol helps the brain in people who have abnormally high cholesterol levels. The results of a study of statins in people with normal cholesterol will be reported soon.

Vascular disease disrupts nerve cell circuits that are necessary for decision making, memory, and speech. The result is memory impairment that looks very much like Alzheimer's and may occur along with it but has a slightly different course.

How Vascular Disease Damages the Brain

- Clogged vessels means that less oxygen can get to the brain.
- Plaque clogging the arteries can break off, blocking a vessel and causing a stroke.
- Ministrokes easily go undetected and, therefore, untreated.
- High-fat diets cause plaque to build up in the brain.

Despite the link between vascular disease and memory impairment, many people with Alzheimer's disease have no diagnosable cardiovascular complaints. Why? Because vascular disease can impair mental functioning quite subtly, long before it limits physical well-being or shows up on your doctor's radar. You can have blockages in the vessels in your brain or in your neck that are impeding blood flow to your brain yet no heart condition calling out for treatment.

If you have had any small strokes, called transient ischemic attacks, ask your doctor about getting an ultrasound exam of your carotid artery in your neck and possibly of your brain to look for blockages. If those arteries are blocked, you will need treatment, which usually begins with a cholesterol-lowering regimen. Get rechecked three to six months after starting treatment.

To protect the brain from vascular disease, keep cholesterol levels, blood pressure, blood sugar, and weight in the healthy range. This means LDL or "bad cholesterol" should be below 130 mg/dL for most older people. But LDL guidelines vary with risk factors, so check with your doctor about the level that's best for you. For example, in people with diabetes or heart disease, LDL should be below 100 mg/dL.

Richard, a sixty-year-old executive, was initially diagnosed by a neurologist at a memory disorders clinic as having MCI or early Alzheimer's. The news was devastating, particularly since his mother had dementia in her late sixties. When he and his wife went for a follow-up appointment to talk with the neurologist about what he should do, a few more important details came out. Richard complained of feeling tired all the time, probably because his job was so stressful. His wife piped up: "We're both exhausted because his snoring has gotten so bad!" Aha, said the doctor.

It turned out that Richard had sleep apnea, which was successfully treated with a special mask that provides pressured air at night. Richard also needed to talk to the clinic psychiatrist about his stress, and he eventually started an antidepressant and eased his work load a bit. Within a couple of months, his wife reported that he seemed more engaged and able to concentrate better.

He also got motivated to try a strength-building exercise and spent more time teaching his grandson how to play tennis, a sport at which he had competed successfully for years. Final score: His memory improved slightly and stayed stable. The conclusion: His MCI was due to treatable conditions (stress, sleep apnea, sedentary lifestyle) and was not Alzheimer's.

▶ **Consider:** How you treat your heart while you are in your mid-forties or -fifties may set the stage for your future brain health.

Blood Clots: Brain Pollution

Blood is a little like an urban stream, dotted with bits of air bubbles and debris. But in the case of blood, the debris, called emboli, are blood clots and bits of plaque that break free from arteries. When plaque gets into brain vessels, it's called spontaneous cerebral emboli. Occasionally emboli block blood flow, so the less of them in the blood the better. Researchers compared the frequency of spontaneous cerebral emboli in people with dementia (half the group had Alzheimer's disease and the other half had vascular dementia) and healthy individuals in the same age range. After just one hour of ultrasound monitoring, about 40 percent of patients with either form of dementia had spontaneous emboli, while only about 15 percent of the healthy group did.

The study is more evidence linking vascular disease to Alzheimer's. But this study is only one hour in time. We need to know how people with frequent emboli fare over the years. If emboli do cause people to develop Alzheimer's earlier than they would have otherwise, then fighting emboli with low-dose aspirin or blood thinners will probably be part of an Alzheimer's prevention strategy.

In the meantime, ask your doctor how you can lower your vascular risk factors for Alzheimer's. Get help from a dietician to make sure you are eating a healthy, balanced diet that limits fat intake. Get a copy of your last physical exam to see how you scored on cholesterol levels, weight, and waist size and get them checked at each physical. The American Heart Association's Web site has an excellent resource called "Meet the Bad Fats Brothers" in their Diet and Nutrition section (www .americanheart.org) that provides step-by-step advice on selecting the most heart-healthy diets. As we said earlier, you don't want to limit your cholesterol intake severely, but to keep it in the healthy range.

Watch Your Blood Pressure

People who have chronic, uncontrolled high blood pressure, called hypertension, in midlife are more likely than their nonhypertensive peers to develop Alzheimer's disease. The studies are mixed on whether taking medication to control blood pressure lowers the risk of Alzheimer's. But consider this: Hypertension causes vessels in the brain to become stiff, which decreases blood flow to the brain. So it simply makes sense to keep your blood pressure low. But not too low. As with cholesterol, you want a balance; very low blood pressure isn't good for the brain either.

Generally, blood pressure should be close to normal (120/80), or at a level where you don't feel tired, dizzy, or unable to function well. If you feel tired or light-headed when you stand up, you may have very low blood pressure and need to have your medication adjusted. If you have headaches or your eyesight is being affected, then your blood pressure may be too high.

No Smoking

Smoking may harm the brain by increasing a person's risk of having a stroke or by causing lung or other health problems that impair memory. Studies once suggested that smokers were less likely than nonsmokers to have Alzheimer's, but it is possible the smokers simply died younger of other diseases such as cancer. Nicotine can increase attention and short-term memory, and many drugs that mimic nicotine are in development to treat or prevent Alzheimer's. But smoking is not the way to go. Think long term. Quit now.

Strokes and Alzheimer's

Strokes may not cause Alzheimer's directly, but the vascular disease that causes strokes increases the risk of Alzheimer's. Also, strokes can damage the brain, so a person's thinking and memory often decline, at least temporarily. Researchers monitored a large group of people over age sixty-five who were all free of dementia when the study started. After five years, the study participants who had suffered a stroke were the most likely to have memory loss and to process information less quickly.

► DIABETES: ALL-AROUND DANGEROUS

One in five people over age sixty-five has type II (so-called adult-onset) diabetes, and many more are at risk of developing the disease. Middle-aged diabetics are more likely than their nondiabetic peers to develop dementia later in life. One study found that people with type II diabetes were 65 percent more likely to develop Alzheimer's than nondiabetics. But just getting your blood sugar under control doesn't necessarily protect you against the diabetes-Alzheimer's link. In one study, researchers helped diabetics control their blood sugar levels, but the diabetics' mental status didn't improve. The lesson: It's more difficult to clear the fog than to prevent it from rolling in.

How Diabetes Harms the Brain

- Diabetes damages blood vessels throughout the body and increases the risk of stroke.

- When a person has diabetes, cells throughout the body, including the brain, fail to respond to insulin, which means they fail to absorb sugar to meet their energy needs. As a result, cells starve while the concentration of glucose in the blood increases. Also, an enzyme that degrades insulin decreases, which may trigger Alzheimer's changes in the brain.

- Diabetes leads to inflammation in the brain, which increases the risk of Alzheimer's.

There's help and hope, however.

- Diabetics who controlled their cholesterol by taking cholesterol-lowering drugs called statins were less likely to have a stroke, which lowered their risk for developing dementia.

- Many laboratory studies suggest that taking medication to boost insulin sensitivity may help protect the brain from Alzheimer's, though that's still not confirmed.

- Medications used to treat diabetes are also being tested as Alzheimer's remedies. (But one of those drugs, Avandia, may be bad for your heart, studies are now suggesting.)

Metabolic Syndrome

Related to diabetes, metabolic syndrome is a combination of excess fat around the abdomen, high triglyceride levels, low HDL (good cholesterol), high blood pressure, and elevated fasting glucose. In a large study of men and women in their seventies, participants with metabolic syndrome were more likely to develop Alzheimer's during the five-year study than those without the syndrome, but only if they also had high levels of inflammation, as measured by blood tests.

Surprisingly, you don't have to have very high numbers to qualify for the metabolic syndrome label. The American Heart Association and others define it as having three or more of the following conditions:

- Waistline measuring greater than thirty-five inches for women and forty inches for men. For people genetically at risk for diabetes, the measurement is thirty-one to thirty-five inches for women and thirty-seven to thirty-nine inches for men. (This is not your pants size. It's what the tape measure tells you when you measure your waist with the tape against your skin.)
- Triglyceride levels of 150 mg/dL or higher, or taking medication for high triglycerides.
- HDL levels below 40 mg/dL for men and below 50 mg/dL for women, or taking medication for low HDL.
- Blood pressure at or about 130/85, or taking medication for high blood pressure.
- Fasting blood sugar (blood glucose) of 100 mg/dL or higher, or receiving treatment for high blood sugar.

Metabolic syndrome is a controversial diagnosis. Some people argue that it is not a true, separate condition but, instead, a combination of risk factors. Nevertheless, the evidence suggests that even borderline high numbers can combine to put you at risk of developing Alzheimer's and other diseases.

► OBESITY: AS DANGEROUS FOR YOUR BRAIN AS FOR YOUR HEART

Studies are beginning to link being very overweight or obese to developing Alzheimer's. In a group of older women without Alzheimer's, those who were very overweight at age seventy were the most likely to develop Alzheimer's disease ten to eighteen years later. The more overweight a person was, the greater her risk of developing Alzheimer's. Another large study showed that obesity even at midlife is associated with an increased risk of Alzheimer's disease later in life.

The link between Alzheimer's and obesity may be leptin, a hormone secreted by fat cells that has many roles in the brain: It announces that you are full and also boosts learning and memory. Studies suggest that leptin fails to move from the fat cells to the brain as readily in some obese individuals as in nonobese people. Being overweight also increases blood clotting and boosts cortisol levels, which isn't good for brain cells.

Carrying extra pounds around the waist, as opposed to the hips, is particularly dangerous for the heart and the head. The tendency to put weight on around the middle (having the shape of an apple instead of a pear) may be inherited. A study found that women with the most fat around their waist were one and a half times more likely to develop dementia than those with a slimmer waistline.

If you're worried about your waistline, get a measuring tape, lift up your shirt, and measure. If you're a man and it's forty inches or more, or a woman and it's thirty-five inches or more, that's a red flag waving in front of your refrigerator telling you to cut back and go exercise, even if your weight is close to normal. You should also check your body mass index (a measure of obesity) online at www .nhlbisupport.com/bmi.

If you are around people with Alzheimer's, you may be surprised by the link between obesity and dementia for one very good reason: The rate of obesity among this group is actually fairly low because it turns out that people often lose weight before getting diagnosed with Alzheimer's. We strongly recommend eating a healthy diet and exercising to reduce the risk of Alzheimer's and to delay its symptoms.

► EXERCISE FOR THE SAKE OF YOUR BRAIN

A forest of about 100 billion branching nerve cells connect to one another throughout your brain. For your brain to process memories and experiences, those neurons must communicate with one another. But Alzheimer's destroys those connections (synapses). New research is showing us how the brain can operate around that destruction.

Neurons form new connections around the damaged areas, even after the onset of normal age-related declines in mental abilities. How do they perform such magic? With the help of growth factors, protein molecules in the brain cells that help keep the synapses healthy and connected, aid the flow of memory and learning chemicals in the brain, and appear to protect nerve cells against injury.

When adults aged sixty to seventy-nine gradually increased their aerobic exercise over six months, the size of their brain's gray matter (which houses nerve cells) and white matter (which houses the fiber tracts) increased, a study showed. A study of younger adults found that exercising for one hour daily for twelve weeks increased activity in the brain regions adjacent to the memory center. Animal studies suggest that changes in activity are due to new nerve cell connections forming. The participants exercised for five minutes at low intensity, did five minutes of stretching, then did forty minutes of aerobic cycling or running and ten minutes of cool-down exercises.

"Before-and-after" pictures of people who have lost weight or had a makeover are a popular feature of fashion magazines. Doctors like before-and-after pictures too. In fact, one group of researchers took pictures of healthy sixty- and seventy-year-olds before and after they participated in a six-month program of brisk walking. But it wasn't their muscle tone or even their hearts that the doctors wanted to see.

They were looking at the activity levels of different parts of the participants' brains. The brain-imaging pictures revealed that exercise led to an increase in the activity of brain cells, suggesting that those parts of the brain were functioning better than before. Other studies have revealed that more physically fit people have slightly less thinning of their brain tissue in areas normally diminished by age. The denser the tissue, the greater the likelihood that those key connections between brain cells will remain intact.

Memory tests reveal the same good news. In a Japanese study, 70 percent of 265 individuals without Alzheimer's or with MCI who participated in a yearlong exercise program saw improvement in their memory test scores. The participants with MCI showed more improvement than the others.

The bottom line: Studies that follow large groups of people over many years also reveal that people who exercise regularly are less likely than their sedentary peers to develop Alzheimer's. Indeed, regular exercisers over age sixty-five have about half the risk of developing dementia, compared with people who are similar in many ways except the amount that they exercise.

Animals provide us an inside-the-brain view of the benefits of exercise. Rodents that were given an exercise wheel in their cages exercised a lot and had many more new brain cells and better connections between the cells than animals that lived without the wheel. The cell changes appear to have a direct benefit: Animals that exercise are better learners than sedentary animals. In addition, among mice that are predisposed to develop Alzheimer's disease, the ones allowed to exercise have less amyloid plaque. In another animal study, the level of one growth factor, brain-derived neurotrophic factor, increased in the brain's memory center after a week of regular exercise.

How Exercise Helps

- Reduces the chances of developing conditions that may contribute to Alzheimer's, including diabetes, high cholesterol, high blood pressure, and stroke
- Increases blood flow to the brain. (More than one-fourth of the blood from every heartbeat goes to the brain.)
- Triggers the release of brain chemicals, including endorphins, that help improve mood and response to stress
- Stimulates growth factors that help maintain the brain nerve cells
- Promotes new synaptic connections between brain cells

You may be wondering, "Just how much do I have to sweat to get these kinds of benefits?" The general rule is the more regularly you exercise, the better. But always warm up and cool down.

What Qualifies as Regular Exercise

- One half hour *brisk* walk at least five days a week
- Stretching (about ten minutes) on the days you exercise

- Strength training, such as working with weights, at least two to three times a week. (Strength training protects your brain indirectly: Good muscle tone guards against falls and the cascade of events, including hospitalization, that can follow.)

If you rarely or never exercise, start very gradually and build up to the recommended intensity over several weeks. It is better to go slow and steady rather than injure yourself. The Centers for Disease Control has excellent exercise recommendations for older adults. Go to www.cdc.gov, then type "physical activity" in the search box. A new exercise package is coming from the NIA Web site soon!

What Counts as Aerobic Exercise

- Vigorous dance
- Brisk walking
- Hiking
- Bicycling
- Aerobics
- Swimming
- Water aerobics
- Tennis, basketball, or other team sports where you move a lot
- Golf, if you walk the course

Although there is no strong evidence that they help memory, yoga and the Chinese exercises tai chi and qigong may boost concentration and reduce stress. Qigong, which you can do sitting, is quiet and meditative. Tai chi involves following slow, gentle, flowing movements. You can learn both through classes in many areas of the country.

It's Never Too Late to Benefit from Exercise

Among people with dementia, those who exercise do better on memory tests. For people with Alzheimer's, exercise reduces restlessness, improves attention, and elevates mood. However, people with Alzheimer's need to be monitored closely when they exercise, so they don't get lost or become overheated, chilled, dizzy, injured, or exhausted. Also, be prepared for the unintended effects of new-found fitness: They may have more mobility and be able to wander off more easily.

► MEMORABLE MEALS: HOW TO EAT AS IF YOUR BRAIN DEPENDED ON IT

One of the loudest messages you'll get via the media about prevent-ing Alzheimer's is that diet makes a difference, and it may. But as the rest of this chapter shows, so do a lot of other parts of your day. No single food or vitamin is likely to prevent or even delay Alzheimer's, but a healthy diet may help delay the onset or progression of Alzheimer's, and it certainly won't hurt.

Here's what to eat every day, if possible. If you are trying to keep your weight down, go for the low-fat options.

- 2½ cups dark green, leafy vegetables, such as kale and spinach, or dark-skinned vegetables, such as eggplant, brussels sprouts, broccoli, beets
- 2 cups colorful and high-fiber fruits, such as prunes, raisins, strawberries, plums, oranges, red grapes, cherries, raspberries, pomegranate
- 6 ounces whole grains, such as whole-wheat bread or pasta, brown rice, oatmeal
- 5½ ounces protein, preferably beans, egg whites, whey protein, lean meat and poultry, or fish (avoid fish that is high in mercury)
- 3 cups milk, yogurt, and other dairy foods, or foods that sub-stitute for dairy, such as soy milk
- monounsaturated fats, found in olive oil

Other Foods for the Brain

- Apples, apricots, cherries, nonfat yogurt, baked beans, grapes, oranges, oatmeal, and apple juice all are good for maintaining steady blood sugar levels.

- Prunes, raisins, blueberries, spinach, plums, and broccoli are top sources of antioxidants.

- Nuts, salmon, and olive oil provide healthy fats (omega-3s).

► WHAT ABOUT ANTIOXIDANTS?

As the body breaks down food, it releases so-called free radicals, oxygen molecules that bounce around the body damaging other cells and, studies suggest, eventually increasing a person's risk of heart disease, cancer, and possibly Alzheimer's disease. Compounds called antioxidants may protect against some of this cell damage.

Clinical trials comparing the effectiveness of antioxidant vitamins to placebos have found more risks than anticipated for heart patients and no real benefits in delaying the onset of Alzheimer's. Large quantities of antioxidants, as opposed to the levels found in a healthy diet, may interfere with the body's normal immune response to cell damage, among other negative side effects.

Eating fresh fruits, red and orange fruit juices, green tea, and vegetables daily are the best way to get your antioxidants (and a host of other nutrients), in part because you are unlikely to get too high a dose.

The Vitamin E Story

Vitamin E, an antioxidant, was given to people with Alzheimer's to delay progression of the disease but is no longer recommended for this purpose. Its popularity over the past twenty-five years resembles that of a Hollywood starlet. It also resembles other vitamins' stories of fame and misfortune, including the B vitamins.

- In the early and mid-1990s, community surveys found that people who took vitamin E were less likely to develop Alzheimer's, or they got it later in life. Clinical trials also suggested that vitamin E might slow Parkinson's disease and protect against heart disease.

- In 1997 a large clinical trial of people who had moderate Alzheimer's showed that the participants who were given very high doses (2,000 IU per day) of vitamin E didn't decline as quickly as the participants not on vitamin E.

- Although some researchers questioned the study's statistics, this study and prior studies increased the number of Alzheimer's experts and panels recommending high-dose vitamin E to prevent or slow the effects of Alzheimer's.

- Then in 2005, a large clinical trial found that vitamin E did not slow progression of Alzheimer's in people with MCI.

- Also in 2005, a review of multiple studies showed that people with vascular disease or diabetes who took more than 400 IU of vitamin E for seven years face an increased risk of heart failure. Taking vitamin E and C combined also increased their risk of dying prematurely of any cause.

- The bottom line: Extra vitamin E doesn't help the brain or the heart.

▶ THE MEDITERRANEAN WAY

Individual vitamins may not alter your Alzheimer's risk, since it's the diet as a whole and no one nutrient that the brain depends on. One of the most important recent findings on diet and Alzheimer's is that the so-called Mediterranean (think Greece or Italy) diet helps to protect the brain, and it does so in the same way that it protects the heart: by limiting the body's development of plaque, oxidative stress, and inflammation. The diet includes lots of fruits, vegetables, legumes, grains, and olive oil; moderate consumption of wine; and more fish than red meat, which keeps saturated fat and calories in check.

When a multiethnic group of over two thousand residents of New York City followed this diet, the participants who adhered to it most carefully over four years had slightly fewer cases of Alzheimer's disease and overall a slower rate of decline in their thinking and memory than those who were least compliant.

Eating fish even once a week appeared to lower the risk of Alzheimer's by 60 percent, according to one study. You should avoid eating the following fish regularly, however, because they contain high levels of mercury from polluted water: shark, swordfish, king mackerel, and tilefish. To find out about the mercury levels of fish that you or friends catch, check with the local department of fisheries and watch for advisories posted in fishing spots. Good fish picks are salmon, mackerel, sardines, albacore tuna, lake trout, herring, and halibut.

Although the fatty acid in fish, omega-3, has been associated with numerous health benefits, from protecting the adult heart to improving eyesight, it's still unclear whether taking omega-3 lowers the risk of Alzheimer's. In a recent clinical trial, people with mild Alzheimer's derived no benefits from taking omega-3 supplements.

We know, however, that these fatty acids are essential to learning and memory in early development. We've also seen in rats that omega-3s improve brain cell connections and reduce oxidative damage. People with Alzheimer's tend to have low levels of omega-3s in blood and brain tissue.

Other Sources of Omega-3s

- Venison and buffalo if grass-fed
- Some brands of eggs are supplemented with docosahexanoic acid (DHA), the omega-3 fatty acid found in fish
- Canola oil, flaxseed, flaxseed oil, nuts, seeds, and leafy green vegetables such as purslane are all good sources of the type of omega-3 fatty acid contained in plants, called alpha-linolenic acid (ALA)

As with any nutrient, more isn't necessarily better. Large amounts of omega-3s are dangerous. For one, your body uses many different types of fatty acids and taking too much of one type can throw off your body's healthy ratio of fatty acids. Foods with the right ratios are unhydrogenated, unsaturated fats such as oil-based salad dressings, nuts, seeds, fish, mayonnaise, and eggs.

▶ B IS FOR BRAIN

Vitamins B_6 and B_{12}, as well as the B vitamin called folate or folic acid may help protect the brain. Some studies suggest that high doses of vitamins B_1, B_{12}, and folic acid should improve brain metabolism and nerve cell function. However, clinical trials on the beneficial effects of the B family haven't been positive with regard to improving memory.

Folic acid. People with low levels of folic acid may be at an increased risk of developing MCI and Alzheimer's disease, according to a variety of studies. Foods rich in folic acid are broccoli, asparagus, peas, lettuce, beans, orange juice, whole-grain or fortified breads, pastas, and rice.

B_{12}. We know that a deficiency of vitamin B_{12} can cause memory loss, anemia, and nerve damage, and that B_{12} is often low in older people, particularly those with memory problems. However, reversing a B_{12} deficiency does not always clear up memory problems. Still, elderly individuals need to be sure to eat enough foods rich in B_{12}, such as meat, poultry, fish, eggs, milk, and cheese. They may need more B_{12} than younger people do, because they lack sufficient acid in their stomach to release the B_{12} from the food they eat. Heavy drinkers of any age are likely to be low on all nutrients, especially B vitamins and thiamine.

Homocysteine. If the B vitamins do help the brain, it may be by controlling levels of an amino acid in the blood called homocysteine. Having high levels of homocysteine may increase the risk of dementia, heart disease, and stroke. Studies of mice show that excess homocysteine destroys brain cells.

B supplements. At this point it is unclear whether taking folic acid or B vitamins or even lowering homocysteine levels changes a person's risk of getting Alzheimer's or slows the progression of the disease. So play it safe and get your vitamins through the foods you eat. Don't take supplements just for preventing Alzheimer's unless you are deficient in the nutrient.

Daily vitamin supplements optional. Most people do not need a multivitamin if they eat a balanced diet. It's fine if you want to take a multivitamin without iron that provides 100 percent of your recommended daily allowance (RDA) for vitamins and minerals, but a vitamin pill doesn't let you off the hook when it comes to eating a great diet.

▶ CHEERS? THE DEAL WITH ALCOHOL

In the story of Alzheimer's, wine plays the roles of good guy and bad. Heavy alcohol use can cause its own form of acute or chronic dementia. However, in a study of almost 750 people over the age of sixty-five, half of whom had early-stage Alzheimer's, those who had between one and six drinks of any kind of alcohol in a week had a lower risk of developing Alzheimer's disease than those who abstained. It makes sense for women to limit themselves to one drink a day for other reasons, including that alcohol may increase a woman's risk of breast cancer. Among specific types of alcohol, the best research data are for red wine. Other liquors, such as vodka and whiskey, are not as well studied.

Wine in moderation probably helps the brain by increasing levels of resveratrol, procyanadins, and good cholesterol. It may also lower the risk of stroke. However, we don't have enough evidence to recommend starting or increasing your alcohol intake to ward off Alzheimer's disease.

Resveratrol, a chemical found in grape skins, peanuts, and berries, is a type of natural estrogen called phytoestrogen. Animal studies show that it has many beneficial effects, including activating genes that increase life span (longevity genes) and reducing inflammation and free radicals. However, the animals got megaconcentrated doses (the amount found in about fifty bottles of wine daily). So until clinical trials are completed we will not know how much we should be getting or what its risks are. Synthetic resveratrol sold as supplements has not been shown to delay dementia.

EXPENSIVE WORRYING

Concerned that she was becoming forgetful, a middle-aged businesswoman whose mother had Alzheimer's disease decided to try some herbal and vitamin supplements that her friends recommended for memory. She had also read that some natural products might stop memory loss. She first took

(continued)

just one type of vitamin, but when she returned monthly on half-price days for refills, the salesperson convinced her to add a new supplement to her regimen. It wasn't long before she was spending four hundred dollars a month on fifteen separate pills. Now not only was her memory worrying her, but so was her budget.

She finally went for testing at a memory disorders clinic. The tests uncovered no Alzheimer's disease but lots of anxiety about her health. The doctor reassured her that she was not getting Alzheimer's disease and gave her strategies for dealing with her anxiety, including walking every day. The forgetfulness soon diminished and her worries gradually leveled out. Her co-pay on the bill for the memory evaluation cost less than a month of supplements.

We would have also told her: Watch your diet and exercise your mind. You'll feel better mentally and physically. It's a win-win solution.

► CURRY, ANYONE?

Rates of Alzheimer's in India are lower than in the United States. This could be because Indians have a shorter life expectancy and a lower prevalence of the ApoE4 gene. But researchers also wonder if it might have something to do with Indians' love affair with curry. The turmeric in curry contains an anti-inflammatory, antioxidant, cholesterol-lowering compound called curcumin.

A clinical trial is exploring the effects of two different doses of curcumin in patients with early- and middle-stage Alzheimer's disease, to monitor how well it is absorbed, plus its effects, if any, on

- inflammation
- oxidative damage
- cholesterol levels
- thinking and memory
- behavior
- daily functioning

Again, it is premature to buy curcumin supplements since we don't yet know the best—if any—dose. Treat yourself to an occasional curry dinner—if you like curry—or try recipes that call for turmeric, a rather mild spice that goes well with many foods.

► SUPPLEMENTAL SUPPLEMENTS

Many people, including many doctors, take herbs and supplements. They tend to be health-conscious, educated consumers who take advantage of what is now termed "integrative medicine," or medicine that combines both traditional and, by Western standards, untraditional medicine. Most major university medical centers are creating programs of integrative medicine, built on a strong foundation of scientific evidence.

While integrative medicine has many advantages, herbs and supplements may interact with prescription and over-the-counter medications and exacerbate chronic conditions. For example, a woman developed internal bleeding from taking a combination of a prescribed blood thinner along with her self-prescribed approach to Alzheimer's prevention: vitamin E. Take the case of a product called phosphatidylserine (PS) that may help the flow of nerve impulses. PS is an essential ingredient in nerve cell membranes and signal transmission. The PS in over-the-counter products now comes from soybeans, but PS used to come from cow brains until concerns surfaced over mad cow disease. PS has improved the mental abilities slightly in some older people, including those with Alzheimer's, but the study findings are not consistent.

Other supplements, often labeled "mind boosters," contain many different ingredients that may have been shown in some study to have plausible biological benefits to the brain. However, the pills' contents may vary from batch to batch, so you could be fine with one batch and react poorly to another. You should also consider:

- Have the many ingredients been tested together?
- How might they affect or interact with any prescription or over-the-counter medicines you are taking?
- Will you have an allergic reaction to any one of the compounds, or to the preservatives in the pills not listed on the bottle?

▶ HERBAL HEALING?

Roughly 25 percent of modern prescription drugs originated from herbal sources. The Alzheimer's medication Razadyne was originally extracted from a daffodil, for example. Herbs have the potential to provide natural, safe, and effective remedies at a lower cost than prescription drugs, though they can have risks also. Since medical doctors are usually uninformed about herbal remedies, if you are interested in herbs, you may want to seek the advice of an alternative medicine specialist. Many academic centers, such as Harvard University, Duke University, the University of Arizona, and Columbia University, have clinics staffed by doctors trained in alternative medicine.

Herbals have many of the same risks and disadvantages as nutritional supplements:

- Studies have yet to show that they definitely help people with Alzheimer's.

- They may have unknown side effects.

- The FDA requires a company to show through studies that its herbal supplements are effective *only* if the company puts a claim on the product that it treats specific diseases or symptoms.

- The quality and ingredients of herbals are sometimes not what the label claims, so you need to buy herbals through reputable stores.

Do Your Research

How would you feel if your doctor said you need to take five diluted medications? That might be what you're getting in one "natural" supplement pill. Few of these combinations have even been tested. So before you decide to try individual herbal supplements, do your research on the products and always let your doctors know what you are taking. For the most credible information available on herbals, check out:

- The FDA's Web site to learn how it regulates dietary supplements: www.cfsan.fda.gov/~dms/ds-faq.html.

- NIH Office of Dietary Supplements at http://dietary-supplements.info.nih.gov/. Click on "Health Information," then "Full List of Dietary Supplement Fact Sheets."
- www.peoplespharmacy.com. Click on "Herb Library" at left.
- American Botanical Council's Web site: www.herbalgram.org

Myths About Herbals

- Even if a product may not help you, it can't hurt.
- Natural means healthful and safe.
- If the label doesn't list any side effects or cautions, then you know it's safe.
- When a product is recalled, all of the bottles are removed from shelves.

Serious injuries and adverse events are less common with common herbal products than they are with prescription drugs or even aerobic exercise. Still, that is no justification for taking an unproven remedy.

► HERBS THAT MAY HELP THE MIND

Here are a few of the most promising herbs, with Chinese club moss leading the list. But as with all medicines, talk to your doctor or qualified alternative medicine practitioner about the medications' usefulness and side effects for you.

Chinese Club Moss (Huperzine A)

This moss extract has been popular in China for thousands of years for treating fever and other conditions. It is now being used in several countries for memory loss. It appears to work by blocking a brain enzyme cholinesterase that clears up excess acetylcholine, a neurotransmitter in the brain. People with Alzheimer's have too little acetylcholine and could use the extra acetylcholine that cholinesterase normally removes. (Most prescription Alzheimer's medications work the same way.)

In one eight-week study that included people with and without Alzheimer's, thinking and memory functions improved more in people who took the extract than in participants given a placebo. Animal and test-tube studies show that the moss extract may protect brain cells from the ravages of the plaques and tangles that contribute to Alzheimer's. Finally, the moss appears to work as an antioxidant. In an ongoing, rigorous government-run clinical trial, people with mild to moderate Alzheimer's are taking either 200 or 400 micrograms twice daily for six months.

Warnings: Chinese club moss should not be combined with other cholinesterase inhibitors, including the Alzheimer's medications Aricept, Exelon, and Razadyne. Like any cholinesterase inhibitor, it could in theory cause blurry vision, nausea, irregular heartbeat, and sweating, among other side effects. But so far it appears to have minimal side effects.

Ginkgo Biloba Extract

Possibly one of the best studied of the herbs for people concerned about getting Alzheimer's disease, ginkgo is rich in flavonoids and terpenoids, which may reduce inflammation in the brain. Ginkgo may be an antioxidant and increase blood flow to the brain. After some fairly positive studies of ginkgo were published, the news went negative in 2005 when two trials (in people with and without Alzheimer's) showed that gingko was no more beneficial than a placebo. Then a small study in 2006 directly comparing ginkgo with Aricept, a common cholinesterase inhibitor, showed that the two medicines produced similar benefits.

Ginkgo is really being put to the test now: A rigorous, government-run study of about three thousand healthy men and women over age seventy-five is investigating whether 240 milligrams of ginkgo daily will help prevent or delay dementia. The results should be out in 2009. Other studies are investigating the effect of ginkgo on reducing symptoms of vascular disease, which could be important also for people hoping to ward off Alzheimer's.

Warnings: The main concern about ginkgo is that it may increase bleeding among people who take blood thinners or high-dose aspirin, though this has not been clearly demonstrated. It could also cause headaches, nausea, and restlessness, which is the case with most medicines that affect the brain.

Sage

Sage may be one of those herbs that is moving out of the kitchen and into the medicine cabinet, but it's still very iffy. Sage may work as a cholinesterase inhibitor and anti-inflammatory and possibly have some of the positive effects of estrogen on nerve cell growth.

Researchers are studying its effectiveness at improving the mental function of people with mild Alzheimer's disease. In an ongoing study, they are giving sage extract to forty people and then testing their attention, memory, and visual memory. The researchers use a brain-imaging device to see if and how the sage is interacting with brain cells. A small trial in healthy people suggested it may decrease anxiety and increase attention.

Warnings: Sage oil is poisonous, so it shouldn't be ingested or used for aromatherapy. Sage may lower blood sugar. It's not as well studied as the two other herbs we describe, and its long-term safety in Alzheimer's patients is unknown.

► SURGERY'S AFTERMATH

Surgery leaves everyone feeling groggy, out of it, and generally lousy for a while. But for people in their sixties and above, it's worse. Research shows that at least a third of older patients show persistent mild decline on tests of their mental abilities after heart surgery. This is also true for such seemingly routine surgery as orthopedic procedures. The surgery may increase inflammation and the likelihood of plaque breaking loose from inside a blood vessel and traveling to the brain. Some forms of general anesthesia may speed up the formation of plaques in the brain, studies of animals suggest. The risk of surgery or any hospitalization is even greater for people who already have Alzheimer's.

Although this sounds worrying, the evidence is still very preliminary. People who need any surgery should not avoid it, but they should make sure that their surgical team minimizes the risks to the brain. Certain surgical techniques, such as lowering a patient's temperature during surgery and then warming him or her gradually at the end of the procedure, reduce the risk of cognitive impairment following heart surgery. These techniques are not yet routine in general surgical practice. Don't hesitate to ask your anesthesiologist, as well as your surgeon, about these procedures or others. Also, make sure you are treated promptly for infection and pain after surgery, as both may influence how well your brain (and the rest of you) recovers.

▶ IN SUMMARY: YOUR BRAIN-HEALTHY RX

Eat Well

- Eat fruits and vegetables every day and fish that is low in mercury at least once a week. A healthy vegetarian diet is also great for the brain.
- Eat healthy fats; avoid saturated or trans fats.
- If you drink alcohol, limit it to one drink a day for women and two for men.

Move It

- Exercise at least five days a week (daily is better) for at least half an hour (you can break that into ten-minute segments). Walking, dancing, gardening all count.

Weigh In

- Maintain a healthy weight and watch out for an expanding waistline (yours).

Clear the Vessels

- Ask your doctor if you need to take a daily baby aspirin.
- Keep your total cholesterol below 200 and your LDL less than 130.
- Keep your blood pressure in a healthy range for you.
- Keep your fasting blood sugar less than 100 mg/dL.

Use Common Sense

- Treat hearing and vision problems.
- Watch out for side effects or interactions from medications.
- Wear seat belts and bike helmets, and use handrails to avoid falls.

CHAPTER SEVENTEEN

STAYING CONNECTED: KEEPING YOUR BRAIN ACTIVE

It is not enough to add years to one's life: One must also add life to those years.

—JOHN F. KENNEDY

We gave you the first part of our prescription for a brain-healthy lifestyle in the previous chapter and that was the tougher part: Exercise and eat right. Here comes the good news. The very activities that make life interesting and rewarding—learning new things, enjoying friends and hobbies, reducing stress, and increasing plea-surable experiences—can help protect your brain against memory loss. But few of us are pros at having fun, so here are some tips.

▶ PEOPLE POWER: SOCIALIZING IS GOOD FOR YOUR BRAIN

One way to keep your cells communicating is to engage in the prac-tice yourself. In a study of people over age fifty-five, those with larger social networks had smaller declines in thinking and memory function as they aged. When researchers take a group of people and divide them according to how much they interact with others in a way that is meaningful to them, the ones who score toward the very involved end are less likely to develop Alzheimer's than those who are less involved. Research has also shown that having strong social networks minimizes the effect of Alzheimer's-related brain damage on thinking and memory. In fact, in one large study, people whose jobs involved working with or talking with others were less likely to get Alzheimer's than people working alone.

What's behind this link between social and brain networks?

- People with a large group of friends and family are more likely to engage in physical and mental activity, which boosts brain function.

- Very social people may have stronger brain circuits or more easily use alternative circuits when the need arises to remain social after Alzheimer's symptoms have begun.

- Social engagement may reduce effects of stress on the brain, and people with few friends tend to have more stress in their lives.

Don't run out and volunteer someplace or make amends with an annoying relative in an attempt to ward off Alzheimer's. The goal is to find or to maintain relationships that you value and that provide meaning without causing you undue stress. For example, being very involved with your church may provide valuable social and spiritual support, but people who are devout out of a fear of going to hell or of being punished face the same risk of getting Alzheimer's disease as nonaffiliated individuals.

What if you are a bit of a loner by nature and would just as soon go to a museum by yourself or stay home and enjoy the garden? Or if you simply have no time to do anything except go to work and support your family, whom you never see because you work so much? Don't put "getting Alzheimer's" on your list of worries.

- Feeling stressed out or anxious is not great for the brain.

- As is the case with so many possible ways to ward off Alzheimer's, having close social ties is only one possible source of protection for your brain.

- Close relationships are not a guarantee that you won't get Alzheimer's.
- Stimulating leisure activities (see below), such as gardening or going to a museum, are good for your brain even if enjoyed alone.
- Being really engaged in challenging work, unless it contributes to your chronic stress, also protects the brain.

John, a retired school principal, didn't want to leave his wife, Barbara, alone when he volunteered at the after-school program for at-risk children. Since Barbara's diagnosis of Alzheimer's disease, she seemed to have lost interest in everything except making sure he was by her side all the time. John suggested there were younger children at the program who could probably use her help with reading while he led sports activities for the older boys. Barbara was matched with a seven-year-old girl who was too withdrawn to read aloud in class. Barbara started reading to her, even adding her own stories from her childhood. Soon, other girls joined them, attracted to Barbara's stories. John was surprised by her improved mood, self-confidence, and ability to stay with an activity. He was relieved to learn that her memory scores had not declined at her next visit to the doctor and wondered if he could credit the volunteer activity.

► LEISURE TIME: A TIME TO CONNECT (BRAIN CELLS)

Your choice of leisure activities, what you do when you're not working or taking care of your day-to-day chores, makes a difference to your brain. Ask a group of healthy individuals how much they participate in stimulating leisure activities, divide the group into the most active and least active, then see how they perform over the years on tests of their memory and mental abilities. The active group will decline more slowly than the less active group. Research suggests that people who are in the top third for activity are about half as likely to develop early signs of Alzheimer's, compared with the least involved people. This is true after ruling out the effects of participants' age, educational level, illnesses, and depression and how they performed on tests of thinking and memory when the study began—all factors that can affect the likelihood of developing Alzheimer's.

Stimulating leisure activities probably help the brain by building a "cognitive reserve" or extra connections between cells that your brain can turn to as it ages, reducing chronic stress and promoting a healthy lifestyle (when you're busy, you're not sitting on the couch eating junk food!).

▶ **Good to Know:** Four activities—reading, board games, playing musical instruments, and dancing—were the most significant in protecting against dementia in one landmark study.

Animals tipped off researchers to the possibility that an enriched environment protects the aging brain. Rodents that live in stimulating environments (cages with plenty of toys and rodent friends) are less likely to get Alzheimer's than animals living in less interesting circumstances. Moreover, the brains of animals that live in these environments have more neural connections and a growth factor called brain-derived neurotrophic factor, yet they have less amyloid in their brains compared with their colleagues in the boring cages.

NOT ALL MEMORY IS THE SAME

We have many specific types of memory, and each gets strengthened in different ways:

- *Procedural*—your memory for a sequence of tasks, such as steps of a dance. To improve it, learn a new dance, a new software package, or how to program your new cell phone, for example.
- *Visual*—recognizing what you have seen. Try one of the memory games where you have to match names with faces,

(continued)

> or challenge yourself by trying to match the pictures and names of rare animals or plants.
>
> - *Verbal*—remembering what words mean and the names of things. To improve verbal memory, try to memorize something you have to say out loud, such as a speech, poetry, or song lyrics.

► TRY THESE

Remember, everything in moderation is better than any one thing to excess.

- Play sports or cycle or walk on new trails.
- Learn a new strategy game like bocce, board games, chess, or a challenging new computer game.
- Learn a second language or get better at one you already know. Learning sign language is particularly good for your brain as it uses both procedural and verbal skills.
- Dance.
- Read books that challenge you.
- Learn how to use an iPod or program your TiVo.
- Write letters, short stories, a blog, a graphic novel.
- Volunteer at a literacy program.
- Do crossword puzzles.
- Host a salon to discuss current events at your home or meet at a coffee shop.
- Go to a museum or sit in on an art history lecture.
- Get your art, crafts, or a prized pet in shape to show in a competition.
- Take a class, or teach a class. There are Osher Lifelong Learning Institutes (www.usm.maine.edu/olli/national/) throughout the United States, often affiliated with university or continuing care retirement communities, offering people over age fifty-five opportunities to take or teach classes.

- Ask your neighbor how to cook one of the meals you smell wafting from his or her kitchen.
- Use a computer to stay in touch with friends and family, plan outings, do mental exercise games, read the news, and much more.

The list could go on, because it includes anything that engages and challenges you. Watching television is a passive, sedentary activity that doesn't require you to interact (unless your favorite team is up at bat). But watching documentaries, news programs, or quiz shows where you learn new information can boost the brain. (Don't think you have to be busy every minute: Relaxing, avoiding stress, and feeling pampered are important to everyone's quality of life as well.)

If Music Moves You

Learn to play a musical instrument or practice new tunes on an instrument that you used to enjoy but gave up. Check out New Horizon's International Music Association at www.newhorizonsmusic .org/nhima.htm. They help adults of all ages to learn music in an affordable group setting, to attend adult music camps, and to form or join bands of all types. You don't need to know how to play an instrument. It's a twofer—learn or sharpen your music skills and engage with others in a supportive environment.

GO FOR THE NEW, NOT ALWAYS THE TRIED AND TRUE

When looking for stimulating activities, consider ones that don't play to your strengths. If you are an accountant and have never tried drawing in your life, take a drawing class. If you already speak two languages or are very comfortable doing crossword puzzles, then try a manual activity. You need to reach out of your comfort zone to challenge your brain.

Creativity for Any Mind

When Alzheimer's strikes, it can be difficult to maintain your normal brain-enriching activities. A program called TimeSlips (www .timeslips.org), offered at senior day programs and nursing homes, gives people with moderate-stage Alzheimer's an opportunity to be creative and exercise the brain. The participants create stories together using old photographs. The activity boosts the attention span of people with dementia, along with their ability to engage and talk.

Doing Good Is Good for Your Brain

Volunteer work has a variety of benefits for all ages, but studies show that elders may benefit the most. Volunteering decreases depression, which sometimes precedes or accompanies early Alzheimer's, particularly in older people. When researchers studied volunteers with a group called Experience Corps, which trains people over age fifty-five to tutor and mentor children in urban public schools and after-school programs, they found that the older volunteers improved their own planning and organizing skills. Plus, they benefited from the extra exercise and socializing that the volunteer work offered. Experience Corps is in fourteen cities. Check it out at www .experiencecorps.org.

WHO HAS TIME?

Is your reaction to reading that leisure time is good for your brain, "Who has time for leisure?" If so, take a minute and read on for some quick-fix brain tips—how to slip stimulating your senses into your busy day. The idea is to take a minute for yourself and to find pleasure in small things.

- Look out the window and breathe deeply as you search for the first sign of spring or the first star at night.
- Take a minute to admire a baby or cute dog or nice car, or feed someone's meter.
- Plant a garden with no more than five plants.

- Listen to books on tape while you do boring chores.
- Subscribe to the magazine you've been wanting, even if you read only one article or look at the cartoons.
- Set aside ten minutes (you *do* have ten minutes) every day to do one healthy activity that you haven't done enough of *and* that you enjoy: read a book, do yoga, walk briskly around the block, practice an instrument, talk to your best friend, make a new friend. You decide.

Engage Your Senses

Staying active helps the brain in part because stimulating all five senses appears to build those neuronal connections that the brain needs to stay young. It doesn't matter how brief or idiosyncratic the stimuli.

- Slowing down to literally smell the roses—or a nice perfume at the cosmetics counter—gives your sense of smell a mini-workout.
- Visiting a modern art museum, going on a gallery walk, or studying art books at the library is a visual treat that may help you see an image in a new way.
- Singing, particularly in a group, or going to a concert makes the auditory-processing cells in your brain do jumping jacks.
- Join a pottery class to get a real feel for mud!
- Don't just watch the kids make sand castles—join in!
- Try a fruit or vegetable you've never eaten.

▶ **Help Your Senses Stay Sharp:** You can remember only what your brain perceives. Keep your glasses and hearing aid prescriptions up to date and . . . use them!

Daily meditation might also help, by stimulating the part of the brain that handles attention. A form of mind work called mindfulness meditation improves brain and immune function, reduces anxiety, and buffers the effects of stress hormones, such as cortisol, on the brain. But to get the most out of it, you do need to try to do it every day. Look for classes in your community that teach mindfulness meditation, or you can order instructional CDs and tapes through the Internet.

Losing your desire to participate in stimulating leisure activities may be an early sign of memory loss. Because Alzheimer's can go undetected for years, it's hard to know exactly when Alzheimer's begins to change the choices people make or the activities they find doable and enjoyable.

► THE IMPORTANCE OF EDUCATION

Using your brain creates connections between nerve cells that you will rely on as you age or as Alzheimer's depletes the existing supply. Education also introduces you to activities that stimulate the mind, such as reading, going to museums, and discussing issues with friends and colleagues. Less education usually means a lifetime of less-than-challenging jobs.

The more brain connections you establish from years of education and mental stimulation, the bigger your cognitive reserve. If you enter middle age with a good memory and reasoning skills, you stay sharp longer than you would have otherwise.

In a very large study of older female nurses, the participants who had a graduate degree were less likely to decline mentally during the two-year study, compared with women with less education. As a result of challenging their brain, graduates may have laid down a cognitive reserve that protected them in their later years.

In a study of more than one thousand residents of Stockholm, Sweden, participants who had fewer than eight years of formal education were two times more likely to develop Alzheimer's, compared with the participants who had eight-plus years of school. However, a separate, long-term study in the United States showed that quality also counts. African Americans who received an eighth-grade education in the South before desegregation were at higher risk for Alzheimer's than African Americans with the same number of years of education in the then-superior schools of New York City.

Challenging your brain is not a guarantee that Alzheimer's won't eventually make a dent. Even Nobel laureates, such as Dr. George Hitchings, a pioneer in the development of cancer and AIDS drugs, develop Alzheimer's disease. The one comforting thought: Their cognitive reserve probably warded off the disabling effects of Alzheimer's symptoms for many years.

► GYMS FOR THE BRAIN

There are formal programs for people with and without Alzheimer's. People with Alzheimer's, much like stroke or head injury patients, benefit from exercising their brains, but they need their own version of the exercises. In a safe, supportive setting, a few months of memory training can slightly improve the ability of some people in early-stage Alzheimer's to

- recognize faces and names
- provide correct change
- respond to and process information more rapidly
- keep track of time and location

For example, in a small study of people with MCI, half the group participated in twice-weekly, three-and-a-half-hour sessions of activities to boost their thinking, memory, and awareness of their environment, called "reality orientation." They also practiced day-to-day activities such as dressing and washing. By the program's end, the mental abilities of the group that received the training remained stable longer. The people who had the least education benefited the most from the training.

Another twice-a-week program tested on a larger group of people with moderate-stage Alzheimer's disease oriented them to the day of the week and their location; provided hands-on activities that stimulated their senses, such as art and music; engaged them in word games; and helped them reminisce. The group's thinking and memory improved and, most important, they said their quality of life improved.

If you are looking for a brain exercise program for people with Alzheimer's, consider finding a clinical trial that is investigating cognitive training. You can also take cognitive rehabilitation classes offered by centers or health professionals, but they cost hundreds or thousands of dollars and are not covered by insurance.

Here's an example of a brain workout that researchers gave study participants who had Alzheimer's:

- The class met for forty-five-minute sessions twice a week for twelve weeks.

- They practiced techniques for putting a name to a face, such as associating a prominent facial feature with a name (Ned the Nose, for example).

- They practiced recording in notebooks important dates, their medication schedules, and the contact information of family members, friends, and doctors. They reviewed their notebooks twice a day during the study.

- To improve their attention span, they practiced clicking a button in response to yellow boxes that randomly appeared on a computer screen.

Mind Exercises for People Without Alzheimer's

Studies on the benefits of formal brain exercise programs have been mixed. A review of studies showed that strength training and aerobics did more to keep older persons' planning, remembering, and multitasking skills sharp than did a formal brain exercise program. But a large recent study suggested that specific types of cognitive training for healthy older adults may have some mental benefits over a five-year period, with periodic booster sessions. It appears that brain exercise programs can produce short-term improvements, but if you stop practicing, benefits may gradually disappear. The best bet is probably to do exercises for both your brain and your body.

▶ **Tip:** If you are doing brain exercises, ask your family members or friends if they have noticed any improvements in how you are doing on your day-to-day responsibilities and activities.

Learning or sharpening a skill or task boosts everyone's mood, self-confidence, and sense of being in control. Feeling good about yourself improves your memory, especially compared to worrying about failure. So if you or a family member is interested in cognitive training, make sure it is rewarding or confidence building. Everyone, including people with Alzheimer's, thinks more clearly if they feel comfortable about their mental abilities and the limitations they face every day.

One brain game we like for people without Alzheimer's is Nintendo's Brain Age, developed by a neuroscientist. It's fun, is portable, gives instant feedback, has different levels of difficulty, and does not require an Internet connection. But it's a game and not a proven treatment. Other leading training programs developed by scientists—Brain Fitness, Brain Builder, Happy Neuron, Mind Fit, and My Brain Trainer—have their own advantages but require a computer and Internet access. *Neurobics* by L. Katz and M. Rubin was one of the original books in this area.

For more information on healthy brain aging, see www.alz.org/we_can_help_brain_health_maintain_your_brain.asp and dana.org/pdf/other/sharp_learning.pdf.

SIMPLE SOLUTIONS

Write It Down

No matter what your mental state or what you do to improve it, you can't expect to remember everything. So give yourself a break and use memory aids. This is one old-fashioned remedy that can really work. Here are a few tools worth employing:

- Write it down, preferably on a daily planner or in your PDA but not on a little piece of paper that you can't find later. Notes taped up in familiar prominent places may work as well.

- Make an effort to remember. Be quite deliberate about it. That might include repeating aloud or to yourself what you want to remember. For example, if you say, "I'm leaving the keys in my left pocket" as you do it, it will be easier to remember where you put them.

- Create a visual image. If you want to remember to check the back door for a package, visualize the back door. If you are getting ready to go out, visualize the one item you might forget, such as sunglasses or tissues.

- Associate what you are trying to remember with what you already know. When meeting a new person, use the person's name in conversation, think of someone else who has the same name, or think of a word that rhymes with the name, such as Sane Jane.

- Pace yourself. Memorize small segments at a time. To remember a phone number, think of it as three chunks of information. Better yet, store the number in your cell phone or put it on your phone's speed dial.

- Ask your spouse or other family members to help you remember.

- Be consistent. Put your glasses, medications, newspaper, and anything else you use every day in the same place, every day.

- Look for visual cues. To remember where you parked, look for specific landmarks or put something distinctive on your car.

- Keep all your passwords in one (well-hidden) place.

- Record a conversation or take notes if it's something you really need to remember, such as at a doctor's appointment or a meeting with a lawyer.

- Use the alarm on your watch, phone, or clock to remind you of daily appointments.

Each of us has a unique learning or memorizing style. Figure out what works best for you and try to practice it consistently.

Sleep for Your Brain

Your brain turns experiences into memories while you sleep. Chronic sleep deprivation causes Alzheimer's-like symptoms. Too little sleep affects concentration, impairs memory, worsens confusion, and can induce hallucinations, mood swings, and increased sensitivity to pain. To improve your sleep:

- Set a schedule and stick to it to establish your sleep cycle.
- Avoid exercise five to six hours before you plan to go to sleep.
- Eat light and not too late, to avoid heartburn or reflux.
- Avoid caffeine, nicotine, and alcohol.
- Avoid over-the-counter sleep aids and sleeping pills.
- If you can't sleep, get up and listen to music or read something not too exciting but interesting enough to keep your attention.

Don't Distress—De-Stress

When you feel like you're losing your memory, it may just be stress slowing your thinking.

Stress is bad for your brain—the distressing, chronic, long-term kind, not what you feel when you are losing at bridge (or poker), biking up a hill, or getting beat in a game of tennis. The bad stress comes with working too much overtime, having too little help, feeling like everyone needs you and everything is your responsibility, and being unable to meet expectations. For many seniors, this will be the stress of taking care of a relative who has Alzheimer's.

The irony is that people under chronic stress may be more likely to develop Alzheimer's than people who occasionally or rarely feel stressed. In one study, more than one thousand people without dementia were rated for their proneness to psychological distress, and then tested for Alzheimer's disease three to six years later. After controlling for other factors that can cause Alzheimer's disease, the people who were prone to anxiety were two and a half times more likely to develop Alzheimer's disease than the other study participants. Untreated anxiety and depression may have the same effects as chronic stress.

The stress-Alzheimer's link was more apparent in white people than in African Americans. A study of white clergy members found that the clergy most prone to neuroticism, which is a type of anxiety, were also more likely to develop Alzheimer's disease.

We don't fully understand why stress increases the risk of

Alzheimer's, but we do know that it causes your body to release a mix of hormones, including cortisol, that raise blood pressure and increase your risk of having heart disease or a stroke.

Stress Has Many Causes . . .

- Untreated anxiety or depression
- Inadequate or poor quality sleep
- Poverty or financial hardship
- Unsafe living, work, or school environments
- Not enough playtime
- Not enough family time (or too much family time)
- Too much work (or too little work)
- Too many problems, not enough solutions
- Being a family caregiver

. . . and Solutions

- Stress management exercises, which you can learn through classes or books
- Treating the underlying depression and anxiety
- Seeing a counselor or therapist
- Exercising
- Medications
- Participating in spiritual or religious activities
- Practicing tai chi, yoga, meditation
- Improving your quality and quantity of sleep
- Getting help with your care responsibilities

▶ IN SUMMARY

Stay Connected

- Keep your brain active.
- Seek out mentally engaging leisure activities.
- Stay involved with people.

Stay Cool

- Avoid long-term, high levels of stress.
- Seek treatment for any mental health problems, especially depression and anxiety.

PART SIX

► "DOES PERSONALITY CHANGE WITH MEMORY LOSS?" AND OTHER FREQUENTLY ASKED QUESTIONS

CHAPTER EIGHTEEN

OUR TOP 40 QUESTIONS AND ANSWERS

Radio disc jockeys have their Top 40 playlist, and we have a Top 40 list too—of the questions we are most frequently asked about caring for people in the early to middle stages of Alzheimer's. If you have Alzheimer's or are caring for someone who does, these questions have probably been on your mind, too, and you've wondered where to go for a reliable answer.

These aren't the medical questions you jot down to ask your physician but the ones that keep you up at night, worrying about how to deal with Alzheimer's day in and day out. You are not alone in wondering about these things; decades of experience tell us that other people have the same or very similar concerns.

The FAQs fall into six general categories:

1. Five Versions of "Is It Alzheimer's?"
2. The Hows and Whys of Testing
3. Understanding How Alzheimer's Changes Personality
4. Daily Life: Managing Money, Driving, Travel, and Other Basics
5. Getting Others to Understand
6. Protecting Against Alzheimer's

▶ FIVE VERSIONS OF "IS IT ALZHEIMER'S?"

If doctors sometimes have a difficult time diagnosing Alzheimer's correctly, it's even harder for family members.

1. "Isn't it normal to get forgetful when you retire?"
—A sixty-five-year-old-man whose wife is worried about his memory

Our memory begins to decline before retirement age, but most people don't start worrying about memory loss until they retire. Retirees may no longer dismiss their memory lapses as simply the result of being busy and stressed out. Also, they may start wondering if this is the beginning of age-related memory loss. Some people retire because of difficulty with their memory or keeping up at work.

Once you retire and no longer have deadlines at work, you may think it's okay to be forgetful. Actually, the need for a good working memory doesn't change with retirement. You may choose to stop remembering certain facts or figures that are no longer important to you, but you need to be ready to absorb new information for a fulfilling retirement. Retirees and their spouses are well advised to stay involved in stimulating, challenging, and meaningful activities.

So how do you decide what is normal forgetfulness and what isn't? First, listen to your wife. If she notices a significant change in you or complains that you are repeating yourself more than usual, assume she isn't exaggerating or nagging. You, like others, may "forget" or dismiss mild changes in recent memory because it is understandably uncomfortable for you to think about.

Second, ask yourself some difficult questions:

- Have you been more frustrated trying to remember what happened that morning or that minute?

- Are activities that were once easy for you now more difficult or taking longer?

- Are you having more trouble planning, organizing, or paying bills?

- Do you find yourself double-checking yourself more?

- Are you avoiding situations because you are afraid of making mistakes?
- Are memory lapses making you more irritable, frustrated, or unsure of yourself?
- Are you misplacing or losing things more than in the past? (Keys and glasses don't count—we know they enjoy a good game of hide-and-seek.)
- Is it harder for you to follow directions or learn your way to a new place?
- Are you getting lost in familiar places?

If so, it may be time for you and your wife to seek professional advice from your doctor. As with any serious medical condition, it's never a good idea to ignore real memory problems, as much as we'd like them, instead of our keys, to disappear.

2. "Isn't it true that taking too many medicines at one time can make the doctors think you have Alzheimer's?"
—A seventy-five-year-old husband who is worried about his wife

There are more than fifty medications that can cause, albeit rarely, confusion or memory loss. Other medications, particularly at high dosages and particularly in older people, can cause drowsiness, disorientation, or forgetfulness. Your wife may appear sedated or sleepy if the dose of even one medicine is too high for her body's changing ability to use, absorb, and eliminate the medicine. Certain combinations of medications or the combination of medicine and certain chronic diseases can also disrupt thinking. This is why doctors review a patient's prescriptions and over-the-counter medicines as part of any evaluation of a memory problem. And that's why patients or their care providers must give each of their doctors their complete list of medications.

On the other hand, Alzheimer's disease may be causing your wife to dislike or distrust medicines and to insist that the medicines slow her down. If her mental condition was solely related to her medications, the changes would have come on suddenly and would disappear when the medicines are adjusted. People who are overmedicated generally look sleepy all the time. People with Alzheimer's are actually fairly alert and vigilant, until the disease advances.

Even if your wife has Alzheimer's, careful review and monitoring of her medicine cabinet is essential to help her function at her best. Her medicines may be necessary for other conditions, but perhaps the dosage or time of day she takes them can be adjusted to cause fewer problems. As people age, the same dose of a medicine they have taken for years can become too much for their system.

Moreover, people with Alzheimer's can be very sensitive to the effects of medicines, especially antihistamines and some of the older antidepressants. Some drugs also work at cross-purposes with Aricept or other medicines prescribed for Alzheimer's disease. Your pharmacist may be the first person to check with about medication interactions.

If your wife needs to take fewer pills, her doctor will tell you how to decrease the quantity slowly. If you are dissatisfied with the doctor's advice, check with another doctor or pharmacist. Knowing a lot about your wife's medicines, and what problems to watch for, will make you her best advocate.

3. *"Should my wife be tested for Alzheimer's just because she got lost driving?"*   —A sixty-eight-year-old husband

Everyone gets lost sometimes, particularly if she is under stress or preoccupied. To determine if getting lost is a sign of Alzheimer's, ask:

- Does she get lost in new or familiar areas? New locations can be challenging to the best navigators. But people with Alzheimer's get lost in familiar areas also.

- How often does she get lost? More than rarely is dangerous and may be a sign of Alzheimer's.

- Is she quickly able to recognize where she is and find her way? People with Alzheimer's cannot.

- Has her behavior, personality, thinking, communication, or judgment changed in other ways? By the time a person is getting lost as a result of Alzheimer's disease, she is usually showing signs of memory loss in other areas of her life.

Don't hesitate to help your wife get a thorough medical evaluation to determine the cause of her confusion. Even if she does receive a diagnosis of Alzheimer's, it doesn't necessarily mean that her

license will be revoked, though she may need to stop driving to protect her safety and the safety of others.

4. "Can grief cause Alzheimer's? My mom is so confused and
forgetful since my dad died." —A daughter in her forties

In anyone, grief can cause a range of powerful physical and emotional reactions, including confusion and disorientation. Grief does
not cause Alzheimer's, but it may unmask it. Your dad may have been
helping your mom more than anyone realized, and after he died, her
impairments came to light. He was probably meeting her day-to-day
needs, making sure she understood what was going on in the world
around her, and filling in the gaps in her memory or reasoning ability.
Thanks to your dad, she felt normal and even successful.

So losing him is like losing a part of her ability to think, plan, and
remember. She's not used to asking others for assistance, knowing
what she might need, or having others help her. Even if your parents
weren't that close, they may have worked out useful routines as her
subtle memory lapses became problematic.

People with mild to moderate memory disorders are extremely
sensitive to changes in their routine and in the people around them
or their environment. The absence of a primary care provider and
lifelong partner is probably the most disruptive change of all. Your
mom will generally be more confused, disoriented, fearful, or frustrated, and in need of reassurance. She will have a lower threshold
for any stress or further changes in routines.

5. "Isn't it possible my wife was misdiagnosed with Alzheimer's
when it is just depression?" —A husband in his sixties

Depression is a serious and treatable condition, so we don't tend to
dismiss symptoms as "just depression." Depression by itself can
cause changes in mood, thinking, memory, and behavior. Depressed
older adults may not try as hard on tests that assess memory and
thinking. If you question your wife's diagnosis, by all means get a
second opinion from a psychiatrist or psychologist who specializes
in depression and Alzheimer's.

A first episode of serious depression late in life may be a sign
that Alzheimer's is just around the corner. Apathy, loss of initiative,

inability to start or finish projects, or withdrawing from hobbies or activities may be your wife's response to feeling forgetful and fearing she will make mistakes.

Even if your wife's mood and behavior are related to Alzheimer's, she needs a thorough evaluation to sort out her illnesses. She can be treated for both depression and Alzheimer's simultaneously, though most specialists will suggest treating the depression first. Fortunately, the depressive symptoms often respond well to antidepressant medication, supportive therapy, and the addition of enjoyable activities. Ignore cavalier suggestions like, "Of course she is depressed— wouldn't you be depressed if you had Alzheimer's?" The quality of both her life and yours can be enhanced with the accurate diagnosis and treatment of both serious conditions.

▶ THE HOWS AND WHYS OF TESTING

6. "How do I get my father to go to the doctor when he thinks nothing is wrong?"   —A forty-five-year-old daughter

Most people with a memory disorder are not good judges of their own behavior. For example, people with Alzheimer's don't know they repeat themselves a lot, because they genuinely don't remember what they just said.

Your dad may not be intentionally stubborn or even in denial. Instead, he may actually sense something scary, wrong, or different with his thinking and is trying to blame his confusion or mistakes on others. He may complain that people are simply asking too much of him or grumble that all these gadgets (toaster, microwave oven, television, you fill in the blank) are too darn complicated to use anyway.

There are many successful approaches to getting medical help for a resistant, memory-impaired relative. You may need to resort to being cunning, but when it comes to Alzheimer's, the end (proper medical evaluation and care) justifies the means. (And don't forget that *cunning* is not the same as *conning*.) Here are some strategies to try. You know your father, so pick which you think will work best for him.

- Offer to take him to the doctor about a bothersome complaint he has had, such as back pain or fatigue. Point out that new treatments for his ailment may be available.

- Find a doctor he can trust. Ask someone whom he has always admired, say, a neighbor or his lawyer, to recommend one. Or find a doctor with whom he may have something in common— they graduated from the same college, for example.

- If your dad has always refused to see a woman physician or a foreign physician, this is not the time to insist he become open-minded.

- Some spouses suggest to their partner that they both have a physical because they are getting older, for insurance purposes, or to plan for their retirement.

Now for timing: Schedule the appointment for when the office is the least busy and when you or a close, observant relative can go with him. If he has refused to go, don't tell him until the last minute that it's time to go. When he asks where he's going, be matter-of-fact. Try to slip "doctor appointment" in between "running an errand" and "getting lunch" or "going to the golf course." Be sure to bring to the appointment all his current prescription and over-the-counter medicines, and recent medical records of tests, procedures, or hospitalizations.

Before the appointment, alert the doctor or a nurse to your concerns about your dad's memory, why your dad thinks he's going to the doctor, and his resistance to discuss his memory. If you are unable to speak to someone before the appointment, you may need to pass the nurse or doctor a note explaining the situation. Avoid discussing your dad's memory in front of him and let him do the talking during the appointment. Follow up with a phone call to the doctor if necessary, but it's better to get the message to the doctor before the exam.

7. "Why fight him to go to the doctor when only an autopsy can diagnose Alzheimer's?"
—The seventy-four-year-old wife of a man with memory problems

It's true that no diagnosis is guaranteed to be 100 percent accurate, but skilled doctors are finding that their clinical diagnoses are supported by the autopsy about 90 percent of the time. Moreover, autopsies on brain tissue may not reveal any disease that would have been treated differently.

The advantages of diagnosing the cause of memory problems early and accurately are numerous. For one, conditions other than dementia, including congestive heart failure or (rarely) a tumor, can cause memory problems. Certain medicines or combination of medicines impair memory, and when they are eliminated or reduced, memory function improves.

You want to know if it is Alzheimer's, because a thorough medical evaluation can identify the skills and abilities your husband has retained or lost. If you understand the level of his impairment, you are more likely to give him the help he needs. You will also learn how much he can and should do on his own.

If it is Alzheimer's, you need to know because:

- People with Alzheimer's function better when they are getting medical and emotional support designed to address their specific needs.

- Starting treatment early with Alzheimer's medications is important in order to maintain cognition and function.

- Alzheimer's shortens the life span and requires couples to adjust their plans for their future.

- Understanding Alzheimer's helps couples decide together how to best preserve their safety and assets.

- A good physician can encourage couples to decide how to handle sensitive issues, such as who should manage family finances and whether the spouse with Alzheimer's can drive. Getting professional guidance on these emotional questions takes some of the burden and blame off the healthy spouse.

- While they can still make reasoned judgments, people with Alzheimer's need time to think about how they want to live and time to talk with their family about what is important to them.

- Couples may have many things they want to say to each other and do together before disability limits their options.

- Many people with early Alzheimer's are relieved to learn that their memory difficulties are not their fault, that trying harder won't necessarily lead to success, and that it's not a sign of weakness to ask for help.

8. *"What difference does it make if my aunt doesn't know the day and date? She's retired."* —A fifty-one-year-old man

Doctors ask people with memory problems to name the date or day of the week to get a sense of the person's orientation and whether it has changed since the last visit. Doctors also ask patients what town they are in, who the president is, and other seemingly trivial questions.

You may think the doctor is making unfair assumptions about your aunt's general thinking ability just because she can't come up with these specifics. However, this and other information helps the doctor and your aunt determine if her needs for help have changed, from medications to more detailed calendars and digital clocks in her home. Eventually, the specifics of day and date won't be nearly as important for her as distinguishing breakfast time from dinnertime or knowing how to dress appropriately for the weather and season.

At these later stages, digital clocks and calendars won't help, as she will not remember to look at them and will not understand what they mean. You may not know the day and date at all times yourself, but you know where to look for that information. It's hard for families to believe, but giving people with Alzheimer's more technological cues can backfire by making them feel bad that they can't use the new tools. Instead, let your aunt preserve her self-esteem by accepting her well-practiced excuses, such as "I'm retired—I don't keep track of those things anymore."

9. *"What kind of doctor specializes in memory problems? Is there someplace I can send my husband where they are testing medicines for memory loss? Can he stay at the university's clinical center while they study him?"* —A wife in her seventies

Doctors who specialize in memory problems are neurologists, psychiatrists, and geriatricians, and they are usually associated with major medical centers or memory disorder clinics. They would work with but not replace your husband's primary-care doctor.

Although many centers and clinics do test medicines designed to treat memory disorders, they don't have study participants stay at their centers. Doctors have learned that people with Alzheimer's function worse in new or unfamiliar environments, including hospitals, where they are at risk of becoming more confused or even delirious. Much of what we have learned about Alzheimer's is from research done on animals or tissue cultures, not just from studies on people with established Alzheimer's disease.

That said, there are outpatient studies, called clinical trials, of Alzheimer's medications that your husband may be able to enroll in. If he is qualified to participate, he would receive either the medicine being tested or a so-called placebo pill that has no effects. You would bring him periodically to the clinic for checkups, where you would also be asked about his memory and behavior. Unfortunately, most of the medicines now under review are only for people with mild cognitive impairment or early-stage Alzheimer's.

If what you also need is a break from caring for your husband, call your county aging agency or nearest Alzheimer's Association for advice on finding assistance. Three good options for respite care exist:

- A day program for people with Alzheimer's
- A live-in facility that takes people with dementia for short stays
- A caregiver to come to your home, so you can get out for a few hours on a regular basis

When you take a break from your husband, you are helping both of you. Research studies have shown that family caregivers need time away from their relative to protect their own health and retain their capacity and patience to provide the best care.

10. "Is it worth it to get a second opinion? The doctor said my dad's CAT scan was normal, but he just isn't himself anymore."
                                                        —A forty-year-old son

Absolutely. First, no single test, including a CAT scan, which is like a three-dimensional X-ray, can diagnose Alzheimer's. CAT scans actually detect rare, serious, or remediable problems that may be mistaken for Alzheimer's, such as tumors or damage from head injuries.

The red flag in your question is "he just isn't himself anymore." A close family member's observations of changes in a person's functioning, mood, behavior, or personality, and a thorough neurological and physical examination are usually more predictive of early memory impairment than imaging or laboratory studies.

Ask yourself about changes separate from any physical ailments:

- Does he refuse to participate in activities that once were easy for him?
- Have you noticed changes in his personality? Is he more irritable, easily frustrated, suspicious, worried, fearful, or withdrawn?
- Does he check himself more, such as checking if he turned off a light or packed his golf clubs?
- Does he repeat himself, ask more questions, or request more reminders?
- Did these changes develop subtly and slowly, making it difficult to pinpoint when they began?
- Is he making poor decisions or showing a lack of his usual judgment or tact?
- How many people in the family are noticing these changes?

Your answers will probably confirm your initial intuition that you need a second opinion. Asking your dad to undergo a comprehensive evaluation of his memory may be difficult. But an early and accurate diagnosis will help your dad get the help and extra protection he needs. You can feel proud that you put the stoplight in place before an accident happened.

► UNDERSTANDING HOW ALZHEIMER'S CHANGES PERSONALITY

The problems might seem funny, if only they weren't so real.

11. "How can she complain about having nothing to do and get none of the housework done when she is home all day?"
—A husband in his sixties whose wife has early-onset Alzheimer's

People with Alzheimer's have trouble with what is called "executive function"—the ability to plan a series of steps, initiate those steps, and then organize, sequence, and stay on task. Organizing their approach to housework or, eventually, even to getting dressed and performing other personal activities becomes more difficult over time. Part of the problem is that their sense of elapsed time is off-kilter, so your wife may look out a window or dust the same table for hours, then look up with surprise when you return from work. What was an eight-hour day for you may seem like eight minutes or eight days to her.

You want to come home to dinner and a clean house, and your wife wants to feel like a contributing member of the family, much as she did before her illness. But she may have lost the ability to do the work that she once did easily. If her dementia is mild, notes and telephone reminders from you may be all she needs to get through her day. But as the disease progresses, she will need someone, such as a paid companion, to help her do the housework and to keep her safe. If she previously enjoyed her homemaker role, it is worth finding ways to help her do these chores.

As the disease progresses, she will become tired and frustrated more quickly. Thinking and staying on task, no matter how simple the task looks to you, will easily fatigue your wife. Without a structured, predictable routine, which means doing the same activities at the same time and in the same order each day, with regular breaks, she may become anxious and agitated.

12. "Why do people with Alzheimer's make up stories or just tell outright lies? My wife tells everyone I am having an affair with our maid." **—A seventy-three-year-old husband**

Accusations of spousal infidelity and of family members stealing are the most common delusions of both men and women with dementia. Why do they make these false accusations? In the case of your wife, she probably has an irrational fear that you will abandon her in a world that no longer makes sense. She can't keep in her memory why the housekeeper is there or a female neighbor has dropped by, so she comes up with stories that make sense to her at that moment.

You might think that she is telling lies or stories to annoy you, insult you, or make you look bad to family and friends. But her impairment prevents her not only from remembering that you are faithful but also from carrying out any sort of plans, including malicious ones.

Arguing or attempting to be logical with her will not help. She will forget what you said and remember only that you were angry with her. As upsetting as her accusations are, respond calmly and casually to them. Dredge up some old lines from your courting days, like, "You are the only woman in my life—you can depend on me." Distract her with a ride in the car or a request to help you in the yard or the kitchen.

When she accuses you falsely in front of others, say to your guests, "Well, that's a tale for another day," then distract her by showing her something or walking with her. Offer your friends a bargain: "I'll agree to believe only half of what I hear about you if you do the same for me!"

13. "Does Alzheimer's increase your sex drive? My husband demands sex right after we have sex."   —A sixty-one-year-old wife

No, Alzheimer's by itself doesn't increase or decrease sex drive. Your husband probably forgets that he just had sex. He may also forget what is proper behavior in the bedroom or that he needs to consider your feelings. Alzheimer's or frontotemporal dementia may have eroded his inhibition, causing him to act inappropriately or to use crude sexual language. In addition, his need for intimacy may be greater than yours because he is afraid of being abandoned. Or he may just be perseverating (getting an idea stuck in his head) about sex.

You won't be able to convince your husband that "enough is enough." Instead, sleep in another room or stay out of his sight until he is asleep. Also, both of you might enjoy less intimate forms of touching, such as foot rubs or head massages. As difficult as it is, refrain from telling him that his demands are crazy or inconsiderate. He will understand your strong negative feelings but not know how to make it right. Feel free to discuss your problem with an Alzheimer's Association help line volunteer or members of a support group. You may be surprised by how many caregivers have similar experiences.

14. "Why are women with Alzheimer's so hard on their husbands and so nice to everyone else? She even accused me of stealing her underwear."   —A seventy-two-year-old husband

If it is any consolation, men with Alzheimer's can be mean to their spouses as well. People with Alzheimer's get angry for different reasons, including feeling scared, frustrated, and resentful of needing help or losing control. They almost always take out their anger on the person nearest and dearest to them.

Your wife can no longer remember all that you do and have done for her. Because of her own disabilities, she feels that her needs are not being met. You are her care provider, so her problems must be your fault. As she struggles to make sense of a topsy-turvy world, she will say things before thinking about your feelings.

The hardest part about being married to someone with Alzheimer's is separating the disease from the person. You will both be better off if you avoid taking personally her mean behavior. Be mad at the disease together—not angry at each other.

Although it seems odd to the spouse who has just been yelled at, many people in early to middle stages of Alzheimer's behave appropriately and pleasantly during brief social visits, if they are well rested. Instead of resenting her ability to be nice to everyone else, try to appreciate it. You need your friends to enjoy her, as both of you will benefit if you keep up your social contacts. Many husbands like you crave normal adult conversation when their wives are no longer capable of it.

15. "Why does my wife not care about how she looks anymore? She wears the same outfit every day and won't even wash it. She used to be a snappy dresser."   **—A sixty-six-year-old husband**

Most likely she does care and remembers being a snappy dresser. However, hygiene and dress inevitably deteriorate with the progression of dementia. Making and carrying out any decisions become very tough, and that includes picking out an outfit and putting it on. Since her long-term memory is better than her short-term recall, she remembers only that she always wears clothes—not that she might need to change or clean her outfit.

For her to continue to look clean and tidy, someone will need to help her to dress and manage her wardrobe. Making that a priority will help her and you feel better, since you are both accustomed to her looking really nice. Go through your wife's closet and remove everything that is out of season, uncomfortable, and difficult to put on. Hang things that go together on the same hanger, and don't forget the favorite scarf or piece of jewelry. If she needs new clothes, order from a catalog—even if it means returning things that don't fit, it may save time and frustration. Perhaps a woman friend might enjoy helping you and your wife with these wardrobe tasks.

Your daily tasks will include reminding her to take off her pajamas or dirty clothes in order to put on the clean ones. Discreetly toss dirty clothes in the wash, perhaps while she is in the bathroom. Lay her clothes on the bed each day in the order she puts them on, such as underwear on top. You can give her two outfits to choose between. Eventually, she may prefer one type of outfit, such as an attractive sweat suit, that is comfortable and easy to put on.

Let her do as much as she can with encouragement, perhaps showing her how nice she looks in the mirror if she can still recognize herself. When she can no longer fasten buttons or tie her shoes, don't reveal your disappointment. How you take over the task will make a big difference in how she feels about herself. Compliment her often on her retained good looks. Remind her that she is still "the belle of the ball."

16. "Is turning against your grandchildren a symptom of Alzheimer's? Mom has always taken care of my kids while I work, but now they say she's mean and uninterested in them."
—A daughter in her thirties

Turning against people, including family members, is not a specific symptom of Alzheimer's disease. But if she has Alzheimer's, it has shortened her fuse and made it hard for her to be polite and caring. She is frustrated because she is forgetting what she is supposed to do yet wants to do things right. Your mom loves the children in the same way she always has but feels overwhelmed trying to care for them. It's probably time to find a new sitter or someone to help her watch the kids.

Babysitting requires far more patience, vigilance, thinking, memory, attention, planning, and judgment than most people with even moderate Alzheimer's disease can muster. Rational arguments or pleading with your mom to act like a responsible grown-up won't work. Your mother's judgment is not what it once was. She remembers she is an adult, but her behavior may look childlike. Your children respond in kind and the tension escalates.

Your children can be taught to respond appropriately to their grandmother, but they need your help. Get your children and mother together for brief visits to preserve the warm relationship they once had. After your mom no longer has the responsibility of caring for the children, with your encouragement and direction her attitude toward them may improve significantly.

17. "Does personality change with memory loss? My mother was much more outgoing and sympathetic to my problems before, and now she doesn't seem to care about anyone but herself."
—**A thirty-eight-year-old daughter**

Sadly, personality changes are often the first signs of Alzheimer's disease. Your mother may have lost the ability to understand how you feel, even though she still loves you. She may be scared of making mistakes in social situations, so she withdraws to preserve her self-esteem. It's all she can do to understand and monitor her own feelings and reactions. Keep in mind when she seems uncaring that it's the disease talking.

Your mother's self-centeredness is hard on you. Talking to others who appreciated her qualities will help. You may also want to find someone in your family who can fill in for your mom as your older, wiser guide. Consider joining a support group or talking to an Alzheimer's Association counselor for support. Her personality changes may come faster than you can cope with on your own.

Just as she helped you when you were younger, now you can offer her support. You don't have to become her mother, nor will she ever be your child, but you can take satisfaction in helping her meet her needs now, which some children describe as "full-circle care." Part of that is accepting where she is now. She probably does not know that she has withdrawn, and telling her won't help. Instead, remind her that she's a great mom and that you appreciate her. Enjoy what she has to offer, even if it's just the memory of the mother she was.

18. "Why won't my mother make even the simplest decisions about what she wants to eat in a restaurant?"
—**A forty-seven-year-old daughter**

It's hard to watch a confident mother become so indecisive. She would like to be able to make decisions, but because of her disability she can't remember the options long enough to decide between them. You may think she has just given up and doesn't care anymore for her mother-daughter lunches, but she needs and enjoys them now more than ever.

Going out to lunch with a person who has Alzheimer's is more enjoyable if you follow slightly unusual rules of etiquette. If your mother doesn't answer a server's question fairly quickly, just answer for her. Suggest a meal that you know she likes and that she can eat comfortably in public. She may love salads, for example, but if she has trouble getting all that lettuce dripping with great dressing into her mouth, save it for home. If you are unsure what she'll want to eat, ask her to choose between two simple choices, but don't be surprised if she can't even make that decision.

Consider bringing along a small card that states, "My companion has a memory problem. Please address your questions to me," and slip it to the server when he or she seats you.

Order her water right away, as many medications that older people take dry out their mouths. Ask her discreetly a couple of times if she wants more to drink or if she needs to use the bathroom. To make it easier for her to eat, you may also have to arrange or cut up her food, setting some aside if the serving is large.

Taking care of her like this in public will feel odd at first, but she needs help and may even appreciate it. You will probably have to direct the conversation as well, by pointing out people or items of interest in the restaurant, telling her stories from her past, using humor frequently to lighten the mood, and focusing on having fun in the moment.

19. *"Why do people who were such gifted artists like my wife just stop painting? She just got Alzheimer's, but her hands and eyes work fine."* **—A seventy-three-year-old husband**

It's very difficult for family members to watch the people they love give up a profession or hobby that once practically defined who they were. If it's any comfort to you, many great artists, writers, and craftspeople have responded to the onset of Alzheimer's in much the same way. The good news is that you can probably coax your wife to find another way to express herself.

Your wife, like many artists with Alzheimer's, may have stopped painting because she perceives that the quality of her art is not up to her well-remembered standards. Work that once came naturally may now prove difficult and frustrating, as her sense of perspective, and her ability to plan and carry out a painting, may be off.

Don't expect her or push her to continue her painting if it no longer brings her pleasure. Families in your situation have had better success finding other creative outlets for their loved ones. She might enjoy working with clay, making collages, trying simple computer graphic games, or even arranging artwork or photographs for scrapbooks. Inquire at a local adult day center or senior center about art therapists to help her explore a new medium. Don't give up—she may thrive when she finds a new way to express her remaining creative talents.

► DAILY LIFE: MANAGING MONEY, DRIVING, TRAVEL, AND OTHER BASICS

20. "How do I get Dad to let me help with the bills? He's paying some bills three times and ignoring others."
                                                      —A forty-four-year-old son

The ability to pay bills, count change, or use good judgment about money is one of the first skills to deteriorate in people who have Alzheimer's. Your dad may be writing but never recording or mailing his checks, or forgetting that he has just paid a bill. He may be stubborn about letting you take over the bills because the one thing he does remember is that he has always paid the bills. Now that this once routine task confuses and frustrates him, he feels as though he is losing control.

Here are some tips you can try to ease into the role of bill payer:

- Offer to pay the bills with him. Let him sign the checks and be sure to tell him where the money is going, so he won't feel you are cheating him.

- Get him a brightly colored "bills basket," to encourage him to put all the bills in the same place when they arrive.

- Ask him for regular "financial advice" to keep him feeling in the loop.

- Go on regular outings to the bank together, where he might enjoy special attention from the tellers or bank employees.

- You may want bank statements and bills sent to your address, but don't rush to have all of his mail forwarded, since he probably enjoys the ritual of opening his letters, even advertisements.

- If there is any indication, however, that he is responding to mail scams or sending money to questionable causes, you will have to monitor the mail or have everything forwarded to you.

- Talk to the bank about setting up a fail-safe system to protect his money while letting him feel in control. Many banks will agree to call a relative if unusual transactions take place on an older person's account.

You will be walking a delicate line between letting him feel involved and protecting his finances from his mistakes. But your efforts are worth it if both his dignity and his assets are protected. Sadly, he will eventually forget about the bills and let you handle them without complaint.

21. "Why would a retired accountant not file taxes for three years? My husband always took care of our business, but now the IRS is after us and he doesn't seem to care." —A sixty-two-year-old wife

A common first symptom of a memory disorder is neglecting vital responsibilities, such as the bookkeeping, while obsessing over something trivial, such as the thermostat setting. If your husband is suffering from a memory disorder, he may have tried and failed to do the taxes, felt frustrated and embarrassed, and then completely forgotten about the work. If so, he is probably also neglecting other tasks, such as paying bills.

He needs a thorough medical evaluation, and if he is suffering from Alzheimer's, you or someone you trust needs to take over all financial responsibilities immediately. If your husband's paperwork and files are in disarray, you will need to ask the Internal Revenue Service for an extension on your taxes.

Be aware that confronting your husband and asking him to explain his actions will prove frustrating for both of you. He will feel unjustly attacked, and you will feel like he doesn't care. Keep in mind that he simply does not have the ability to remember, organize, or act as he once did. Get frustrated at the disease and not at each other. Just make sure that the uncomfortable task of keeping up with the taxes gets done.

22. *"How do I get my mom to remember to take her medicine? I fill those daily pillboxes for her each week, but she takes every kind of pill except what the doctors prescribe."* —A daughter in her forties

Your mom is not taking the medicine that her doctor prescribes either because she doesn't value traditional medications or she is showing signs of cognitive impairment. Mismanaging medicines is one of the main reasons individuals must give up living alone or unsupervised. There are many obstacles that may be getting in the way of your mother taking her medication:

- She can't keep track of time, so she may not think to take her morning medications in the morning.
- She forgets why the medicines are needed, or she doesn't think she needs the pills because she is not in pain.
- She thinks she has an illness from long ago, so she takes what worked for that condition.
- She may even have little stockpiles of the medication, which can become her security object. Clearing it out of her house will only encourage her to go get more. (This can happen with alcohol as well.)

Some children put up signs in their parent's house to remind him or her to take their pills, but the parent forgets to look at the signs. Others call at specific times to remind their parent to take their pill, only to be left dangling while the parent goes in search of the pillbox. Devices on the market to encourage compliance with medical regimens are not designed for people with Alzheimer's. What use is a bell to remind you to take a pill if you can't remember what the bell is for? In other words, there are a million ways to lead her to water, but she may not drink—or at least not from the right trough—unless someone is there to remind and supervise her.

23. *"Isn't it better for someone with Alzheimer's to stay at home?"*
—The seventy-year-old sister of a woman with Alzheimer's disease

Moving is tough for everyone, particularly for people with Alzheimer's. In their own home, they may know where everything is and
how to get around. When they move to a new home, they have trouble learning and remembering its layout. However, as Alzheimer's
progresses, even familiar surroundings may seem unfamiliar.

Like others, your sister may prefer to stay in her own home for as
long as possible. But people with Alzheimer's face real risks when
they live alone in a home that is not Alzheimer's-proof or with family members who can't keep a close eye on them. Your sister may
forget to turn off the stove, take her medicines, or lock doors, for example. She may become frightened by imagined and real risks, such
as being robbed, in part because she has lost reasoning or judgment
about how to respond to dangerous situations. She may simply feel
overwhelmed by routine house chores and responsibilities.

Because Alzheimer's robs people of their ability to adjust well to
new environments, it's better to move your sister or to hire help for
her before the disease progresses. That will give paid care providers
a chance to get to know and feel connected to her before she becomes very impaired.

What not to do: Frequent moves between homes, such as staying
for two weeks with you and then two weeks with a daughter, is almost always worse than settling in at one place and establishing a
routine. The goal is to make your sister feel secure and "at home"
wherever she is, and that requires being near people who know and
understand her and her disability.

24. *"Why does the doctor insist that my dad stop driving just because he has Alzheimer's? He is a much better driver than my mom."*   —A forty-eight-year-old son

Driving is one of the toughest losses faced by people with Alzheimer's.
Yet by the time they are diagnosed, people with Alzheimer's often
have become lost while driving on familiar routes or had fender
benders and unexplained accidents. The doctor probably diagnosed problems in your dad that make him a risky driver yet are
still very subtle.

The doctor is concerned about your dad because Alzheimer's quickly robs even experienced drivers of the ability to respond appropriately to a new or sudden situation on the road. Indications off the road that your dad may not be ready for the unexpected include having difficulty starting, planning, or organizing an activity or having trouble using routine objects like the toaster or coffeemaker.

If you or your dad questions the doctor's judgment, check out the excellent tools available at www.thehartford.com/alzheimers and www.thehartford.com/talkwitholderdrivers/worksheets/main .htm for assessing driving skills, or ask for a driving test at the Department of Motor Vehicles or a driving evaluation from an occupational therapist. Your dad may not agree to testing unless he gets considerable support from you and your mother. You also have to be able to live with the test results, whether you agree with them or not.

Before giving up driving, many people with Alzheimer's limit their drives to short, familiar routes in the daylight at times when traffic is minimal. However, you can't depend on your dad to know if and when he can safely drive. Monitor him carefully, even if he has passed a driving test.

Now is the time to look at options to reduce your parents' dependence on their car. Some possibilities to consider are delivery services, taxi charge accounts, church volunteer drivers, and a paid companion for part of the day to drive and escort your parents to activities or appointments. Unfortunately, these options may be expensive or inconvenient. They are, however, far less expensive, emotionally and financially, than an accident.

25. "How can I get my grandmother to stop going to the grocery store every day to buy the same thing? How can I teach her to make a list?"   **—A teenage granddaughter**

Your grandmother probably has problems with short-term or recent memory. She doesn't remember shopping yesterday, and her most vivid memory is that she needs one item, so off she goes. Going to the grocery store is also one part of her daily routine that she enjoys.

Early in the course of Alzheimer's disease, people lose their thinking-ahead and list-making skills. Even if she was a very good planner and shopper before, she can no longer do either. Telling her not to buy something won't help, because she can't remember your good advice. And reminding her that she already has a house full of tissues will only embarrass her.

Instead, take the kinder approach, which is to help her with what she can't do and encourage her to do what she can. If she lives alone, make sure her food is stored properly and old food is tossed out. If she is collecting large quantities of the same items, discreetly re-move them before they block her movement. If you are willing and have the time, take her shopping once a week. An outing with a lov-ing granddaughter may be the high point of her day, and it will offer you two the opportunity to become closer. To ensure your visit is successful, try these basic steps:

- Call to remind her you are coming.
- Make a shopping list together before you head out.
- At the store, as much as possible let her make her own selec-tions.
- Don't argue with her in front of others.
- Remind her gently that she already has certain items.
- Discreetly put excess items back.
- If she insists, point out that you don't have enough money to buy more than one of each item "this time."

26. "Isn't it a good idea to take all those trips we have been putting off, now that my wife was just diagnosed with Alzheimer's?"
—A husband in his sixties

You'll want to make the most of your time together, whether it's on trips or at home. If both of you are really eager to travel and are up to the task of planning a trip, go now before her disease progresses. But make sure the trip will suit her. People with Alzheimer's, even in the early stage, often get tired easily and are quickly overstimulated and upset by noise, large crowds, or too much activity.

Here are some tips you won't find in your typical guidebook that are sure to make your trip more enjoyable.

Before You Go

- Plan a trip that involves more watching than participating. Good choices are activities where she can set her own pace, such as going to a museum but skipping the guided tour. Bridge and golf may be out, but an evening of cards with you or hitting balls at a golf driving range may be fun. Attend a lecture, but don't expect her to be able to talk about it over lunch afterward.

- Consider inviting along an understanding couple or woman friend, if you would both enjoy the company. Another woman could accompany your wife while you go off on an adventure, or even assist her in the ladies' room or help her pick out nice outfits on a shopping spree.

- Plan to avoid rush hours, either on the road or at airports and train stations.

- Assume you will have to keep track of all logistics. If your wife objects because she was always the trip planner, tell her it's your turn this time.

- To help her avoid the embarrassment of being stumped by simple questions from strangers, discreetly hand out small cards stating that your wife has a memory disorder and questions should be addressed to you. You could give them to waiters, chambermaids, tour guides, and new friends.

Packing

- If you've never packed for your wife, ask for some help from a daughter or woman friend.

- Include a security object, like a favorite sun hat, purse, pillow, or pictures of her grandchildren or pets, to make strange places feel like home.

While Traveling

- Establish a predictable routine, even if you are doing different activities or are in different places every day. Plan your showers, naps, and meals for the same time each day.

- If possible, stay in the same hotel or cottage for your entire vacation and get to know your locale, instead of destination hopping.

- Schedule more breaks or downtime than you would have in the past. You might want to enjoy an outing in the morning, then catch a nap or stay poolside for the afternoon.

- Allow longer times to do everything—from getting ready to enjoying meals.

- Try going for regular walks in the morning to get her oriented and to talk about your day.

- Offer her no more than two choices, whether it's items on the menu for dinner or activities to do that day. She may have more trouble making decisions while traveling than she did in the familiar routine of home.

- If she gets uncharacteristically irritable or withdrawn, she probably needs a rest or a change of scenery.

Alzheimer's doesn't just rob people's memory of what they did this morning or five minutes ago. It can also steal a person's sense of self and sense of self-worth. So compliment your wife often and chat about other trips you two took together.

Finally, try not to judge the success of the trip by what she remembers of it. For people with Alzheimer's, you can create great moments but not necessarily new great memories. She will remember having fun with you even if she doesn't remember the where or when of the trip. For yourself, enjoy remembering those times during your trip when life felt a little like the good old days.

27. "Should I tell my brother with Alzheimer's that our other brother just died? What if he forgets it or asks why our other brother doesn't come around anymore?"   —A seventy-one-year-old man

Yes, your brother deserves to know that his brother died, especially if it just happened. He may not respond as he would have before developing Alzheimer's, but he should be given a chance to talk about his brother and to mourn with close family members. If telling your brother about the death is too difficult for you, ask someone else in the family to tell him.

His ability and desire to attend the funeral or memorial service will depend on his comfort with traveling, crowds, and sitting quietly for what may feel like a long, emotional event. Don't assume, however, that he is too fragile to be included in all the activities.

Regardless of whom they recognize, many people with Alzheimer's delight in the social aspects of a funeral and the other activities surrounding the death of a close family member. Their poor memory and inability to comprehend death serve as a protective shield from the stresses and grief that overwhelm healthy individuals. A woman at the funeral of her husband may wish he were there to admire the lovely flowers but show no grief that he is dead. She simply doesn't connect the service to her husband's death.

Be prepared for your brother to forget that your other brother just died. Rather than reminding him, which may cause him new grief each time he hears it, treat what your brother says as reminiscing. So you might acknowledge that "Yes, Bill was like that" or "Yes, I always wanted to be as cool as you and Bill." You don't have to agree that your dead brother is still alive to respond lovingly to your brother's remarks.

For example, a man with Alzheimer's repeatedly asked his wife why his parents, who had died, didn't visit when they lived just down the road. She finally decided to answer each time with, "Oh, they were here, and they asked about you and sent you their love." It always reassured him and made him smile.

28. "How do I get my mom to go to a support group for family members? She really needs to go because she is losing it with my dad." —A daughter in her forties whose father has Alzheimer's

It's best not to point out to your mom that she "needs" a group or that she is losing it with your dad. She is frustrated by the changes in her life partner and probably feeling somewhat rotten about herself as well. But going to a support group is a big and difficult step for her. She may be facing some of the common roadblocks to attending support groups, which include:

- Not knowing what to expect. Many older individuals think of support groups as encounter or therapy groups.
- Not wanting to talk about loved ones or their own feelings with a group of strangers.
- Worrying that talking about their loved one, or even just going to a support group, is disloyal.
- Being too busy, too tired, or not having a sitter to cover her time away.

During support group meetings, participants generally describe problems they are having and ask the others how they have handled similar situations. The tone is not doom and gloom—there are tears, but there is also humor, encouragement, and friendship. No one is required to confess anything, and group members generally respect confidences.

When you investigate groups that she may want to join, you will probably discover that some are just for spouses or just for women or men, but most have a mix of participants. Some have speakers, sponsor educational forums, or get involved in fund-raising or advocacy for research. Others operate more like a seminar than a support group. Most don't expect participants to make every meeting.

Your mom may be more willing to attend a support group if you tell her:

- about someone you know who benefited from a group.
- that many people come to their first meeting insisting they are not "the support group type."
- that the group will simply help her learn more about how to take care of your dad. Many wives at first won't consider the importance of taking care of themselves, though she will learn more about that through the group as well.
- that you will go with her to a meeting, or she could take a friend, neighbor, or other family member.

If she still decides against joining a formal Alzheimer's support group, there are other options, such as supportive Listservs or chat rooms sponsored by the Alzheimer's Association. Your mother may want to attend educational events for families of people with Alzheimer's. She may also find other women whose husbands have Alzheimer's, by attending a bridge club, Sunday-school class, or women's golf club. Don't give up—there are many ways for your mom to get the support she will need to cope with your dad's illness.

29. "Are there groups for people with memory problems? How could I get my mom to try it?"   —A thirty-six-year-old son

There are groups for people with mild to moderate memory disorders, and some metropolitan areas offer a wide selection of programs and services. Many Alzheimer's Association chapters sponsor groups that meet formally for six to eight weeks and then informally to socialize after that.

The time to suggest to your mom that she check out a group is when she complains or hints that she is looking for something to do, or that her friends don't visit much, or that she is lonely. Tell her that you heard about a group that is forming and may interest her. She can meet individually with the group leader to learn about their program and see if it is right for her.

If she joins the group, she will probably like it and find the other members supportive and interesting. She will have a chance to talk about her frustrations and successes and to listen to others' stories. The participants will together laugh at themselves as they grieve their losses. They may never learn one another's names, but they will probably recognize one another as friends. There may be lots of repetition of themes in the meetings, but few will complain about being bored.

Yes, it's worth it to find the right group for your mom and to encourage her to try it sooner rather than later. But know that she will need gentle reminders, encouragement, and perhaps someone like you to go with her, until it becomes part of her routine or even the highlight of her week or month.

▶ GETTING OTHERS TO UNDERSTAND

Explaining Alzheimer's to friends and family, including to those who have Alzheimer's, is never easy and always important.

30. *"How do you get your friends to understand that just because you have Alzheimer's, you're not deaf and dumb?"*
—**A sixty-year-old woman with Alzheimer's**

It might surprise people who don't have the disease, but this is a very common and devastating problem for people with early Alzheimer's. Friends and family make wrong assumptions about your capabilities, which makes trying to adapt to Alzheimer's even more difficult.

Here are some pointers on what to say. Your friends will probably follow your husband's or children's example, so start with family first. Explain very directly that

- although you repeat yourself because you can't remember who has heard your stories, Alzheimer's doesn't make you deaf or dumb (speaking loudly, for example, is completely unnecessary)

- you still enjoy going out, say, to dinner, museums, shows, or shopping, but you do better in familiar places earlier in the day or with a companion

- you would appreciate rides to places and reminders about events

- hosting or coordinating activities has become too stressful, but you would enjoy helping with them

- you hope everyone can ignore your mistakes and laugh with you at the crazy things we all do, to varying degrees, as we age

For more advice, contact the Alzheimer's Association about joining an early-stage Alzheimer's support group, either online or in person, where you'll get lots of tips (and sympathy) from other members. The association also has materials illustrating how to talk to and offer dignified help to people with Alzheimer's.

31. *"How can I explain to my five-year-old why his grandmother keeps calling him by his father's name?"*
—**A thirty-three-year-old daughter-in-law**

Answer his questions simply and matter-of-factly. Children often surprise adults with their acceptance of differences. You will probably succeed by explaining that Grandmother's memory isn't working as well as it used to. Since she once had a little boy just like him, she gets their names mixed up. He will be happy to hear that she loves him very much and is eager to play, even when she gets names mixed up. You might need to add that, like anyone, Grandmother's feelings get hurt if she is teased or treated rudely when she makes mistakes.

This is a good time to talk to him about other changes in his grandmother that he may have noticed. Explain that his grandmother's brain (her "thinker" inside her head) has new problems, much like the legs of a person in a wheelchair. She doesn't need a wheelchair, but she does need help from her family to figure things out. Reassure your son that this kind of brain trouble is sad, but it happens only to older people, not to children or their parents (hopefully).

Encourage your son to ask you questions about his grandmother. Read him *Wilfrid Gordon McDonald Partridge* by Mem Fox. At five, he's just the right age for this wonderful story about a grandparent's memory loss.

32. *"How do I get my brother's children to understand that he can't live alone anymore?"*
—The seventy-six-year-old sister of a man with Alzheimer's

Problems related to Alzheimer's are sometimes invisible to occasional visitors, so you may need to spell out what you are seeing. A casual observer may not realize, for example, that your brother is sleeping in his clothes, eating spoiled food, taking outdated medicines, or afraid to leave his house. His children might not know if he has forgotten how to use his power tools correctly, how to call for help, or how to spot a financial scam. These problems are easy to hide and embarrassing to talk or hear about.

Your brother's children may even feel that their father should move but, for a variety of reasons, are not making it happen. They may not want to acknowledge that their father is no longer the strong man they remember, or they may not be ready to face his resistance to moving. The burden of caring for him or paying for his care may be stopping them. You need to find out what the roadblocks are and help his children overcome them. If the children won't listen to you, ask your brother's neighbors, friends, other family members, and doctors to take up the cause.

33. *"Is denial a symptom of Alzheimer's? I can't convince my dad to go to an adult day program because he won't admit he has a memory problem."*
—A forty-six-year-old son

Both the person with Alzheimer's and his family members can be in denial about the disease. But denial isn't the issue with your dad. Instead, he probably just forgets that he forgets and that he has Alzheimer's. As your dad's disease progresses, he will be even less able to evaluate his abilities objectively, but he may also forget that he doesn't want to go to the day program.

Your dad's most vivid memory is of himself as a healthy individual. In his mind, he neither looks nor behaves like the old people at the center; instead, he is a man in his prime who must deal with a nagging son or other family members. Don't wait for your dad to admit he has a memory problem or ask to go to the program—it won't happen.

To coax him to go with you to the center, focus on the positives. Instead of telling him what he can't do, such as stay home alone, re-mind him about what he enjoys, even if it's just eating lunch. Then explain that the program offers those activities and, equally impor-tant, the staff needs his help. Many people in day programs think they are there to help out. Few participants ever said, "Oh, yes, I would love to go to an adult day center."

Before bringing your dad to the center, make sure it has truly stimulating activities that won't insult his intelligence or abilities, and that the staff are caring, professional, and experienced at taking care of people with Alzheimer's.

34. "How do you get one parent to believe the other one has a memory problem?"
—A son in his fifties who is worried about his mother's memory

The illness of a husband or wife is particularly difficult because you are seeing someone you care about suffer and, at the same time, your support system disintegrates. As a result, one spouse often covers for, excuses, or denies signs of decline in the other, especially symptoms with scary, uncertain, or overwhelming consequences. Your parents may also be trying to protect you or to avoid burdening you. Such an effort to appear normal is exhausting.

It sounds as though your dad won't believe that your mom has a memory problem. Instead of asking him to face up to the facts, you may have better success if you first focus on helping your dad meet your mom's health needs. Eventually, after you have gained his trust, try telling your dad that you

- see changes in your mom that worry you
- both need to know what is going on, so that you can do everything possible to help your mom
- understand his desire to shield her from tests and the possibility of a frightening diagnosis
- are willing to find the appropriate doctor and set up an appointment that is convenient for all three of you
- are not jumping to conclusions but just gathering information
- are open and willing to seek a second opinion, if necessary
- will not treat her with any less respect or dignity if she has a memory problem

Finally, remind your dad how he and your mom always made sure you got prompt medical attention. Now it's your turn to return the favor. Instead of being argumentative, appreciate that your position as the son will make your experience of her symptoms different from that of your father. Trust that the doctor will use everyone's perspectives when diagnosing your mom and developing treatment options.

35. "Why won't my mom's doctor take my calls? Mom has him completely fooled."   —A daughter in her thirties

The doctor apparently believes that your mom's memory and judgment are fine and is protecting your mom's legal right to privacy. If it is any consolation, you are not alone. Not having access to a family member's medical information is a common frustration for family caregivers. And patients' abilities to fool their doctors is one of the main reasons Alzheimer's goes undiagnosed all too often in the early stages.

You may think your mother is showing signs of Alzheimer's, but she isn't complaining about her memory to the doctor, and her doctor isn't picking up the cues or testing her memory. The doctor may not have enough time, as dealing with your mother's other chronic conditions or perceived health concerns may take up the entire office visit. Many people with early memory loss look and sound fine in a brief office visit, fooling even a cautious doctor. Your mom may believe that her memory is fine because she can vividly remember events from fifty years ago. She forgets that she forgets.

How to get a foot in the door? First, ask your mother if you can accompany her to the doctor because *you* have questions or worries about how to help her maintain her health. When you get to the office, alert the nurse that you are with your mother because you have sensitive questions about her health (see question #6 for the how-to details). Your mom may initially be angry that you are butting into her business, but if she does in fact have a progressive memory disorder, she will eventually forget the event.

More important, you will have protected her from the many risks associated with untreated or undiagnosed Alzheimer's, including poor money management, getting lost, driving dangerously, and more.

► PROTECTING AGAINST ALZHEIMER'S

Many people wonder if there are ways to guard their own or their loved ones' brains against Alzheimer's.

36. "Is there anything I can do now to keep from getting Alzheimer's like my mom and her mom?"   —*A forty-nine-year-old daughter*

It is scary to watch such devastating losses in the women in your family and wonder if you are next. While there is no magic vaccine or prevention (at least not yet), you can take care of your body and brain in ways that may slow the arrival of Alzheimer's, if not actually stop it.

According to some studies, people with high blood pressure and cholesterol levels are more likely to get Alzheimer's than their healthier peers. So what's good for your heart is probably good for your head. Doing challenging and novel activities is also good for your mind. Find games or other activities that keep you engaged and stimulated.

You have probably heard all too often that you should avoid stress—but for most of us that would require hiding under our blankets or hiring a full-time housekeeper and a private helicopter to get us to work on time. But you can try to identify and deal with at least some of the sources of stress in your life. If you have a stressful job you hate, you can look for a better one. If you are taking care of elderly parents and young children, call a family meeting to ask for some practical assistance.

Here are some other ways you can try to ward off Alzheimer's by being good to yourself:

- Seek treatment for anxiety or depression.

- Exercise regularly.

- Get enough sleep.

- Eat a healthy, low-fat diet that includes weekly servings of fish high in omega-3 fatty acids.

- If you drink, drink moderately. One small alcoholic drink (one ounce of alcohol, four ounces of wine) a day may even protect against Alzheimer's.

- Take a multivitamin without iron but know it doesn't substitute for a healthy diet.

- Stay connected to people and groups that are important to you.

- Participate in a memory disorders study to stay up to date on new treatments and preventative measures.

- Try stress management techniques, such as yoga.

You may know people who have done most of the items on this list and have still developed dementia. Instead of giving up, concentrate on the immediate benefits of improving your overall quality of life and hope it will also make a difference for your future.

37. "Should we throw out our aluminum pans? I heard that aluminum can cause Alzheimer's." —A thirty-five-year-old mother

Researchers are investigating whether any metals, including aluminum, play any role in Alzheimer's. However, no one has proved that using cookware, deodorants, or cans that contain aluminum cause Alzheimer's. As you read articles and listen to news stories about Alzheimer's, you will hear about many links between what you ingest on a day-to-day basis, such as aluminum or even some medications, and memory loss. Unfortunately, nothing as simple as avoiding aluminum cookware will prevent a memory disorder. Stay tuned but skeptical about any simple causes or solutions to this complex and common illness.

38. *"How can my eighty-year-old dad be able to run a mile a day and still have Alzheimer's? I thought exercise preserved the brain."*
—A fifty-four-year-old son

Although exercise protects the brain and almost every other organ in our body, it is unlikely that any one activity by itself will ever prevent Alzheimer's. Still, if your dad weren't such an avid runner, his memory, thinking, mood, attention, and sleep would probably have deteriorated further. Many people with Alzheimer's have excess energy but limited physical capacity or endurance to discharge that energy. As a result, they are more likely than your dad to suffer from agitation, depression, balance problems, and behavioral disorders that make caring for them a challenge.

Your dad has probably always been a high-energy guy who enjoyed exercise. As other parts of his life and identity give way to Alzheimer's, he can still enjoy the familiar routine and self-esteem that running provides. Few people with Alzheimer's are disabled in all areas of their life, and they need to be reminded of what they can do, not what they are losing. So cheer your dad on and make sure he's running where he won't be at risk of falling or getting lost.

39. *"Isn't it a good idea to try a new hobby when you get Alzheimer's? My wife doesn't have a bad case and I think she'd better 'use it or lose it.'"*   —A husband in his sixties

In a perfectly rational world, if a disability or illness required that you give up a hobby, you would simply fill your time with a new activity. Unfortunately, however, Alzheimer's is not part of the rational world. Your wife may be scared to try anything new, because remembering how to do even familiar tasks is so difficult. Alzheimer's can make beginning a new activity or carrying out a multistep process seem impossible. She will need encouragement to pursue a new hobby, or even to continue her old ones, because she is probably aware of her disability and eager to appear normal.

When considering activities for her, avoid fast-paced classes, competitive games that require speedy responses, or new technical skills like needlework or photography. Instead, suggest an activity that is similar to something she enjoyed before developing Alzheimer's and, even better, something the two of you like to do together.

- She may enjoy going to a garden club with friends who understand and won't put her on the spot, but she may not want to take gardening or golf lessons with a new teacher or group.

- She might enjoy hitting golf balls with you or an old friend at a driving range instead of playing an entire game.

- If she enjoyed a volunteer job, ask another understanding volunteer to work with her.

- Consider delivering meals-on-wheels to needy individuals. You can drive, and she can take the meals to the door.

A diagnosis of Alzheimer's should not put a halt to pleasurable hobbies or useful activities. Rather, consider it an opportunity—even if not a sought-after one—to find new paths to old pleasures. But because Alzheimer's is a progressive disease, remember that your wife will need more support and guidance over time.

40. "Are there some classes my grandmother could take to improve her memory?"   —A twenty-year-old college student

Classes for sharpening and improving memory skills have become somewhat common at community centers, senior centers, and local colleges. Some are based on valid research about how memory works; others verge on pop psychology.

Healthy adults of all ages can learn new skills to improve their memory. But people with Alzheimer's need special classes. If your grandmother's Alzheimer's has progressed, she won't be able to remember the mnemonics or other strategies that many classes teach. Even if she is in the moderate stage, regular classes may prove difficult and frustrating for her.

However, a thorough evaluation will reveal her level of impairment and what skills she has retained. The doctor can then suggest memory strategies or special classes for her, including credible classes or clinical trials of cognitive stimulation or cognitive training from an Alzheimer's research center.

If she is very aware of and concerned about her memory loss, she will be motivated to succeed—but only if an experienced instructor is careful to build up her self-esteem instead of wearing it down. People with Alzheimer's or any diagnosed brain disorder are extremely vulnerable to the frustration that comes with trying hard and getting little in return. For example, her quality of life will not improve if she spends hours trying to remember her grandchildren's names, only to forget them at the next family get-together when she wants to appear like her old self.

If memory instruction isn't for her, find other classes or activities she might enjoy, such as taking a cooking class with you or joining a film society or a zoo trip with the grandchildren. Staying active, engaged, and connected to people will keep her mind working at its maximum capacity, with a smile on her face.

RESOURCES

ORGANIZATIONS

Alzheimer's Association
www.alz.org
   The Alzheimer's Association is the leading voluntary organization devoted to promoting Alzheimer's research and supporting people who are affected by Alzheimer's. Call its Contact Center (800-272-3900) anytime to speak with multilingual, trained professionals about caring for people with Alzheimer's, finding help in your community, or participating in research studies. Its Web site hosts numerous resources. Check out its online support and discussion groups for people with early-stage or early-onset Alzheimer's and their family members at http://alzheimers.infopop.cc/eve; research updates at www.alz.org/alzheimers_disease_clinical_studies.asp; help finding care at www.alz.org/carefinder and SNAP for Seniors, national online dementia-specific senior housing database.
   This is the best dementia-specific interactive search engine for care options throughout the United States. Publications available by calling the Alzheimer's Association include *Money Matters: Helping the Person with Dementia Settle Financial Issues* and Green-Field Library annotated reading lists, which include a 2006 reading list on early-stage and early-onset dementia.

Alzheimer's Disease Education & Referral Center
www.nia.nih.gov/alzheimers
   Part of the National Institute on Aging, this site offers explanations of research findings and clinical drug trials. You'll also find a list of federally funded Alzheimer's Disease Research Centers. Call 800-222-2225 for their free packet of information for caregivers (and ask to be added to the *Connections* newsletter mailing list). Call 800-438-4380 to talk to an agency information specialist if you don't have online access or you would like specific topical materials mailed to you.

Alzheimer's Disease International
www.alz.co.uk/havedementia
   This group provides excellent information for people with dementia, including tips for early-stage dementia.

Alzheimer's Foundation of America
www.alzfdn.org
> This national nonprofit Alzheimer's service organization sponsors educational forums and memory screenings. It has a free quarterly caregiver newsletter and a telephone support network.

AARP
www.aarp.org/families.caregiving
> AARP is the leading nonprofit, nonpartisan membership organization in the Unites States for people age fifty and above. It has excellent information on its Web site about all aspects of family caregiving, including advice on juggling a job and caregiving.

American Association for Geriatric Psychiatry Foundation
www.gmhfonline.org/gmhf
> This group offers help finding a geriatric psychiatrist while also providing information on Alzheimer's and caring for a person with Alzheimer's. For information specific to Alzheimer's, click on "Consumer/Patient information." Also go to www.aagponline.org/prof/position_caredmnalz.asp for a document titled "The American Association of Geriatric Psychiatry Position Statement: Principles of Care for Patients with Dementia Resulting from Alzheimer Disease" (July 2006), which describes the level of care patients and their families should expect from their physician.

National Association of Professional Geriatric Care Managers
www.caremanager.org
> The group provides information on what geriatric care managers do and how to find one.

National Association for Home Care and Hospice
www.nahc.org/consumer/home.html
> This group helps patients, including people with Alzheimer's, get medical, social, or daily activities assistance.

National Adult Day Services Association
www.nadsa.org
> The group provides information on adult day services, including for people with Alzheimer's. On its Web site, you can see listings of adult day services in your community.

Leeza's Place
www.leezasplace.org
> The Leeza Gibbons Memory Foundation sponsors community centers in Florida, New York, and California for people with early-stage dementia and their families. The Web site lists free materials on caregiver stress.

BOOKS, ARTICLES, AND OTHER PUBLICATIONS

About All Aspects of Alzheimer's and Other Dementias

The 36-Hour Day: A Family Guide to Caring for Persons with Alzheimer Disease, Related Dementing Illnesses, and Memory Loss in Later Life, 4th ed., by Nancy L. Mace and Peter V. Rabins (Baltimore: Johns Hopkins University Press, 2006). A very comprehensive overview of Alzheimer's, particularly useful for information on the psychiatric or behavioral symptoms of moderate- to late-stage Alzheimer's.

Perspectives. E-mail lsnyder@ucsd.edu for free e-mail editions of this excellent newsletter, which offers information on coping, group programs for people with early-stage Alzheimer's, research updates, and more.

The Pleasure Was Mine by Tommy Hays (New York: St. Martin's Press, 2006). A wonderful novel about a Southern family's experience with Alzheimer's.

Wilfrid Gordon McDonald Partridge by Mem Fox (La Jolla, CA: Kane/Miller, 1995). A story for preschoolers about Alzheimer's disease.

About Brain Health

The Memory Prescription: Dr. Gary Small's 14-Day Plan to Keep Your Brain and Body Young by Gary Small with Gigi Vorgan (New York: Hyperion, 2005). The book, written by a researcher and his wife, provides practical advice on possible ways to keep your brain fit.

For People with Early-Stage Dementia

Taking Action: A Personal & Practical Guide for Persons with Memory Loss (2007). Go to www.alzco.org for ordering information. A workbook for people with early-stage memory loss, published by the Rocky Mt. Alzheimer's Association.

What Happens Next? Free downloadable and print versions from nia.nih.gov/Publications/WhatHappensNext.htm.

About Caregiving

Surviving Today and Revising Tomorrow by Molly Wood Tully and Mary Ann Blotzer (1993). A booklet written by two wise wives of men with Alzheimer's. Available from the Alzheimer's Association of Greater Washington, 11240 Waples Mill Road, Suite 402, Fairfax, VA 22030; 866-259-0042. $3.00 plus tax and $2.75 shipping.

As Memory Fades by Dr. Geri Richards Hall (2006, revised). An excellent booklet written by an advanced nurse-practitioner with tips on how to respond to problem behaviors related to memory loss. Available at www.centeronaging.uiowa.edu/archive.

Caregiving Strategies (2003). A DVD offering excellent advice for families caring for people with moderate-stage Alzheimer's at home. It is available for sale from www.hcinteractive.com.

Alzheimer's Early Stages: First Steps for Family, Friends and Caregivers, 2d ed., by Daniel Kuhn (Alameda, CA: Hunter House, 2003).

Pressure Points: Alzheimer's and Anger by Edna Ballard, Lisa Gwyther, and T. Patrick Toal (2000). Available from www.dukefamilysupport .org (go to "Links/Resources" on left, then "List of Publications"); $8.00 prepaid. While you're at the site, check out the brochure *When Anger Gets Too Much: Wait a Minute* and sign up for the center's newsletter, the *Caregiver*.

A Dignified Life: The Best Friends Approach to Alzheimer's Care: A Guide for Family Caregivers by Virginia Bell and David Troxel (Deerfield Beach, FL: Health Professions, 2002).

Far Away and Still Caring (National Institute on Aging, 2006). This online booklet has information for long-distance caregivers. www.niapublications.org/shopdisplayproducts.asp?id=29&cat= Caregiving.

"The Top Ten Things Caregivers Don't Want to Hear . . . And a Few Things They Do" by Carol Levine, director of the Family and Health Care Project at the United Hospital Fund and family care provider. The article is great for families and their well-meaning friends. www.uhfnyc.org/pubs-stories3220/pubs-stories_show.htm ?doc_id=417469.

What if It's Not Alzheimer's? A Caregiver's Guide to Dementia by Lisa Radin and Gary Radin (Amherst, NY: Prometheus, 2003). A valuable caregiver's guide on frontotemporal dementias.

"Being in One Place at a Time: Working and Caregiving." This article published on the Johnson & Johnson Web site offers insights on how to manage your "real" job and caregiving job at the same time.

www.strengthforcaring.com/manual/18/368/ being-in-one-place-at-a-time.html.

You Are One of Us: Building Church/Clergy Connections to Alzheimer's Families by Lisa Gwyther (1995). This 100-page paperback book offers hints for clergy and church members about how to understand, respond to, and offer help to church members living with Alzheimer's disease and their families. $5.00 at www .dukefamilysupport.org.

Talking to Alzheimer's: Simple Ways to Connect When You Visit with a Family Member or Friend by Claudia J. Strauss (Oakland, CA: New Harbinger, 2002). This book describes how to have successful visits and conversations with family members or friends who have Alzheimer's.

Learning to Speak Alzheimer's: A Groundbreaking Approach for Everyone Dealing with the Disease by Joanne Koenig Coste (Boston: Houghton Mifflin, 2004). The author is a professional nurse whose husband had early-onset Alzheimer's disease.

"Family Conversations with Older Drivers." Offers tips on how to help older people "retire" from driving. www.thehartford.com/ talkwitholderdrivers.

About Helping People with Alzheimer's Who Can't Be at Home

The Baby Boomer's Guide to Nursing Home Care by Eric M. Carlson and Katharine Bau Hsiao, published by the National Senior Citizens Law Center, 2006. www.nsclc.org; click on "Consumer Info."

"Respite for Persons with Alzheimer's Disease or Related Dementia" (2002). This fact sheet, prepared by the National Respite Center and Resource Network, describes respite options for people with Alzheimer's and their care providers. www.archrespite.org/ archfs55.htm.

Moving a Relative with Memory Loss: A Family Caregiver's Guide by Laurie A. White and Beth Spencer (2000). A specific and compassionate booklet about how to prepare for and cope with the move of a close family member to a residential or nursing facility. Available at www.whisppub.com/bookstore.htm.

The Alzheimer's Health Care Handbook: How to Get the Best Medical Care for Your Relative with Alzheimer's Disease, In and Out of the Hospital by Mary S. Mittelman and Cynthia Epstein (New York: Marlowe & co., 2003). Good tips on how to help people with

Alzheimer's while they are in the hospital and on how to communicate with doctors.

About Caring for the Caregiver

The Caregiver HelpBook: Powerful Tools for Caregivers, 2d ed., from Legacy Caregiver Services, 2006. Excellent strategies for how family caregivers can take care of themselves. www.legacyhealth.org/body .cfm?id=87.

"Financial Steps for Caregivers: What You Need to Know About Money and Retirement," published by the Women's Institute for a Secure Retirement. www.aoa.gov/prof/aoaprog/caregiver/WISER.pdf.

Personal Accounts from People With Alzheimer's and Family Members

No More Words: A Journal of My Mother, Anne Morrow Lindbergh by Reeve Lindbergh (New York: Simon & Schuster, 2002). The daughter of the famous aviators tells about caring for her mother, who had Alzheimer's, at the end of her life.

Alzheimer's, a Love Story: One Year in My Husband's Journey by Ann Davidson (New York: Carol Publishing, 1997). This book gives Davidson's perspective on early-stage and early-onset Alzheimer's. See also her follow-up book, *A Curious Kind of Widow: Loving a Man with Advanced Dementia* (McKinleyville, CA: Daniel & Daniel, 2006).

Speaking Our Minds: Personal Reflections from Individuals with Alzheimer's by Lisa Synder (New York: W. H. Freeman, 2000).

Partial View: An Alzheimer's Journal by Cary Smith Henderson (Dallas: Southern Methodist University Press, 1998). A photo-essay written by a history professor with moderate-stage, early-onset Alzheimer's disease. An award-winning photojournalist contributed black-and-white photographs of Dr. Henderson in his home over one year of his illness.

Alzheimer's from the Inside Out by Richard Taylor (Baltimore: Health Professions, 2006). A psychologist's story about his life with early-stage Alzheimer's disease.

My Journey into Alzheimer's Disease by Robert Davis (Carol Stream, IL: Tyndale House, 1989). A minister who was diagnosed with Pick's disease (only on autopsy) describes his experiences and his view of the responses of his church.

From Odd Behavior to a Difficult Diagnosis by Sandra G. Boodman
    (2007). An informative description of one couple's journey to
    solve the "medical mystery" of frontotemporal dementia (FTD),
    also known as Pick's disease. www.washingtonpost.com/wp-dyn/
    content/article/2007/07/09/AR2007070901320.html?sub=AR.

WEB SITES

All Aspects of Alzheimer's

www.alzforum.org. Popular with scientists, the Web site reports on scien-
    tific findings from basic research and clinical trials. It has public
    research databases and hosts discussion forums.

Especially for People with Early-Stage Dementia and Their Families

www.clinicaltrials.gov. This government-run site describes federally and
    privately supported clinical dementia research studies, including
    their purpose, who may participate, locations, and contact infor-
    mation.

www.pbs.org/theforgetting. This site grew out of the 2004 PBS documen-
    tary *The Forgetting*, which was based on David Shenk's book of
    the same name. At the site, you'll also find coping tips for people
    with Alzheimer's and for their families.

Family Caregiving

www.caregiver.org. Run by the not-for-profit Family Caregiver Alliance,
    this is the single best site for current educational materials for
    caregivers. Download the free overview of residential care options
    and information on publicly funded caregiver support programs in
    each of the fifty states and the District of Columbia at http://
    caregiver.org/caregiver/jsp/content_node.jsp?nodeid=1274.

http://alzheimer.wustl.edu/adrc2/alzheimerlist/. Supported by the Washing-
    ton University Alzheimer's Disease Research Center, this site offers
    access to the Alzheimer List (AL), an e-mail-based support group
    for family caregivers of people with memory loss. You can get

definitive and authoritative responses to your questions from seasoned professionals associated with Alzheimer's Disease Research Centers. Dr. Geri Richards Hall, a nurse-practitioner, and Dr. Jason Karlawosh, a bioethicist, geriatrician, and Alzheimer's researcher, answer questions on medical, ethical, and nursing care issues.

www.longtermcare.gov. The Web site of the government's National Clearinghouse for Long-Term Care Information provides information and resources to help people plan for future long-term-care needs.

www.agelessdesign.com or www.alzstore.com. These sites offer advice and products for making homes safer for people with Alzheimer's. You can also order *In Search of the Alzheimer's Wanderer* by Mark L. Warner (2006), which has information on how to prevent a person with Alzheimer's from wandering.

www.buildingbetterhealth.com. Supported by Consumer Health Interactive. On the left side of the page, click on "Medical Info" and then on "Health Info, A–Z," and you'll find interesting topics on Alzheimer's care.

www.caregiversmarketplace.com. The Caregivers Marketplace is a free program that provides cash back on caregiving products, such as blood pressure monitors for home use, nutritional supplements, diapers, and more, that are not typically covered by insurance or Medicare.

www.medicare.gov. The official site for people on Medicare, the site lets you compare nursing homes and find the latest changes in the Medicare Prescription Part D benefit.

www.fullcirclecare.org. Developed by the Triangle J Council of Governments, Area Agency on Aging in North Carolina, this site for family caregivers has an excellent section on Alzheimer's and easy-to-follow information on seeking and using home- and community-based services and benefits.

www.getpalliativecare.org. Sponsored by the Center to Advance Palliative Care, the site provides information about palliative care and dementia, and about how to find palliative care experts. (People with early- and middle-stage Alzheimer's may have other diseases that require palliative care.)

General Health and Information on Alzheimer's

www.mayoclinic.com/health/alzheimers/AZ9999. The Mayo Clinic provides information on Alzheimer's and MCI from Alzheimer expert Dr. Ronald Peterson.

www.medlineplus.gov. The National Institutes of Health site provides information about federally and privately supported clinical research, including information about specific trials and recent trial results as well as current disease-specific information.

www.nihseniorhealth.gov. An easy-to-use site with material on all major health conditions affecting older people. This site is particularly useful to people who are new to Web searches.

www.healthinaging.org. Run by the American Geriatrics Society, the site offers information on finding a geriatrician, taking care of elders at home, and more. At www.healthinaging.org/agingintheknow, you'll find a helpful list of questions to ask a geriatrician or your doctor about various conditions or tests.

www.ec-online.net. Elder Care Online is a family caregiver and consumer site of the Alzheimer's Research Forum. It provides an online supportive community for all care providers. You can read articles about caregiving, join in the conversations in the chat rooms, and even pick up some pretty good jokes!

www.quackwatch.com. With the goal of combating health-related frauds, myths, fads, fallacies, and misconduct, Quackwatch lets you check out claims that sound too good to be true.

Memory Disorders Other than Alzheimer's

www.lewybodydementia.org. Sponsored by the Lewy Body Dementia Association.

www.ftd-picks.org. Sponsored by the Association of Frontotemporal Dementias.

www.apdaparkinson.org. Sponsored by the American Parkinson Disease Association.

www.stroke.org. Sponsored by the National Stroke Association.

Alternative Medicine

http://nccam.nih.gov/health. Run by the government's National Center for Complementary and Alternative Medicine, this site offers current critical reviews, research updates, and suggestions on all complementary and alternative therapies. You can sign up for its e-mail newsletter.

www.herbalgram.org. The American Botanical Council's site has up-to-date information on herbal medicine.

Insurance, Including Medicare

www.shipusa.org/Find_a_State_SHIP.html. Every state plus Puerto Rico
and the Virgin Islands has a state agency that provides consumers
with information about Medicare Part D and other health insurance concerns. This site helps you get information about your
state's program, called State Health Insurance Assistance Programs (SHIP).

www.benefitscheckup.org. The National Council on Aging's interactive site
provides personalized information on benefits programs for seniors
with limited income and resources. It includes more than 1,550
public and private benefits programs from all fifty states and the
District of Columbia. Before you start, see benefits QuickLINK
from the AARP Foundation.

www.aoa.gov. Run by the government's Administration on Aging, the site
offers many useful tools. To get to the Alzheimer's information,
click on "Elders and Aging" at the top of the page, then click on
the "Alzheimer's Resource Room." (AOA also runs the Eldercare
Locator, which links older people with services in their community. Call 800-677-1116 or check out www.eldercare.gov/
Eldercare/Public/Home.asp.)

www.medicarerights.org. The Medicare Rights Center helps older adults
and people with disabilities get health care. The site provides excellent information on Medicare, and has a special Web seminar
on "Planning and Coordinating Care for People with Alzheimer's."

Legal Information, Including Advance Directives

www.abanet.org/elderly/toolkit/home.html. The American Bar Association Commission on Legal Problems of the Elderly offers excellent free advance planning guides and tools for conversations with
family members. You can download the guides from the site.

www.naela.com. The National Academy of Elder Law Attorneys offers information on finding a specialist in elder law for families with
considerable assets that need managing or considerable family
conflicts that need resolving.

www.caringinfo.org. Part of the National Hospice and Palliative Care Organization, this site has advance directive forms and excellent
information on advance care planning and end-of-life care.

www.vtethicsnetwork.org/Forms.htm. Run by the Vermont Ethics Network, this site has information on advance directives, including a

worksheet designed to help you think about your values as they relate to medical care decisions.

http://caringcommunity.org/taxonomy/page/or/82. Supported by the Community Network for Appropriate Technologies, the site offers information on advance directives, including a values survey, downloadable advance directive forms, and guides for how to talk about this sensitive issue.

Alzheimer's Disease Centers (ADCs)

The National Institute on Aging funds Alzheimer's Disease Centers at major medical institutions across the United States. A state-by-state listing is below. Some ADCs have satellite facilities, which offer diagnostic and treatment services and research opportunities in underserved, rural, and minority communities.

ALABAMA

Alzheimer's Disease Research Center
University of Alabama
Sparks Research Center
1720 7th Avenue South, Suite 650K
Birmingham, AL 35233-7340
www.uab.edu/adc
205-934-3847
e-mail: dmarson@uab.edu

ARIZONA

Arizona Alzheimer's Disease Center/Sun Health Research Institute
Banner Alzheimer's Institute
901 East Willeta Street
Phoenix, AZ 85006
www.azalz.org/
602-239-6525

ARKANSAS

University of Arkansas for Medical Sciences
Alzheimer's Disease Center
Donald W. Reynolds Department of Geriatrics
4301 West Markham, Slot 808
Little Rock, AR 72205-7199
http://alzheimer.uams.edu
501-603-1294

CALIFORNIA

Stanford University
Stanford/VA Alzheimer's Disease Center
Department of Psychiatry, 5550
401 Quarry Road, C305
Stanford, CA 94305-5717
http://alzheimer.stanford.edu
650-852-3287
e-mail: amott@stanford.edu

University of California, Davis
Alzheimer's Disease Center
4860 Y Street, Suite 3700
Sacramento, CA 95817-4540
http://alzheimer.ucdavis.edu
916-734-5496

University of California, Irvine
Alzheimer's Disease Research
Center
Gillespie Neuroscience Research
Facility, Room 1113
Irvine, CA 92697-4540
www.alz.uci.edu
949-824-5847

University of California, Los Angeles
Alzheimer's Disease Center
10911 Weyburn Avenue, Suite 200
Los Angeles, CA 90095-1769
www.adc.ucla.edu
Information on research studies
and clinical trials: 310-206-6379

University of California, San Diego
Alzheimer's Disease Research
Center
Department of Neurosciences
UCSD School of Medicine
9500 Gilman Drive (0624)
La Jolla, CA 92093-0624
http://adrc.ucsd.edu
858-622-5800
e-mail: adrc@ucsd.edu

University of California, San Francisco
Alzheimer's Disease Research
Center

350 Parnassus Avenue, Suite 706
San Francisco, CA 94143-1207
http://memory.ucsf.edu
415-476-6880
e-mail:adrc@memory.ucsf.edu

University of Southern California
Alzheimer's Disease Research
Center
Health Consultation Center
1510 San Pablo Street, HCC643
Los Angeles, CA 90033
www.usc.edu/dept/gero/ADRC
213-740-7777
e-mail: uscadrc@usc.edu

FLORIDA

Florida Alzheimer's Disease Research Center/Byrd Alzheimer's Institute
15310 Amberly Drive,
Suite 320
Tampa, FL 33647
www.floridaadrc.org
866-700-7773
Director's e-mail:
hpotter@byrdinstitute.org

GEORGIA

Emory University
Alzheimer's Disease Center
Neurology Department
101 Woodruff Circle, #6000
Atlanta, GA 30322
www.med.emory.edu/ADC
404-728-6950

ILLINOIS

Northwestern University
Cognitive Neurology and
Alzheimer's Disease Center
Feinberg School of Medicine
675 North St. Claire, Galter
20-100
Chicago, IL 60611
www.brain.northwestern.edu
312-908-9339
e-mail: CNADC-Admin@
northwestern.edu
Director's e-mail: mmesulam@
northwestern.edu

Rush University Medical Center
Alzheimer's Disease Center
Armour Academic Center
600 South Paulina Street, Suite
1028
Chicago, IL 60612
www.rush.edu/radc
312-942-2362

INDIANA

**Indiana University School of
Medicine**
Indiana Alzheimer Disease
Center
Department of Pathology and
Lab Medicine
635 Barnhill Drive, MS-A-138
Indianapolis, IN 46202-5120
http://iadc.iupui.edu
317-278-5500
e-mail: iadc@iupui.edu

KENTUCKY

University of Kentucky
Alzheimer's Disease Center
Sanders-Brown Center on Aging,
Room 101
800 South Limestone Street
Lexington, KY 40536-0230
www.mc.uky.edu/coa/
859-323-6040

MARYLAND

Johns Hopkins University
Alzheimer's Disease Research
Center
Division of Neuropathology
558 Ross Research Building
720 Rutland Avenue
Baltimore, MD 21205-2196
www.alzresearch.org
410-502-5164

MASSACHUSETTS

Boston University
Alzheimer's Disease Center
Bedford VA Medical Center
GRECC Program (182B)
200 Springs Road
Bedford, MA 01730
www.bu.edu/alzresearch
617-638-5368
e-mail: decart@bu.edu

Massachusetts General Hospital/ Harvard Medical School
Alzheimer's Disease Research Center
114 16th Street, Room 2009
Charlestown, MA 02129
http://madrc.org
617-726-3987

MICHIGAN

University of Michigan
Alzheimer's Disease Research Center
Department of Neurology
300 North Ingalls, Room 3D15
Ann Arbor, MI 48109-0489
www.med.umich.edu/alzheimers
734-764-2190
e-mail: neuro-ADresearch@med.umich.edu

MINNESOTA

Mayo Clinic
Alzheimer's Disease Research Center
Department of Neurology
200 First Street, SW
Rochester, MN 55905
http://mayoresearch.mayo.edu/
mayo/research/alzheimers_center
507-284-1324
e-mail: mayoADC@mayo.edu

MISSOURI

Washington University School of Medicine

Alzheimer's Disease Research Center
Department of Neurology
4488 Forest Park Avenue, Suite 130
St. Louis, MO 63108-2293
http://alzheimer.wustl.edu
Research participation and questions: 314-286-2683
Education and rural outreach: 314-286-2882 or 286-0930

NEW YORK

Columbia University
Alzheimer's Disease Center
630 West 168 Street, P&S 15-402
New York, NY 10032
www.alzheimercenter.org
212-305-1818

Mount Sinai School of Medicine
Alzheimer's Disease Research Center
Department of Psychiatry
One Gustave Levy Place, Box 1230
New York, NY 10029-6574
www.mssm.edu/psychiatry/adrc
212-241-8329

New York University
Alzheimer's Disease Center
ADRC, Millhauser Labs
560 First Avenue
New York, NY 10016
www.med.nyu.edu/adc
212-263-8088

NORTH CAROLINA

Duke University Medical Center
Joseph and Kathleen Bryan
Alzheimer's Disease Research
Center
2200 West Main Street,
Suite A-230
Durham, NC 27705
http://adrc.mc.duke.edu
866-444-2372 (toll free)

OREGON

**Oregon Health and Science
University**
Aging and Alzheimer's Disease
Center CR 131
3181 SW Sam Jackson Park
Road
Portland, OR 97239-3098
www.ohsu.edu/research/
alzheimers
503-494-6976

PENNSYLVANIA

**University of Pennsylvania
School of Medicine**
Alzheimer's Disease Center
Department of Pathology and
Laboratory Medicine
HUP, Maloney 3rd Floor
36th and Spruce Streets
Philadelphia, PA 19104-4283
www.uphs.upenn.edu/ADC
215-662-7810

University of Pittsburgh
Alzheimer's Disease Research
Center
Department of Neurology
3471 Fifth Avenue, Suite 811
Pittsburgh, PA 15213-2582
www.adrc.pitt.edu
412-692-2700

TEXAS

**University of Texas,
Southwestern Medical Center**
Alzheimer's Disease Research
Center
Department of Neurology
5323 Harry Hines Boulevard
Dallas, TX 75390-9036
www.utsouthwestern.edu/
alzheimers/research
214-648-9376

WASHINGTON

University of Washington
Alzheimer's Disease Center
VA Puget Sound Health Care
System
Mental Health Services, S-116
1660 South Columbian Way
Seattle, WA 98108
www.depts.washington.edu/
adrcweb
206-277-3281

APPENDIX A: STAGES OF SYMPTOM PROGRESSION IN EARLY THROUGH MODERATE ALZHEIMER'S DISEASE

By Lisa Gwyther, M.S.W, ACSW

This isn't a tool that doctors use for staging patients, but it should give family members an idea of what happens to people with Alzheimer's as the disease progresses. Doctors use other tests for determining what stage the patient is in.

FIRST STAGE (MILD OR EARLY STAGE)— LASTS TWO TO FOUR YEARS LEADING UP TO AND AFTER DIAGNOSIS

Symptoms and Examples

- Recent memory loss—repeats stories and questions.
- Confusion about places—gets lost on way to work; arrives at wrong time or place.
- Loss of spontaneity—becomes withdrawn and uninterested.
- Mood / personality changes—becomes anxious about symptoms; avoids people.
- Poor judgment—makes bad decisions.
- Takes longer with routine chores—forgets grocery list; loses things; constantly rechecks calendar or clock.
- Trouble handling money and paying bills—forgets which bills are paid.

SECOND STAGE (MODERATE OR MIDDLE STAGE)— LASTS TWO TO TEN YEARS AFTER DIAGNOSIS

Symptoms and Examples

- Increasing memory loss and confusion, shorter attention span—can't remember visits even though the visitor just left.
- Problems recognizing close friends and / or family.
- Repetitive movements.
- Restless, especially in late afternoon and at night—may get up at night and wander.
- Perceptual-motor problems—difficulty getting into a chair, setting table for a meal.
- Difficulty organizing thoughts or thinking logically—mixes up day and night.
- Can't find right words—makes up stories to fill in memory blanks.
- Problems with reading, writing—can't follow written signs.
- May be suspicious, irritable, fidgety, teary, or silly—may accuse children of stealing, spouse of infidelity.
- Loss of impulse control—curses, tactless, may undress at inappropriate times or in wrong place.
- Gains and then loses weight—forgets when last meal was eaten, may gradually lose interest in food.
- May see or hear things that are not there.
- Needs full-time supervision.

THIRD STAGE (LATE OR SEVERE STAGE)— LASTS ONE TO THREE YEARS

The third stage, which we don't discuss in this book, is when the person's abilities deteriorate significantly and nursing-home care may be required.

APPENDIX B: SAMPLE INFORMED CONSENT FORM (AND HOW TO READ BETWEEN THE LINES)

The following is an informed consent form for the clinical trial of a fictitious drug, Nerve Factor XY-162, with our comments *[italicized in brackets]* explaining what everything means. Consent forms vary from study to study, but they all, by law, must contain the same core information.

ICF Version Date: 7/10/07 *[the date that the study was last reviewed by the ethics committee]*

ICF Expires Date: 7/10/08 *[when the study's ethics committee permit will expire]*

THE CLINICAL TRIALS GROUP
[PEOPLE RUNNING THE SHOW]
CONSENT FOR RESEARCH:

A MULTI-CENTER, RANDOMIZED, DOUBLE-BLINDED, PLACEBO-CONTROLLED TRIAL OF NERVE FACTOR XY-162 TO SLOW THE PROGRESSION OF ALZHEIMER'S DISEASE

Principal Investigator: J. Smith, M.D.

IRB Registry # 1111-11
[That multiline, ALL CAPS mouthful is the title. Don't ignore it. It summarizes the entire study. "Multi-center" means that different centers are conducting the same study in different parts of the country or world—a good thing, because it means the drug will be tested on more people under a variety of conditions.
"Randomized" and "placebo-controlled" mean all participants have a chance of getting either a placebo or the drug, Nerve Factor XY-162: the name of the drug is fictitious, but many experimental drugs have names with numbers in them. "Double-blinded" tells you that neither the participants nor the researchers know who is receiving the placebo and who gets the treatment until the study's over.]
[The following introduction describes who is paying for the study. Potential conflicts of interest, such as the trial doctor getting paid to do the study or

owning stock in the company that makes the drug, should also be outlined in the introduction.]

DESCRIPTION AND PURPOSE OF THE TRIAL

You are being asked to participate in an investigational drug research study to test Nerve Factor XY-162 in the treatment of Alzheimer's disease (AD). *["Investigational" means the study drug is still being tested in research studies and is not approved by the U.S. Food and Drug Administration (FDA) for the treatment of Alzheimer's.]* The purpose of this study is to determine the safety, tolerability, and effectiveness of Nerve Factor XY-162 in treating or slowing the progression of AD. You were selected as a possible participant because of the memory problems you have been experiencing and because you have been diagnosed with AD. *[If the diagnosis in the consent form seems incorrect, notify both the doctor overseeing the study and your regular doctor. Unscrupulous trial directors may write down whatever diagnosis fits the study criteria in order to get participants in the study.]*

Nerve Factor XY-162 is a drug that in mice appears to lower amyloid levels in the brain. Nerve Factor XY-162 can be obtained only through this trial. Little is known about whether this agent can affect the memory problems associated with AD. *[If the description of the drug's effectiveness is sparse, as it is here, ask the trial doctor whether more evidence of the drug's potential is available. When little information exists, that usually means no one has studied the drug or the pharmaceutical company is not publicizing the information. Trial directors who are studying a drug developed by a pharmaceutical company receive a book called the Investigator's Brochure, which describes all of the animal and human studies conducted by the company to date. Unfortunately, many doctors are either too busy to read this brochure or are not trained to understand the data in it. Some doctors simply take the company's word on the drug's safety record because they don't want to challenge the company and risk losing its financial support.]*

If you agree to participate, you will be one of approximately 400 subjects enrolled in the study at about 40 sites in the United States. *[Find out how many people have already enrolled. It's usually safer to be subject #301 than subject #1, since doctors will have learned more about the drug. For example, in one study researchers reduced by half the dose of a promising Alzheimer's drug after a participant had a stroke.]* A total of 10 to 15 subjects from the Clinical Trials Group will participate in this study. This is a randomized and double-blinded 1:1 study, which means that each participant will have an approximately equal chance (like the flip of a coin) of being assigned to receive either the active study drug (Nerve Factor XY-162) or placebo (a pill with no active drug) for a period of 18 months. Neither you nor the study personnel will know if you are receiving Nerve

Factor XY-162 or placebo. In the event of a serious side effect, the identity of the study drug or placebo can be determined immediately. *[You should ask how immediate is "immediately." Usually this means within a few hours, but it can be as long as twenty-four hours. Ask your doctor what mechanisms are in place to access the information in emergencies, including on holidays.]*

The study will include eight clinic visits during a period of approximately 21 months from the first to last visit. *[The number of visits stated in the consent form is usually an optimistic estimate. Plan on a few more visits.]* You must have a person, your care provider (spouse, relative, or friend), who is willing to:

- Accompany you to all of the study visits
- Monitor your taking of the study drug
- Communicate changes in your health to the study doctor over the period of this study

During this study, Dr. Smith and her staff will be monitoring your condition.

If you decide to take part in the trial, Dr. Smith and/or a study team member will perform tests to determine whether you can take part in the study. You will not be considered eligible for the study until you and/or your legally authorized representative and your care provider have signed the consent form. You will be asked about any medication you are currently taking. You will undergo a screening assessment including medical history, physical examination, tests of your memory and thinking skills, an electrocardiogram (EKG) (a tracing of the electrical activity of the heart) and blood tests. Both you and your care provider will be asked about prescription medications (medications your doctor has prescribed) and over-the-counter medications (medications, vitamins, and other remedies you may buy at the store) that you are currently using and/or may have used in the past 30 days. About one tablespoon of your blood will be drawn by needle stick from a vein in your arm to determine if there are any problems that might prevent you from participating in the study or that could be responsible for any changes in your condition throughout the study period. This visit will take approximately two hours. *[The key word here is "approximately." Plan for the visits to take longer than the consent form states. Bring magazines and snacks with you. Unless the clinic is understaffed or inefficient, the longer the visit, the more comprehensive the exam.]*

If you qualify for this study, you and your care provider will return to the clinic at approximately the same time for your remaining seven visits. Each follow-up visit will generally last approximately two hours. The final visit will last approximately three to four hours.

Baseline Visit (Visit 2)

[During this visit you start on either the medication or placebo, which are both referred to as the "study drug."]

If the screening visit proves that you are eligible for this study, you will undergo what is called the baseline evaluation. This visit will take approximately two hours. The study staff will assess your memory, attention, vocabulary, mood, behavior, and motor function to determine what is considered "normal" for you. Your vital signs (blood pressure, heart rate, temperature, and breathing rate) and weight will be checked, and you will receive enough study drug to last until your next visit.

Approximately two tablespoons of your blood will be drawn to run a variety of tests, including to extract DNA (genetic material) to assess your apolipoprotein (ApoE) gene type. There is evidence that ApoE gene type may influence the rate of Alzheimer's disease progression or a subject's response to treatment. You will not receive any results from this blood collection, and the results will be kept confidential. This test is voluntary. If you do not wish to have your genetic material tested and stored, you may still participate in this study. *[Most Alzheimer's researchers want blood samples for genetic testing, even if it's not a genetics study.]*

_____ "I agree to allow the DNA testing to determine my ApoE gene type."

_____ "I do not agree to allow the DNA testing to determine my ApoE gene type."

We will collect your Social Security number in order to track information about your use of medical services and health-related expenses. We will also use relevant information from administrative records such as Medicare or Medicaid to learn more about your health-related expenses. Information gathered from Medicare and Medicaid will be used for research purposes only and will be kept strictly confidential. This portion of the test is voluntary. If you do not wish to have your Social Security number collected, you may still participate in the study.

_____ "I agree to provide my Social Security number to the investigator."

_____ "I do not agree to provide my Social Security number to the investigator."

If you agree to participate in this clinical research study, you will be enrolled in one of two possible study groups. One group will receive placebo for the duration of the study. The other group will receive Nerve Factor

XY-162 for the duration of the study. You will be assigned to one of these two groups randomly (such as by a flip of a coin) and will have an equal chance (one to one) of being enrolled in either group. At the end of the visit, you will be given a bottle of study tablets. You will take one tablet once a day in the evening. At each study visit, the study team will supply you with enough study tablets to last until the next visit. At each visit you will return the bottle and all unused study tablets from the previous visit. *[Do not hold on to study pills or try to break them open to see inside; you may get dropped from the study for violating the study protocol. The amount of medication you are asked to take may change during the course of the study, if, for example, the researchers are trying to see what dose works best or if the drug needs to be increased gradually.]* During each visit, the study team will review how you should take the study tablets.

Nerve Factor XY-162 and placebo tablets will be blinded *[neither you, the study team, nor the study doctor will know which study group you are in]*. However, if a medical emergency occurs, the study doctor can make the information available to emergency personnel.

Visit 3
[Side effects that come on quickly will probably show up by this visit, within two to six weeks of starting the drug. You should discuss them with the doctor and clinic staff, who will want to investigate all of your concerns and may ask you to undergo additional testing, such as blood tests.]
This visit will occur six weeks after you begin taking the study drug. You should bring any remaining study drug and the drug bottle with you to this and all remaining visits. This will serve as a safety visit to ensure that you are not having problems taking the study drug. The visit will include a review of side effects, and approximately one teaspoon of blood will be drawn by needle stick to measure your liver function. You will be given the study drug that you'll be taking for the next six weeks. This visit will take approximately one hour.

Visits 4–8
[Throughout the study, the staff will run many tests on you, checking, for example, your blood pressure, liver function, blood-cell count, and kidney function. Even if the test results are normal, ask how they compare to results from your last visit. "Normal" covers a wide range and most doctors take action only if the values are two to three times above the normal range. You don't want your results to be heading in the wrong direction.]
Each of these visits will also include measurements of your blood pressure and heart rate, a brief physical examination, as well as evaluations of your memory and thinking skills and your functional abilities *[your ability to do daily chores and basic activities such as bathing and dressing]*. Approximately one teaspoon of your blood will be drawn at Visits 4, 5, and 6 to measure

kidney and liver function. Approximately one tablespoon of blood will be drawn at Visit 7 to measure cholesterol and liver function and for other routine blood tests. Each of these visits will take approximately two hours. You will receive enough of the study drug to last until your next visit at Visits 4, 5, and 6. The study drug will not be supplied beyond the study period. *[Even though you have signed the form agreeing that the drug will not be available beyond the study period, after the study is over, you can ask to participate in an "open-label extension study" so you can continue to get the drug. Often by the end of the study the company has decided to continue offering the drug.]* You will be asked to bring your drug bottle and any unused drug each time you return for a visit throughout the remainder of the study.

Please inform Dr. Smith of any other drugs or remedies (prescription or over-the-counter medications) you take or might take while you are in this study. Also inform Dr. Smith if you have any of the possible side effects listed below, or any other unexpected or unusual symptoms.

GENETIC RESEARCH, DNA SAMPLES, AND DATA STORAGE

At Visit 2, your blood will be drawn by needle stick for ApoE testing and potential DNA storage. This testing is done for research purposes only—the results of the analysis will be kept confidential and you will never be given the results. This study does not involve genetic testing for diagnostic purposes; the research is aimed at developing such testing for the future but cannot currently provide any meaningful information to study participants. There will be no direct linkage of results with your name. This test is voluntary. If you do not wish to have your genetic material tested, you may still participate in this study. If you are concerned about a potential genetic disorder, you should discuss this with your regular doctor and you and your doctor may choose to test specifically for it. This would require additional blood samples and would NOT be part of this research project.

Additionally, you are being asked to store a DNA sample for possible future genetic studies. There will be no direct linkage of stored DNA samples to your name. The DNA will be stored at X Co. (a for-profit company) for at least five years and may be used for future genetic studies in the field of aging. Storage of samples is voluntary; if you do not wish to have your genetic material stored, you may still participate in this study.

Please indicate below whether or not you agree to allow your sample to be kept for future research by initialing the line next to your choice: *[Note that this form asks if they can store your blood for later use. You will be asked to sign other forms referring to blood tests as well.]*

_____ "I agree to allow my sample to be used for future research on Alzheimer's disease and/or aging."

_____ "I agree to allow my sample to be used for future research to study human diseases or disorders *other* than Alzheimer's disease and/or aging."

_____ "I do not agree to allow my samples to be used for future research."

X Co. will keep your data and it may be shared with other researchers in the future. *[Sharing your information will help researchers to learn more about Alzheimer's. Samples, with your name and all identifying information removed, can be stored indefinitely and sometimes sold to companies and other researchers. Ask if saying no will jeopardize your participation in the ongoing trial and if not, feel free to say no. In all cases, ask any questions you have.]* The purpose of our sharing these data and samples is hopefully to understand Alzheimer's better and to find a treatment for the disease. We may also share your information with a biotechnology company in the future. If this occurs, your name will not be revealed to the company. Your genetic information thus may or may not have significant therapeutic or commercial value.

RISKS AND BENFITS

[Don't assume that everything you need to know about the possible risks and benefits is listed in the consent form. Only the most common or serious risks are listed. Most side effects don't become widely known until after the drug has been on the market for at least a year. If you have time and are concerned, ask the study coordinator if you may talk with other participants about their experiences.

Even if the trial drug has only a number and no name, you can still plug that number into an Internet search engine and read about the compound. Find out how often the drug or procedure has caused dangerous side effects and whether any subgroups, such as people with diabetes or heart disease, are particularly susceptible to side effects. You can even schedule a brief appointment with the doctor to talk about the findings published in the Investigator Brochure, which describes:

- *The safety risks of the drug that emerged in animal and human studies*
- *The number of research participants who have taken the drug, including healthy individuals and people with Alzheimer's*
- *The longest period of time participants have been on the drug and the highest dose used*
- *Other uses for the drug*
- *The frequency of the most common side effects*

Find out how long the clinic staff will monitor your side effects after the trial ends or in case you drop out for any reasons. Finally, you should know the signs of unwanted side effects before they occur.]

In this trial your condition will be closely monitored. It is possible that by participating your condition may improve and that this trial may be helpful in developing a new therapy for others with similar illnesses. These benefits cannot be guaranteed. You may not benefit from participating in this study. Your condition may remain the same or get worse. For the subjects in the placebo group, no benefits can be expected. However, this study may lead to the development of effective strategies for slowing the decline of thinking skills and daily functioning in patients with AD, and may also provide information on the safety and benefits of Nerve Factor XY-162 therapy. Access by other researchers to the data and biomaterials, such as DNA and blood samples, generated by this study may stimulate research furthering the development of AD prevention and treatment strategies.

The most frequent side effects of Nerve Factor XY-162 are upset stomach, constipation, gas, stomach pain, diarrhea, nausea, and rash. More occasionally, they can include muscle aches, muscle weakness, and changes in liver function. Serious side effects that can occur in patients taking Nerve Factor XY-162 include meningitis, inflammation of the brain's coverings, hepatotoxicity, which is damage to the liver, and possible death. *[Don't panic when you see "risk of death" on the form. It's in most ICFs for experimental drugs, and many of the safest drugs on the market today included this language in their original consent forms.]* During the study, your doctors will monitor you for side effects by taking blood tests to monitor your liver function. You must promptly report any headaches, fever, neck stiffness, vomiting, blurring, or dizziness. We will monitor you closely for the occurrence of any side effect, and the study drug will be promptly stopped if there appears to be an adverse reaction. The researchers will stop giving participants the drug if they experience significant side effects thought to be related to the use of Nerve Factor XY-162.

There may be unforeseeable risks associated with the use of Nerve Factor XY-162. You have the right to ask any questions concerning the potential and/or known hazards of this trial at any time. Should you, as a result of taking part in this trial, be harmed in any way, you will receive emergency or other medical treatment. During the trial, you will be told if additional information is discovered that may affect your willingness to continue in this trial.

[Many trials are notoriously slow to inform subjects of such developments, in part because team members disagree over how to interpret new research findings and ethics committees take too long to act. Doctors will answer participants' questions about the trial drug, so participants or their care providers

should ask the doctor every three or four months if new information has emerged on the drug. You can also check the Internet. Bottom line: Select a trial run by a doctor who, by going to meetings and reading journals, keeps up on the latest research. Probably the best indicator of this is a doctor who has been running lots of clinical trials for five to ten years and has published review articles or speaks frequently on the topic of the trial. Doctors who participate with the Alzheimer's Disease Cooperative Study (https://adcs.ucsd.edu) are a safe bet.]

Blood will be drawn from your arm by needle stick. This is a standard method for obtaining blood and is briefly painful. Associated risks include minimal discomfort and/or bruising. Other possible, though rare, effects can include infection, excess bleeding, clotting, light-headedness, or fainting.

A risk of being in the study is that you may become tired or frustrated when being asked questions about your Alzheimer's disease. If this occurs, you are free to take a break. You must also contact Dr. Smith or the study staff before starting any new medications. You can contact her at (111) 111-1111.

ALTERNATIVE TREATMENT

[This section will tell you if you are allowed to start a new drug besides the trial drug during the trial, which most studies do permit. Always tell the clinic staff about any changes in your medications, including over-the-counter drugs and supplements.]
Other medications are available as alternatives to treat AD. To date, there are five FDA-approved drug therapies for this condition: Cognex (tacrine), Aricept (donepezil hydrochloride), Razadyne (galantamine), Exelon (rivastigmine), and Namenda (memantine). Thus, alternatives to participation in this study include use of tacrine, donepezil, galantamine, rivastigmine, memantine, or no treatment. If you participate in this study and already take tacrine, donepezil, galantamine, or rivastigmine, you may continue taking it during the study. However, starting tacrine, donepezil, galantamine, memantine, or rivastigmine at any point during the course of the study is not permitted.

Your other choices are:

1. To stay under the care of your present physician, who may decide to try you on one of the currently approved medications listed above.

2. To find another study using another investigational drug, a drug that is being tested to see if it is effective for Alzheimer's disease.

COSTS

The sponsor, X Co., is providing Nerve Factor XY-162 free of charge to participating research subjects. The sponsor will pay all costs associated with being in this study. You or your insurance company will be charged or held responsible for the costs of your routine care, the care you would have received if you were not in this study. *[Note that any routine care that isn't related to the study will be charged to your insurance.]*

CONFIDENTIALITY

[Here you will learn who will have access to data collected on you during the trial and how the data will be stored and your records protected.]
This section explains how personal health information collected about you for the study may be used. Your personal health information includes, but is not limited to, information that was collected for your entry into the study and information that is collected during the study.

The purpose of collecting this information is to allow the study staff and Dr. Smith to conduct the study, to evaluate the study drug, and to analyze the study results.

Study records that identify you will be kept confidential as required by law. Federal Privacy Regulations provide safeguards for privacy, security, and authorized access. The sponsor, government agencies, FDA and other regulators, or their representatives will review your research record. The monitors or auditors *[people hired by the pharmaceutical company to audit the books; it is standard for them to have full access since they are the ones who collect the data from the researchers and send them to the company for analyses]* will have access, while at ABC Hospital, to your research record and case report forms (CRFs) to verify that data is being obtained properly and transcribed accurately from the research record to the CRFs. For records that leave ABC, the case report forms, you will be assigned a unique code number and you will not be identified by name, Social Security number, address, telephone number, or any other direct personal identifier. The key to the code will be kept in a locked file in Dr. Smith's office. Therefore no personal identifying information will be available on CRFs that leave ABC. For example, if results of the study are published in a medical book or journal or presented at meetings for educational purposes, neither your name, nor any other personal health information that specifically identifies you, will be used in those materials.

In addition, your records may be reviewed in order to meet federal or state regulations. *[This is standard, since there are many people who oversee studies. Government-agency representatives audit about 20 to 30 percent of all sites participating in an industry-supported study.]* Dr. Smith and/or her staff may provide personal information to outside reviewers when these reviewers are at the site. Outside reviewers may include representatives from the Food and Drug Administration or the Institutional Review Board. *[This is standard.]* If your research record is reviewed by any of these groups, they may also need to review your entire medical record.

The study results will be retained in your research record for at least six years or until after the study is completed, whichever is longer, or forever. At that time, either the research records will be destroyed, or your name and other identifying information will be removed from the study results at ABC. Any research information in your medical record will be kept indefinitely. The medical research information gathered from this study will be reported to the sponsors, but you will not be identified by name. This information may be further disclosed by the sponsor of this study to government agencies around the world (where they seek to market the drug). If disclosed by the sponsor, the information is no longer covered by federal privacy regulations.

Results of tests and studies are done solely for this research study. They are not a part of your regular care with your primary doctor and will not be included in your medical record. Your permission for review of confidential information, your research record, by study staff or outside reviewers such as monitors or auditors is given by signing this document.

If you decide not to give permission for the release of your personal health information for the study, you will not be able to participate. This is because the study staff and/or Dr. Smith would not be able to collect the information needed to evaluate the study drug, Nerve Factor XY-162.

You may ask to see and copy your personal health information related to the study. You may also ask to correct any study-related information about you that is wrong. You may have to wait until the end of the study to see your study records, so that the study can be organized properly. *[Ask how long after the trial ends that will be, and whether you can see some of your results before then.]*

COMPENSATION FOR INJURY

[Consent forms state that if a participant is injured as a result of being in a trial, the doctor running the trial will not cover any expenses the participant incurs as a result of those injuries, nor will the center or university where the trial is taking place. The doctor will make sure the participant receives medical care, but the bills will be charged to the insurance company, and the participant must cover any expenses not covered by his or her plan. However, if a pharmaceutical company is helping to fund the trial, which is frequently the case, the company, on request from the doctor, may cover the participant's expenses rather than risk loss of goodwill. If a government agency is funding the trial, the participant's expenses will not be covered.]

All forms of medical findings and treatments—whether routine or investigational—involve some risk of injury. In spite of all safety measures, you might develop medical problems from participating in this study. You must report any suspected illness or injury to the study doctor immediately. If such problems take place, the Clinical Trials Group will provide emergency medical treatment and will assist you in getting proper follow-up medical treatment. The study will not provide compensation for research-related injury. If you have a medical or study-related question, or feel you have had a research-related injury, you may contact Dr. Smith at (111) 111-1111 or page her at (111) 111-1111. *[Test this pager to see if it works and keep the number on hand.]*

Being a part of this study while pregnant may expose the unborn child to significant risks. Therefore, pregnant women will be excluded from the study. If you are a woman of childbearing potential, a blood-pregnancy test will be done (using one teaspoon of blood drawn from a vein by needle stick), and it must be negative before you can enter this study. If you are sexually active, you must agree to use appropriate contraceptive measures for the duration of the study. Medically acceptable contraceptives include: 1) surgical sterilization; 2) approved hormonal contraceptives (such as birth-control pills, Depo-Provera, or Lupron Depot); 3) barrier methods (such as a condom or diaphragm) used with a spermicide; or 4) an intrauterine device (IUD). If you do become pregnant during this study, you must inform your study physician immediately.

For men, the treatment used in this study could affect your sperm and could potentially harm a child that you may father while on this study. If you are sexually active, you must agree to use a medically acceptable form of birth control in order to be in this study. Medically acceptable contraceptives include: 1) surgical sterilization; or 2) a condom used with a spermicide.

IMMEDIATE NECESSARY CARE

Immediate necessary care is available if you are injured because of your participation in this study. However, in the event of a study-related injury, there is no provision for free medical care or monetary compensation from your physicians.

Further information concerning this and your rights as a subject in research can be obtained from the Institutional Review Board at (111) 111-1111. *[Don't call this number for medical questions; use it if you want to file a complaint about the doctor or study.]*

VOLUNTARY PARTICIPATION/WITHDRAWAL

[This is key to clinical trials: You can leave a trial anytime. Don't sign up unless you plan on making a serious commitment, but if you need to quit, you can. Before deciding to leave, have a frank discussion with the doctor about your concerns. You will also want to find out if you need to taper off of your drugs slowly or can stop cold turkey. Before you leave, plan to have one or two clinic visits to be checked for side effects and to let the staff complete their paperwork.]

You may choose not to be in the study, or, if you agree to be in the study, you may withdraw from the study at any time. If you withdraw from the study, no new data will be collected for the study purposes unless the data concern an adverse event related to the study. If such an adverse event occurs, we may need to review your entire medical record. All data that have already been collected for the study purposes, and any new information about an adverse event related to the study, will be sent to the study sponsor.

Your decision not to participate or to withdraw from the study will not involve any penalty or loss of benefits to which you are entitled, and will not affect your access to health care at ABC. If you do decide to withdraw, we ask that you contact Dr. Smith in writing and let her know that you are withdrawing from the study.

The study physician, Dr. Smith, X Co., the Institutional Review Board (IRB), or the Food and Drug Administration can stop your participation in this study without your consent. Dr. Smith may stop your participation if it is determined to be in your best interest or if you fail to follow her or her study staff's directions. If you drop out of the study or your participation is discontinued by Dr. Smith, the sponsor, the IRB, or the FDA, you will be asked to return to complete a final safety evaluation and an evaluation of your memory and thinking performance. You must return all unused study tablets and the empty bottle. This final evaluation will include all of the procedures normally performed at Visit 8.

If you agree to allow your blood to be kept for research, you are free to change your mind at any time. We ask that you contact Dr. Smith in writing and let her know that you are withdrawing your permission for your blood to be used for research. Her mailing address is listed above. Any unused blood will have all identifying information removed that would link the sample to you. The sample may then be used for other research, but no one will be able to relate those research results to you.

TO BE SIGNED BY THE RESEARCH SUBJECT

"The purpose of this study, the procedures to be followed, and the risks and benefits have been explained to me. I have been allowed to ask questions I have, and my questions have been answered to my satisfaction. I have received the "Patient Product Information" sheet for Nerve Factor XY-162. I have been informed that I may contact Dr. Smith at (111) 111-1111 or Joe Smith, the study coordinator, at (111) 111-1111, to answer any questions I may have during the study. I may also page Dr. Smith at (111) 111-1111. I have read this consent form and agree to be in this study with the understanding that I may withdraw at any time. I have been told that I will receive a signed copy of this consent form."

[As the study progresses, you will get six or seven revisions of the consent form. File them someplace safe, as you may need them in an emergency.]

_____   _____

Signature of Subject   Date

_____   _____

Signature of Care Provider   Date

_____

Relationship to Subject

_____

Care Provider Name, Printed

_____   _____

Signature of Legal Representative   Date

_____

Relationship to Subject

_____

Legal Representative Name, Printed

_____

"I confirm that I have explained the nature, purpose, and foreseeable effects of the trial to the person(s) named above."

_____

Signature of Individual Obtaining Consent *[staff member]*

_____

Individual Obtaining Consent Name, Printed

[All Alzheimer's trials require both the study participant and the care provider to sign the form. The legal representative can be the participant's next of kin or

someone to whom the participant has given medical power of attorney. Next of kin is normally the spouse, or if there is no spouse, the eldest son or daughter. After the forms are signed, any reliable care provider who knows the participant well can take the participant to the clinic appointments.]

ACKNOWLEDGMENTS

We are very grateful to our editor, Hope Dellon, and our agent, Joelle Delbourgo, who provided invaluable assistance from start to finish. We also want to thank our colleague Tori DeAngelis, who helped write two chapters.

P. Murali Doraiswamy would like to thank the following: Dr. K. Ranga Krishnan for fifteen years of invaluable mentorship; Drs. Dan Blazer and Everett Ellinwood for their support over the years; Dr. Mohan Chilukuri, Dr. Mustafa Husain, Daran Thomas, Dr. Jeffrey Petrella, Dr. James Blumenthal, Dr. John Beyer, Dr. Kenneth Gersing, Dr. Cecil Charles, Dr. Rima Kaddurah-Daouk, Dr. James MacFall, Dr. David Steffens, Hala Husn, LisaLynn Kelley, Marilyn Aiello, Mae Burks, and Caroline Hellegers for their support and collaboration; Geeta Anand for introducing me to Joelle Delbourgo when this project was just an idea in my mind; Peter Guzzardi, Dr. Gary Small, and Dr. Dev Devanand for their invaluable insights; the NIH, AFAR, various professional and patient advocacy groups, and several pharmaceutical companies for supporting my research, speaking, and consulting over the years; Rebecca Levine for her assistance on one chapter; and the incredibly talented Karen Baar, M.P.H., for helping turn my two-page concept sheet into a brilliant proposal. Dr. Doraiswamy would also like to acknowledge that he owns shares in Sonexa Therapeutics, which does not yet have any products for clinical use.

Lisa P. Gwyther gratefully acknowledges the invaluable inspiration and support of Edna L. Ballard, M.S.W., the Joseph and Kathleen Bryan Alzheimer's Disease Research Center and the Center for the Study of Aging and Human Development at Duke University Medical Center.

INDEX